Vascular Anomalies

Editors

MARCELO HOCHMAN
LARA WINE LEE

DERMATOLOGIC CLINICS

www.derm.theclinics.com

Consulting Editor
BRUCE H. THIERS

October 2022 • Volume 40 • Number 4

ELSEVIER

1600 John F. Kennedy Boulevard • Suite 1800 • Philadelphia, Pennsylvania, 19103-2899

http://www.theclinics.com

DERMATOLOGIC CLINICS Volume 40, Number 4
October 2022 ISSN 0733-8635, ISBN-13: 978-0-323-94041-2

Editor: Stacy Eastman
Developmental Editor: Karen Justine Solomon

Dermatologic Clinics (ISSN 0733-8635) is published quarterly by Elsevier Inc., 360 Park Avenue South, New York, NY 10010-1710. Months of publication are January, April, July, and October. Business and editorial offices: 1600 John F. Kennedy Blvd., Suite 1800, Philadelphia, PA 19103-2899. Customer service office: 11830 Westline Drive, St. Louis, MO 63146. Periodicals postage paid at New York, NY, and additional mailing offices. Subscription prices are USD 429.00 per year for US individuals, USD 1,035.00 per year for US institutions, USD 469.00 per year for Canadian individuals, USD 1,071.00 per year for Canadian institutions, USD 525.00 per year for international individuals, USD 1,071.00 per year for international institutions, USD 100.00 per year for US students/residents, USD 100.00 per year for Canadian students/residents, and USD 240 per year for international students/residents. International air speed delivery is included in all *Clinics* subscription prices. All prices are subject to change without notice. **POSTMASTER:** Send address changes to *Dermatologic Clinics*, Elsevier Health Sciences Division, Subscription Customer Service, 3251 Riverport Lane, Maryland Heights, MO 63043. **Customer Service: 1-800-654-2452 (U.S. and Canada); 314-447-8871 (outside U.S. and Canada). Fax: 314-447-8029. E-mail: journalscustomerservice-usa@elsevier.com (for print support); journalsonlinesupport-usa@elsevier.com (for online support).**

Reprints. For copies of 100 or more, of articles in this publication, please contact the Commercial Reprints Department, Elsevier Inc., 360 Park Avenue South, New York, New York 10010-1710. Tel.: 212-633-3874; Fax: 212-633-3820; Email: reprints@elsevier.com.

The *Dermatologic Clinics* is covered in *MEDLINE/PubMed (Index Medicus), Current Contents/Clinical Medicine, Excerpta Medica, Chemical Abstracts,* and *ISI/BIOMED.*

Contributors

CONSULTING EDITOR

BRUCE H. THIERS, MD
Professor and Chairman Emeritus, Department
of Dermatology and Dermatologic Surgery,
Medical University of South Carolina,
Charleston, South Carolina, USA

EDITORS

MARCELO HOCHMAN, MD
Director, Hemangioma & Malformation
Treatment Center, Affiliate Professor of Plastic
Surgery and Otolaryngology–Head and Neck
Surgery, South Carolina, USA

LARA WINE LEE, MD, PhD
Associate Professor, Departments of
Dermatology and Dermatologic Surgery, and
Pediatrics, Medical University of South
Carolina, Charleston, South Carolina, USA

AUTHORS

SHOMOUKH ALSHAMEKH, MD
Children's Hospital of Philadelphia,
Department of Dermatology, Philadelphia,
Pennsylvania, USA

LAURA ANDREWS, MSCR
Medical Student, College of Medicine, Medical
University of South Carolina, Charleston, South
Carolina, USA

KELLY ATHERTON, MSCR
College of Medicine, Medical University of
South Carolina, Charleston, South Carolina,
USA

SUSAN J. BAYLISS, MD
Professor, Division of Dermatology,
Department of Medicine, Washington
University in St. Louis School of Medicine,
St Louis, Missouri, USA

SHAYLA BERGMANN, MD
Associate Professor, Director of Pediatric
Nonmalignant Hematology, Division of
Pediatric Hematology-Oncology, Medical
University of South Carolina, Charleston, South
Carolina, USA

MARIA GNARRA BUETHE, MD, PhD
Department of Dermatology, SUNY Downstate
Health Sciences University, Brooklyn, New
York, USA

SARA S. CATHEY, MD
Clinical Geneticist, Clinical Genetics Division,
Greenwood Genetic Center, North Charleston,
South Carolina, USA

M. IMRAN CHAUDRY, MBBS
Department of Neurosurgery and
Neuroendovascular Surgery, Prisma Health,
Greenville, South Carolina, USA

COLLEEN H. COTTON, MD
Department of Dermatology and Dermatologic
Surgery, Medical University of South Carolina,
Charleston, South Carolina, USA

AUSTIN N. DEHART, MD
Clinical Faculty, Division of Pediatric
Otolaryngology-Head and Neck Surgery,
Phoenix Children's Hospital, Phoenix,
Arkansas, USA

ALEXA DEMAIO, BS
Medical University of South Carolina, College
of Medicine, Charleston, South Carolina, USA

KARLA ESCOBAR, BS
Department of Dermatology, Henry Ford
Health, Detroit, MI, USA

DOV CHARLES GOLDENBERG, MD, PhD
Associate Professor, Plastic Surgery Team
Coordinator at Hospital Israelita Albert
Einstein, Division of Plastic Surgery,
Director of Pediatric Plastic Surgery and
Vascular Anomalies Clinic, Director of the
Residence Program in Plastic Surgery,
Hospital Clínicas da Faculdade de Medicina da
Universidade de São Paulo, Sao Paulo, SP,
Brazil

LAMIAA HAMIE, MD, MS
Department of Dermatology, Division of
Pediatric Dermatology, Medical College of
Wisconsin, Milwaukee, Wisconsin, USA

DIVINA JUSTINA HASBANI, MD
Department of Dermatology, American
University of Beirut Medical Center, Beirut,
Lebanon

HARRIET HINEN, MD
Department of Dermatology and Dermatologic
Surgery, Medical University of South Carolina,
Charleston, South Carolina, USA

JONATHAN HINSHELWOOD, MD
Department of Radiology, Prisma Health,
Greenville, South Carolina, USA

MARCELO HOCHMAN, MD
Director, Hemangioma & Malformation
Treatment Center, Affiliate Professor of Plastic
Surgery and Otolaryngology–Head and Neck
Surgery, South Carolina, USA

MARLA N. JAHNKE, MD
Department of Dermatology, Henry Ford
Health, Detroit, MI, USA

LARA WINE LEE, MD, PhD
Associate Professor, Departments of
Dermatology and Dermatologic Surgery, and
Pediatrics, Medical University of South
Carolina, Charleston, South Carolina,
USA

JULIE LUU, BS
University of the Incarnate Word School of
Osteopathic Medicine, San Antonio, Texas,
USA

JOHN MCALHANY, MD
Medical University of South Carolina,
Charleston, South Carolina, USA

CHRISTINA NEW, MD
Division of Pediatric Hematology-Oncology,
Medical University of South Carolina,
Charleston, South Carolina, USA

KARAN PANDHER, MD
Department of Dermatology, Henry Ford
Health, Detroit, MI, USA

THUY L. PHUNG, MD, PhD
Associate Professor and Medical Director,
Department of Pathology, University of South
Alabama, Mobile, Alabama, USA

GRESHAM T. RICHTER, MD
Department Chair, Department of Pediatric
Otolaryngology-Head and Neck Surgery,
Arkansas Children's Hospital, University of
Arkansas for Medical Sciences, Little Rock,
Arkansas, USA

AUBREY L. ROSE, MS, CGC
Certified Genetic Counselor, Clinical Genetics
Division, Greenwood Genetic Center, North
Charleston, South Carolina, USA

LEONID SHMUYLOVICH, MD, PhD
Assistant Professor, Division of Dermatology,
Department of Medicine, Washington
University in St. Louis School of Medicine, St
Louis, Missouri, USA

CHELSEA SHOPE, MSCR
Medical Student, College of Medicine, Medical
University of South Carolina, Charleston, South
Carolina, USA

MICHAEL J. WATERS, MBBS
Department of Neurosurgery and
Neuroendovascular Surgery, Prisma Health,
Greenville, South Carolina, USA

RICARDO YAMADA, MD
Medical University of South Carolina,
Charleston, South Carolina, USA

RAFAEL FERREIRA ZATZ, MD
Board Certified Plastic Surgeon, Medical
Assistant at the Pediatric Plastic Surgery and
Vascular Anomalies Clinics, Division of Plastic
Surgery, Hospital Clínicas da Faculdade de
Medicina da Universidade de São Paulo, Sao
Paulo, SP, Brazil

Contents

> Before the development of the International Society for the Study of Vascular Anomalies (ISSVA) classification system in 1996, nomenclature used to describe vascular lesions was inconsistent and imprecise. This since widely adopted system stratifies vascular anomalies into vascular malformations and tumors. Vascular tumors involve abnormal proliferation of vascular cells and are further classified as benign, locally aggressive/borderline, or malignant. Vascular malformations are lesions of defective vascular morphogenesis with quiescent endothelium and are named according to their vessel composition, and subdivided into simple; combined, of major named vessels; and syndrome-associated malformations. The updated 2018 ISSVA criteria are referenced in this review.

> Vascular malformations are developmental disorders involving the blood and lymphatic vasculature. The study of vascular malformations is a complex and rapidly evolving field with new understanding and insights into the clinical, histopathology, and molecular basis of these lesions. Diagnostic classification of vascular malformations is based on their unique clinical, radiologic imaging, histologic, and molecular characteristics. This article follows the published classification of the International Society for the Study of Vascular Anomalies. It describes characteristic histopathologic findings in tissues of vascular malformations and information on known genetic causes.

> Vascular tumors are neoplasms of endothelial cell origin. These tumors comprise a broad and complex group of vascular anomalies. Diagnostic classification of these lesions is based on their unique clinical, radiologic imaging, histopathologic, and molecular characteristics. This article follows the published classification of the International Society for the Study of Vascular Anomalies. It describes characteristic histopathologic findings in vascular tumors and information on known genetic causes.

> Vascular tumors and malformations encompass a spectrum of pathology that varies widely in presentation, severity, and treatments. Although typically a clinical diagnosis, accurate classification of lesions is often challenging. Imaging plays an integral role in confirming the clinical diagnosis, determining the extent of disease and

planning treatment strategies. Ultrasound and MRI constitute the backbone of diagnostic imaging in vascular anomalies; however, other modalities such as radiography, computed tomography, and conventional angiography can play a role in certain situations.

Various clinical disciplines defend the modality of therapy available to them (eg, medical vs surgery) when, in fact, multi-modality therapy is usually in the best interest of the patient. The aim of any modality of treatment is to obtain the best possible result for a given patient. To successfully achieve that aim for infantile hemangiomas (IH) and all vascular anomalies, defining what is meant by the best possible result and by when to achieve that, the result needs to be defined. Perhaps more important is to make a determination of what is an acceptable result. The impact of a 1-cm IH of the nasal tip is different from that of the same exact lesion on the thigh. The functional import of a 5-mm IH involving the lower eyelid is potentially very different from the same lesion involving the upper eyelid. These examples highlight that variables, such as size and location, are important. What is considered acceptable as a result of treatment of the nasal tip and upper eyelid IH is different from that for the corresponding thigh and lower lid lesions.

Infantile hemangiomas (IHs) are the most common benign vascular tumors of childhood. They develop during the first few weeks of life and naturally progress by proliferating over several months before they involute and resolve South Carolina; this renders them inconsequential in many cases, but sometimes IHs can have detrimental consequences on function and disfigurement. Hence, systemic propranolol has become a crucial element in IH management, alongside various other medical, procedural, and surgical options that aim to promote their quicker resolution and prevent and alleviate complications.

This article explores what is known regarding infantile hemangioma (IH) genetics. Despite a great deal of research on this topic, the relationship between IH genetics and pathogenesis has yet to be understood. This article also outlines the appropriate work-up and management of syndromes associated with specific presentations of IH.

Vascular tumors are classified into three categories by the International Society for the Study of Vascular Anomalies (ISSVA): benign, locally aggressive/borderline, and malignant. Many of these tumors are rare, cutaneous in nature, and present in childhood. The characterization and delineation of these distinct vascular tumors is an evolving area of clinical research. The diagnosis of these lesions relies on history and clinical presentation, location, histologic appearance, immunohistochemistry, and more recently, associated genetic mutations. This article provides a brief, yet comprehensive overview of all cutaneous vascular tumors currently recognized by the ISSVA, including presentation, diagnosis, and treatment.

Capillary Malformations

Karla Escobar, Karan Pandher, and Marla N. Jahnke

Capillary malformations (CMs) are the most common vascular anomalies, composed of enlarged capillaries and venules with thickened perivascular cell coverage in skin and mucous membranes. These congenital anomalies represent an error in vascular development during embryogenesis. Most of the CMs occur without any syndromic findings; the association between CMs systemic anomalies in some patients, however, makes the recognition of additional syndrome features critical. Some genetic disorders discussed, which feature CMs, include Sturge–Weber syndrome, diffuse CMs with overgrowth, Klippel–Trenaunay syndrome, CLOVES syndrome, among others. This article can aid clinicians in better identifying CMs and associated syndromes and provide consistent terminology to facilitate interdisciplinary management.

Venous Malformations: A Journey Through Their Multifaceted Clinical Presentations

Maria Gnarra Buethe, Susan J. Bayliss, and Leonid Shmuylovich

Venous malformations are the most common congenital vascular malformations. Because venous malformations can be complex, difficult to treat, and associated with late complications, it is important to know the basics of the different types of venous malformations and clinical differential diagnosis. Patients with complex lesions may be best served by a specialty vascular anomalies clinic.

Arteriovenous Malformations

Shomoukh AlShamekh

Arteriovenous malformations (AVMs) are a group of high-flow congenital vascular malformations. They are characterized by abnormal shunting of the blood supply from fast-flow feeding arteries to low-resistance draining veins via a cluster of aberrant blood vessels termed a central nidus. They are often sporadic but can be associated with syndromes. AVMs are of the most challenging vascular malformations to diagnose and manage and often lead to significant morbidity and mortality. Early diagnosis by recognizing clinical features and experienced multidisciplinary team management is essential to minimize and avoid later complications. This article focuses on clinical findings and natural history of AVMs.

Genetic Causes of Vascular Malformations and Common Signaling Pathways Involved in Their Formation

Aubrey L. Rose and Sara S. Cathey

The identification of the genetic causes of vascular malformations is improving understanding of pathogenesis of these lesions and also informing potential opportunities for treatment. Somatic activating mutations affecting RAS/MAPK and PIK3/AKT/mTor pathways are implicated in all types of vascular malformations. Pathogenic variants associated with vascular lesions may be germline or somatic. Next-generation sequencing technologies allow identification of lower level mosaic mutations than was achievable with standard Sanger sequencing. Best practice strategies to identify underlying genetic mutations in vascular malformations are influenced by the tissues involved and the type of vascular lesion.

The treatment of vascular malformations and vascular anomalies is often complex, combining various approaches in the art of medicine to provide best outcomes and quality of life for these patients. Treatment may include but is not limited to the following: local control with compression garments and attire, pain control, surgical procedures and debulking, laser therapy, sclerotherapy, and medical management. In this article, the authors discuss the aspects of medical management, visiting the history of medical treatment, and the recent utilization and success of enzymatic pathway inhibitors, specifically sirolimus and new therapies that hold promise for the future for these patients.

Recommendation for the surgical approach to vascular anomalies is rapidly evolving. From an isolated approach, surgery is best seen nowadays as an adjunctive tool in multidisciplinary management. Several studies focusing on targeted therapy based on genetic findings were published, and their use in clinical practice is on the way.

Lasers are a safe and effective tool for the treatment of vascular anomalies. There are many laser options available. Matching laser parameters with the characteristics of the vasculature in these lesions can selectively deliver energy to the abnormal tissue. This can lead to reduction in size and symptoms of vascular malformations and hemangiomas.

Vascular anomalies are highly variable in their angioarchitecture, location, and flow dynamics. An individualized, multidisciplinary approach to treatment is required, focusing on improving patient quality of life. With appropriate percutaneous or endovascular treatment, patient satisfaction following interventional therapy is generally high, acknowledging that a complete cure may not always be possible.

DERMATOLOGIC CLINICS

SERIES OF RELATED INTEREST

Medical Clinics
https://www.medical.theclinics.com/
Immunology and Allergy Clinics
https://www.immunology.theclinics.com/
Clinics in Plastic Surgery
https://www.plasticsurgery.theclinics.com/
Otolaryngologic Clinics
https://www.oto.theclinics.com/

DERMATOLOGIC CLINICS

FORTHCOMING ISSUES

January 2023
Cutaneous Oncology Update
Stan N. Tolkachjov, Editor

April 2023
Diagnosis, Staging, and Identification in Dermatosurgery
Susan C. Taylor, Editor

July 2023
Dermatologic Diseases in Skin of Color
Susan C. Taylor, Editor

RECENT ISSUES

July 2022
Food and Drug Administration's Role in Dermatology
Markham C. Luke, Editor

April 2022
Pediatric Dermatology Part II
Kelly M. Cordoro, Editor

January 2022
Pediatric Dermatology Part I
Kelly M. Cordoro, Editor

SERIES OF RELATED INTEREST

THE CLINICS ARE NOW AVAILABLE ONLINE!
Access your subscription at:
www.theclinics.com

Preface
Vascular Anomalies: Current State

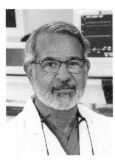 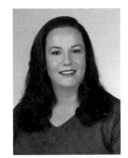

Marcelo Hochman, MD   Lara Wine Lee, MD, PhD

Editors

The field of vascular anomalies has changed over the last 15 years with a deeper understanding of pathophysiology and genetics leading to improvement in therapies. Clearly, the use of an accepted terminology and nomenclature system has led to improved communication across specialties. Multimodality therapy has thus become the norm through increased multispecialty involvement and cooperation. The validity of various treatments (laser, medical, surgical) is becoming less an issue of controversy, and the timing of each in the natural history of various anomalies is becoming clearer. The purpose of this issue is to summarize the current knowledge and serve as a handy reference for the clinician taking care of patients afflicted with these anomalies. Our hope is that the information in this issue becomes rapidly outdated with continued advances.

Marcelo Hochman, MD
Hemangioma & Malformation Treatment Center,
Charleston, SC, USA

526 Johnnie Dodds Boulevard, Suite 202, Mt
Pleasant, SC 29464, USA

Lara Wine Lee, MD, PhD
Department of Dermatology & Dermatologic
Surgery
Department of Pediatrics
Medical University of South Carolina
135 Rutledge Avenue; 11th Floor
Charleston, SC 29425, USA

E-mail addresses:
DrHochman@facialsurgerycenter.com
(M. Hochman)
winelee@musc.edu (L.W. Lee)

Dermatol Clin 40 (2022) xi
https://doi.org/10.1016/j.det.2022.07.003
0733-8635/22/© 2022 Published by Elsevier Inc.

Vascular Anomalies
Nomenclature and Diagnosis

Laura Andrews, MSCR[a], Chelsea Shope, MSCR[a], Lara Wine Lee, MD, PhD[b,c,*],
Marcelo Hochman, MD[d]

KEYWORDS

• Vascular anomaly • Vascular malformation • Vascular tumor • ISSVA • Nomenclature

KEY POINTS

- The 1996 ISSVA classification stratified vascular anomalies into vascular malformations and proliferative vascular lesions (tumors), and has been continually revised as new information is acquired, with the most recent revision in 2018.
- Vascular tumors represent an abnormal proliferation of vascular cells that may be classified as benign, locally aggressive/borderline, or malignant.
- Vascular malformations arise from defective vascular morphogenesis with quiescent endothelium.
- Simple vascular malformations derive their names from their constituent vessel type; combined vascular malformations are those composed of 2 or more vascular malformations associated in a single lesion, and vascular malformations of major named vessels may affect lymphatic vessels, veins, or arteries.
- In syndrome-associated vascular malformations, the lesions may be linked to other anomalies, the majority of which involve overgrowth.

In the past, a lack of logical and consistent nomenclature posed a considerable obstacle to the understanding and diagnosis of vascular lesions.[1] Old classifications were often overly descriptive and complex.[1] Frequently, the term *hemangioma* was used as an indiscriminate term to describe any kind of vascular tumor. It is well known that erroneous classification leads to increased likelihood of improper diagnosis and treatment.[2] Although sometimes possessing similar names and appearance, vascular lesions often differ in prognosis, morbidity, and optimal management techniques. Misdiagnosis may lead to improper treatment leading to suboptimal results and unnecessary family stress.[3,4] Vascular lesions occur in a wide range of age groups and affect various organs, and thus are seen by numerous medical specialists; this further highlights the need for use of common terminology across specialties.[5] In their 1982 article, Mulliken and Glowaki[6] described a binary system based on histologic composition, including the presence or absence of increased mitotic activity and rate of endothelial cell turnover. This binary system divided vascular anomalies into masses or malformations.[2] This binary classification was later adopted by the International Society for the Study of Vascular Anomalies (ISSVA).[7] The 1996 ISSVA

[a] College of Medicine, Medical University of South Carolina, 135 Rutledge Avenue, 11th Floor, Charleston, SC 29425, USA; [b] Department of Dermatology & Dermatologic Surgery, Medical University of South Carolina, 135 Rutledge Avenue 11th Floor, Charleston SC 29425, USA; [c] Department of Pediatrics, Medical University of South Carolina, 135 Rutledge Avenue, 11th Floor, Charleston, SC 29425, USA; [d] Hemangioma & Malformation Treatment Center, 526 Johnnie Dodds Boulevard, Suite 202, Mt Pleasant, SC 29464, USA
* Corresponding author. Department of Dermatology & Dermatologic Surgery, Medical University of South Carolina, 135 Rutledge Avenue 11th Floor, Charleston SC 29425.
E-mail address: winelee@musc.edu

Dermatol Clin 40 (2022) 339–343
https://doi.org/10.1016/j.det.2022.06.007

classification stratified vascular anomalies into vascular malformations and proliferative vascular lesions (tumors), and has been continually revised as new information is acquired, with the most recent revision in 2018. These revisions have included the addition of diseases/conditions, as well as identification of a large number of causative genes.[5] This classification system has been adopted internationally and is widely used in practice. In general, ISSVA classifications reserve the term *vascular mass* for vasoproliferative lesions with increased endothelial cell turnover, whereas *vascular malformation* is used to describe lesions of defective vascular morphogenesis with quiescent endothelium.[2]

VASCULAR TUMORS

Vascular tumors are a subset of vascular anomalies that represent an abnormal proliferation of vascular cells that may be classified as benign, locally aggressive/borderline, or malignant.[7] The term *hemangioma* is included in the descriptive nomenclature for specific vascular tumors that exhibit typical morphologic characteristics and conform to known natural histories.

BENIGN

Infantile hemangioma is a benign proliferation of endothelial cells that typically appears and begins to grow within the first few weeks of life.[8,9] This is in contrast to congenital hemangioma (CH), which are fully formed at birth.[2] CH is a rare, benign proliferation of capillaries that are separated by abnormal fibrotic stroma with overlying epidermal atrophy and loss of dermal adnexal structures.[10] Other types of rare, acquired hemangiomas include spindle cell hemangiomas (SCH), named for their proliferations of cavernous blood vessels with spindled areas in the subcutaneous tissue,[11] and epithelioid hemangiomas (EH), which are vasoformative tumors composed of well-formed vascular channels of epithelioid endothelial cells.[12] Other benign tumors named for their characteristic proliferative patterns include tufted angiomas; pyogenic granulomas, also known as lobular capillary hemangiomas; hobnail, microvenular, anastomosing, glomeruloid, papillary, and acquired elastic hemangiomas; as well as intravascular papillary endothelial hyperplasia, cutaneous epithelioid angiomatous nodules, and littoral cell hemangiomas of the spleen.[7,13]

LOCALLY AGGRESSIVE OR BORDERLINE

Kaposiform hemangioendothelioma are rare tumors named from its growth pattern, which resembles Kaposi sarcoma (KS), also associated with lymphangiomatosis and sheetlike growth.[14] Other tumors termed *hemangioendotheliomas*, include retiform, composite, and polymorphous hemangioendotheliomas. These neoplastic proliferations of endothelial cells are again named for their proliferative patterns.[7] As the name suggests, papillary intralymphatic angioendotheliomas, also known as Dabska tumors, are rare intravascular proliferations of "hobnail" endothelial cells that form intraluminal papillary projections with associated lymphatic vessels.[15] KS, on the other hand, is named for the dermatologist who first described these tumors, Moritz Kaposi.[16] KS is a vascular proliferation in the dermis that resembles lymphatic endothelium[16] and is associated with inflammatory and spindle cells.[17]

MALIGNANT

Although malignant tumors are rare, the 2 most common subtypes in this classification group are angiosarcoma and epithelioid hemangioendothelioma.[7] Angiosarcoma is a highly aggressive neoplastic proliferation of vascular (angio-) endothelial cells (-sarcoma, indicating malignant tumor of connective or nonepithelial tissue).[14] These tumors are uncommon in adult and pediatric patients alike, accounting for only 0.3% of all pediatric sarcomas. Risk factors include radiation, long-standing lymphedema, and heritable diseases such as neurofibromatosis 1 and Klippel-Trenaunay syndrome (KPS).[18] Epithelioid hemangioendothelioma (EHE), has features of EH as the name suggests, as well as angiosarcoma, with variable subcutaneous fat involvement. EHE most commonly arises in the liver of middle-aged patients and is rarely seen in children.[19,20]

VASCULAR MALFORMATIONS

Vascular malformations represent the subset of vascular anomalies that are nonneoplastic in nature. These malformations are composed of dysplastic vessels lined by abnormal endothelium lacking in normal smooth muscle layers and supporting cells.[21] As their name suggests, these lesions represent badly (mal-) formed vessels. Vascular malformations are present at birth, although they may not become apparent until later in life and typically grow proportionally with the patient or in response to trauma, infection, and hormonal changes.[2] Vascular malformations may be composed of capillaries, lymphatic vessels, veins, arteries and veins, or other combinations thereof

Table 1
Combined vascular malformations

CVM	CM + VM	Capillary-venous malformation
CLM	CM + LM	Capillary-lymphatic malformation
CAVM	CM + AVM	Capillary-arteriovenous malformation
LVM	LM + VM	Lymphatic-venous malformation
CLVM	CM + LM + VM	Capillary-lymphatic-venous malformation
CLAVM	CM + LM + AVM	Capillary-lymphatic-arteriovenous malformation
CVAVM	CM + VM + AVM	Capillary-venous-arteriovenous malformation
CLVAVM	CM + LM + VM + AVM	Capillary-lymphatic-venous-arteriovenous malformation

and are named accordingly. Furthermore, they are divided into simple, combined, malformations of major named vessels, and syndrome-associated malformations based on the vessels they contain.[7] In the following sections, the classification and nomenclature of various vascular malformations are detailed.

SIMPLE

Simple vascular malformations derive their names from their constituent vessel type (capillaries, lymphatic vessels, venous vessels, or a combination). Venous malformations (VMs) represent the most common vascular malformation, accounting for between one-half to two-thirds of all vascular malformations encountered clinically, with a prevalence of 1%.[2,22] VMs result from errors in vascular embryogenesis. The vast majority, greater than 90%, are sporadic in origin, with hereditary forms occurring in less than 10%. VMs are present at birth, although they may not always be clinically apparent. The clinical course of VMs depends largely on anatomic location.[22] Variations of VMs exist and include common VMs, familial cutaneo-mucosal VM, blue rubber bleb nevus (bean) syndrome, glomuvenous malformation, cerebral cavernous malformation, familial intraosseous vascular malformation, verrucous VM, and others.[7]

Capillary malformations (CMs), affect cutaneous and mucosal surfaces, without impacting deeper structures. CMs include nevus simplex (also known as a *salmon patch*, *angel kiss*, or *stork bite*), which affects the midline of the head and may lighten and disappear, generally before 5 years of age. However, CMs generally persist throughout life, with darkening and thickening over time.[23] Additional categories of CMs include cutaneous and/or mucosal CM (also known as port-wine stain), which can be syndromic or non-syndromic, reticulate CMs, CM of CM-AVM, cutis marmorata telangiectatica congenita, and others.[7]

Lymphatic malformations (LMs) are low-flow vascular malformations consisting of dilated lymphatic channels and cystic spaces. The incidence of LMs ranges from 1 in 16,000 to 1 in 2000; they are usually apparent at birth or within the first few years of life. Areas of the body rich in lymphatics, especially the head and neck (up to 75%), are most frequently affected.[24] LMs are subdivided into common (cystic) LMs, which are further split into macrocystic, microcystic, and mixed cystic LMs; generalized lymphatic anomalies; LM in Gorham-Stout disease; channel type LM; acquired progressive lymphatic anomaly; and primary lymphedema, among others.[7]

Arteriovenous malformations (AVMs) are fast-flow vascular malformations involving an abnormal connection between primitive feeding arteries and draining veins without a normal intervening capillary network.[25] This aberrant connection results in shunting of blood away from normally supplied tissue with potential for ischemic pain, ulceration, or hemorrhage.[2] AVMs are usually congenital but may not become evident until early childhood. The majority of AVMs are sporadic in origin; however, they may also present as part of hereditary hemorrhagic telangiectasia (HHT), capillary malformation-arteriovenous malformation (CM-AVM), and other syndromes. Congenital arteriovenous fistulas (AVFs) similarly represent a focal connection between an artery and vein and can be sporadic, or part of HHT, CM-AVM, and others.[7,23]

COMBINED

Combined vascular malformations are those composed of 2 or more vascular malformations associated in a single lesion; these may include multiple simple VMs, VMs of major named vessels, or a combination of both. It is possible to have a cutaneous CM associated with an underlying VM, LM, or AVM, or a VM with an LM.[23] The combined vascular malformations include CVM, CLM,

CAVM, LVM, CLVM, CLAVM, CVAVM, and CLVAVM. Descriptions of their nomenclature are described in **Table 1**.

Of Major Named Vessels

Vascular malformations of major named vessels are also known as *channel-type* or *truncal* vascular malformations.[2] These anomalies may affect lymphatic vessels, veins, or arteries. The term malformation encompasses anomalies of the vessel's origin, course, number, length, diameter, valves, communication, or persistence.[7]

Associated with Other Anomalies

Some vascular malformations, both simple and/or of major named vessels, can be linked to other anomalies. The majority of the additional anomalies involve overgrowth, or global or regional excess of growth compared with an equivalent body part or age-related peer group, of the soft tissue and/or bone.[21,23] Many of these syndromes associated with vascular anomalies now have identified causal genetic mutations. This knowledge allows the various syndromes to be viewed as a spectrum of disease, rather than distinct entities.

Phosphatidylinositol-4,5-bisphosphate 3-kinase catalytic subunit alpha gene (PIK3CA)-related overgrowth spectrum (PROS) encompasses a heterogeneous group of disorders associated with overgrowth. These disorders are caused by a somatic mosaic in the PIK3CA.[21] Included in this spectrum are macrocephaly-capillary malformation (M-CM/MCAP), KTS, CLOVES syndrome (congenital lipomatous overgrowth, vascular malformations, epidermal naevi, scoliosis/skeletal, and spinal syndrome) and CLAPO syndrome (capillary vascular malformation of the lower lip, LMs of the head and neck, asymmetry and partial or generalized overgrowth).[7] Other syndromes in this category are Parkes-Weber syndrome, Sturge-Weber syndrome, Proteus syndrome, Maffucci syndrome, microcephaly-CM, and Servelle-Martorell syndrome, among others.[7]

Provisionally Unclassified

A small number of vascular anomalies remain provisionally unclassified. As described in the 2018 ISSVA guidelines, these include intramuscular hemangioma, angiokeratoma, sinusoidal hemangioma, acral arteriovenous tumor, multifocal lymphangioendotheliomatosis with thrombocytopenia/cutaneovisceral angiomatosis with thrombocytopenia, PTEN (type) hamartoma of soft tissue/angiomatosis of soft tissue, and fibroadipose vascular anomaly.[7]

CLINICS CARE POINTS

- Vascular anomalies are categorized as either vascular malformations or vascular tumors.
- Vascular tumors are abnormal proliferations of vascular cells. These are benign, locally agreesive/borderline, or malignant.
- Vascular malformations (VMs) are lesions of dysplastic vessels lined by abnormal endothelium and are named for their vessel type. VMs are categorized as simple, combined, or syndrome-associated.
- There are a small number of vascular anomalies that remain to be classified.

DISCLOSURES

The authors have no conflicts of interests to disclose and no funding sources to report.

REFERENCES

1. Jackson IT, Carreño R, Potparic Z, et al. Hemangiomas, vascular malformations, and lymphovenous malformations: classification and methods of treatment. Plast Reconstr Surg 1993;91(7):1216–30.
2. Monroe EJ. Brief Description of ISSVA Classification for Radiologists. Tech Vasc Interv Radiol 2019;22(4):100628.
3. Nosher JL, Murillo PG, Liszewski M, et al. Vascular anomalies: a pictorial review of nomenclature, diagnosis and treatment. World J Radiol 2014;6(9):677–92.
4. MacFie CC, Jeffery SL. Diagnosis of vascular skin lesions in children: an audit and review. Pediatr Dermatol 2008;25(1):7–12.
5. Kunimoto K, Yamamoto Y, Jinnin M. ISSVA classification of vascular anomalies and molecular biology. Int J Mol Sci 2022;23(4):2358.
6. Mulliken JB, Glowacki J. Classification of pediatric vascular lesions. Plast Reconstr Surg 1982;70(1):120–1.
7. ISSVa classification of vascular anomalies ©2018 international society for the study of vascular anomalies. Available at: issva.org/classification. Accessed February 28, 2022.
8. Mulliken JB, Fishman SJ, Burrows PE. Vascular anomalies. Curr Probl Surg 2000;37(8):517–84.
9. Chang LC, Haggstrom AN, Drolet BA, et al. Growth characteristics of infantile hemangiomas: implications for management. Pediatrics 2008;122(2):360–7.

10. North PE, Waner M, James CA, et al. Congenital nonprogressive hemangioma: a distinct clinicopathologic entity unlike infantile hemangioma. Arch Dermatol 2001;137(12):1607–20.

11. Nimkar A, Mandel M, Buyuk A, et al. Spindle cell hemangioma of the lung: a case report. Cureus 2022;14(1):e21191.

12. Huang X, Chalmers AN. Review of wearable and portable sensors for monitoring personal solar UV exposure. Ann Biomed Eng 2021;49(3):964–78.

13. Baselga E, Wassef M, Lopez S, et al. Agminated, eruptive pyogenic granuloma-like lesions developing over congenital vascular stains. Pediatr Dermatol 2012;29(2):186–90.

14. Hinen HB, Trenor CC 3rd, Wine Lee L. Childhood Vascular Tumors. Front Pediatr 2020;8:573023.

15. Fanburg-Smith JC, Michal M, Partanen TA, et al. Papillary intralymphatic angioendothelioma (PILA): a report of twelve cases of a distinctive vascular tumor with phenotypic features of lymphatic vessels. Am J Surg Pathol 1999;23(9):1004–10.

16. Radu O, Pantanowitz L. Kaposi sarcoma. Arch Pathol Lab Med 2013;137(2):289–94.

17. Cesarman E. Kaposi sarcoma. Nat Rev Dis Primers 2019;5(1):10.

18. Ferrari A, Casanova M, Bisogno G, et al. Malignant vascular tumors in children and adolescents: a report from the Italian and German Soft Tissue Sarcoma Cooperative Group. Med Pediatr Oncol 2002;39(2):109–14.

19. Sardaro A, Bardoscia L, Petruzzelli MF, et al. Epithelioid hemangioendothelioma: an overview and update on a rare vascular tumor. Oncol Rev 2014; 8(2):259.

20. Rosenberg A, Agulnik M. Epithelioid hemangioendothelioma: update on diagnosis and treatment. Curr Treat Options Oncol 2018;19(4):19.

21. Martinez-Lopez A, Salvador-Rodriguez L, Montero-Vilchez T, et al. Vascular malformations syndromes: an update. Curr Opin Pediatr 2019;31(6):747–53.

22. Cooke-Barber J, Kreimer S, Patel M, et al. Venous malformations. Semin Pediatr Surg 2020;29(5):150976.

23. Wassef M, Blei F, Adams D, et al. Vascular anomalies classification: recommendations from the international society for the study of vascular anomalies. Pediatrics 2015;136(1):e203–14.

24. Kulungowski AM, Patel M. Lymphatic malformations. Semin Pediatr Surg 2020;29(5):150971.

25. Uller W, Alomari AI, Richter GT. Arteriovenous malformations. Semin Pediatr Surg 2014;23(4):203–7.

Histopathology of Vascular Malformations

Thuy L. Phung, MD, PhD

KEYWORDS

• Vascular anomalies • Histopathology • Vascular malformations • Molecular pathogenesis

KEY POINTS

- Vascular malformations are classified into distinct categories based on their clinical, structural and biological characteristics.
- Clinico-pathologic correlation is important to arrive at the correct diagnosis.
- Identification of key driver mutations leads to better insight into disease pathogenesis and new therapeutics.

Abbreviations	
AVM	Arteriovenous malformation
BRBNS	Blue rubber bleb nevus syndrome
CM	Capillary malformation
GLA	Generalized lymphatic anomaly
GSD	Gorham-Stout disease
GVM	Glomuvenous malformation
HHT	Hereditary hemorrhagic telangiectasia
KLA	Kaposiform lymphangiomatosis
KTS	Klippel-Trénaunay syndrome
LM	Lymphatic malformation
SWS	Sturge-Weber Syndrome
VM	Venous malformation
VVM	Verrucous venous malformation
H&E	Hematoxylin and eosin

INTRODUCTION

Vascular malformations are a complex and rapidly evolving field. Correspondingly, classification of these disease entities is also evolving, reflecting new insights and understanding into the clinical, pathogenesis, and molecular basis of these lesions. This article follows the International Society for the Study of Vascular Anomalies classification,[1] and describes key tissue histologic characteristics of vascular malformations.

CAPILLARY MALFORMATIONS
Cutaneous and Mucosal Capillary Malformations

Capillary malformation (CM, port-wine stain) can occur in isolation or as part of a syndrome, such

Department of Pathology, University of South Alabama, 2451 University Hospital Drive, Moorer Building, Room 133, Mobile, AL 36617, USA
E-mail address: tphung@health.southalabama.edu

Dermatol Clin 40 (2022) 345–355
https://doi.org/10.1016/j.det.2022.06.008

as Sturge-Weber syndrome (SWS). It presents as pink to violaceous macules and patches, and may darken and become thickened over time. CM exhibits different histologic features depending on the age of the lesion. In early lesion, the changes are subtle because of minimal dilation of capillaries in the dermis.[2,3] As the lesion progresses, blood vessels in the papillary and upper reticular dermis gradually enlarge with red blood cell congestion and dermal fibrosis (**Fig. 1**). Vessels in port-wine stain are capillaries, small veins, and postcapillary venules. The vessels are lined by a single layer of flattened endothelial cells, and the vascular wall becomes thickened because of increased blood flow. In some cases, there are thickening and nodularity of affected skin area with complex dermal changes, including increase in collagen and elastin and hair follicle changes.

Cutis Marmorata Telangiectatica Congenita

Cutis marmorata telangiectatica congenita is a genodermatosis with autosomal-dominant inheritance. It is characterized by skin patterning of reticulate network of dark violet–blue blood vessels, spider-like telangiectasia, and venous lakes.[4] The lesions are segmental or unilateral, occurring frequently on the limbs, trunk, and face or scalp. Histologic features of cutis marmorata telangiectatica congenita includes dilation of capillaries and veins in the dermis (**Fig. 2**). In some cases, there is proliferation of vascular channels.

Hereditary Hemorrhagic Telangiectasia

Hereditary hemorrhagic telangiectasia (HHT) is an autosomal-dominant vascular disorder characterized by numerous punctate telangiectases in the skin and mucous membranes. HHT is caused by mutations in endoglin (*ENG*) in HHT1, or activin A

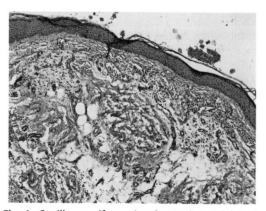

Fig. 1. Capillary malformation (port-wine stain) with dilated capillaries in the upper dermis and edema around blood vessels. H&E stains. X100.

receptor type II-like kinase-1 (*ACVRL1, ALK1*) in HHT2.[5] Skin pathology shows dilated thin-walled blood vessels in the upper dermis. The vessels are capillaries and venules, and are lined by a single layer of flattened endothelium by electron microscopy.[6]

LYMPHATIC MALFORMATIONS
Common Lymphatic Malformations

Lymphatic malformations (LM) consist of a wide spectrum of vascular anomalies affecting the lymphatic system. Most LM are present at birth or during early childhood, often affecting soft tissues. LM is classified as macrocystic, microcystic, or mixed type.[1] LM shows microscopic features of variably-sized lymphatic channels with a single layer of thin endothelium (**Fig. 3**). Some vessels have no vascular wall, whereas others have irregular smooth muscle wall.[7] The lumen may appear empty or contain pale white proteinaceous lymph fluid, lymphocytes, and macrophages. Red blood cell extravasation into lymphatic lumen is observed and may lead to misidentification of such vessels as venous channels. Hemorrhage and thrombi may be present because of spontaneous bleeding, trauma, or communication of lymphatic channels with the venous system. Large macrocystic LM can have thickened and fibrotic vessel walls. PROX-1 and VEGFR-3 are reportedly more sensitive than D2-40 in identifying large lymphatic channels in LM.[8] D2-40 immunostain is a useful biomarker in identifying small lymphatic vessels. Somatic activating mutations in *PIK3CA* are found in some LM.[9,10]

Generalized Lymphatic Anomaly

Generalized lymphatic anomaly (GLA) falls under complex lymphatic anomalies category, which also includes Gorham-Stout disease (GSD), channel-type LM, and kaposiform lymphangiomatosis (KLA). There is diffuse systemic lymphatic anomaly in GLA with multi-organ involvement.[11] Lymph fluid effusions in the thorax and abdomen, and bone defects can lead to significant morbidity.

Affected tissues in GLA show abnormal lymphatic vessels that are diffuse, involving soft tissues and multiple organs, including lung, liver, intestine, and bone. GLA lesions are composed of numerous variably sized lymphatic channels that infiltrate into surrounding tissues (**Fig. 4**).[7] In bones, there are abnormal lymphatic vessels in the medulla and cortex. Both cortical and medullary trabeculae are thin with increased number of osteocytes. The intertrabecular stroma is fibrotic with some lymphocytic infiltrate. Abnormal lymphatic vessels are seen in periosseous soft

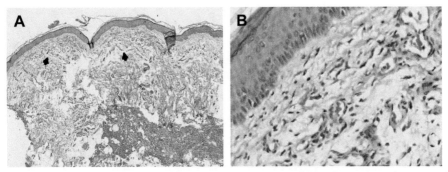

Fig. 2. Cutis marmorata telangiectatica congenita. (*A*) Prominent small blood vessels in the upper dermis (*arrows*). (*B*) Dilated delicate capillaries in loose myxoid stroma. H&E stains. (*A*) X20, (*B*) X100.

tissue. Lymphatic endothelial cells have large nuclei, some of which have "hobnail" appearance with protrusion of cell nuclei into the lumen. Endothelial cell hyperplasia and papillary structures are present. The cells are positive for the lymphatic marker podoplanin by immunostain with D2-40. Somatic pathogenic mutations in *PIK3CA* and *NRAS* (p.Q61R) have been identified in GLA.[12,13]

Kaposiform Lymphangiomatosis

Kaposiform lymphangiomatosis (KLA) is a systemic and aggressive lymphatic anomaly, frequently involving thoracic and abdominal tissues, including lungs, mediastinum, spleen, gastrointestinal tract, and bone. Severe coagulopathy and intralesional hemorrhage are common morbidities of KLA. Whole exome sequencing has identified a somatic mutation in *NRAS* (p.Q61R) in lesional tissue in 10 of 11 individuals with KLA, thus strongly implicating this mutation in the pathogenesis of the disease.[14] Somatic pathogenic mutation in *CBL* gene (*CBL* c.2322 T > G:p.Y774*) has also been identified in a patient with KLA, who does not have *NRAS* mutation.[15]

KLA has unique histologic features with multiple areas of infiltrative spindle-shaped lymphatic endothelial cells without obvious vascular lumen.[7] There is usually minimal cytologic atypia or mitosis. There are hemosiderin and abundant red blood cell extravasation. Abnormal dilated lymphatic vessels are present. In the lungs, spindled cell proliferation occurs in the interlobular septa and around bronchovascular bundles and pleura. The spindled cells are positive for lymphatic markers D2-40 and PROX-1. Spindled endothelial cells are also found in kaposiform hemangioendothelioma and Kaposi sarcoma. However, these two entities have different clinical presentation from KLA.

Gorham-Stout Disease

Gorham-Stout Disease (GSD), also known as "vanishing bone disease," is a complex lymphatic anomaly characterized by the proliferation of lymphatic vessels in soft tissue and bone with progressive bone destruction or osteolysis, leading to cortical bone resorption and replacement by fibrous tissue. Somatic pathogenic mutations in

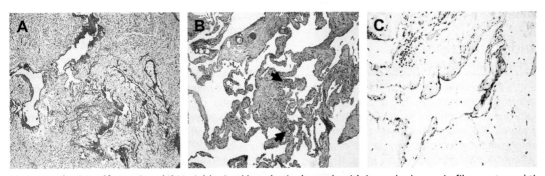

Fig. 3. Lymphatic malformation. (*A*) Variably sized lymphatic channels with irregular lumen in fibrous stromal tissue. (*B*) Large abnormal lymphatic channels with valves and aggregates of lymphocytes (*arrows*). (*C*) Lymphatic endothelium is positive for podoplanin (D2-40 immunostain). H&E stains and immunostains. (*A*) X20, (*B*) X40, (*C*) X200.

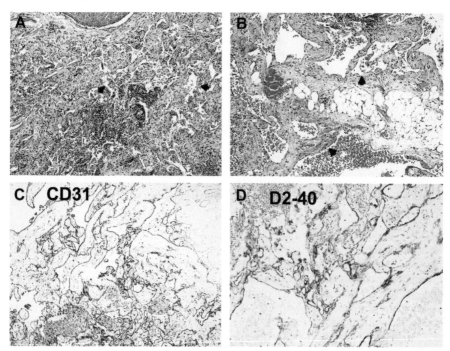

Fig. 4. Generalized lymphatic anomaly. (*A*) Soft tissue with numerous irregularly-shaped and tortuous vascular channels (*arrows*) and clusters of lymphocytes. (*B*) Abnormal vessels with variably thickened muscle wall (*arrows*) and hemorrhage. (*C, D*) The vessels are positive for CD31 and lymphatic marker D2-40 (*brown staining*). H&E stains and immunostains. (*A*) X40, (*B*) X100, (*C*) X40, (*D*) X200.

KRAS (p.G12V and p.Q61R) have been identified in GSD.[16,17]

Affected tissues show that lymphatic vessels, which are not typically present in normal bones, are seen in medullary and cortical bones.[18] There are numerous abnormal lymphatic vessels, and cortical bone is partially or completely destroyed. Abnormal vessels are also present in the periosteum and surrounding soft tissues. There is increased activity of osteoclasts and osteoblasts with new bone formation and bone marrow fibrosis. Lymphatic vessels have thin wall lined by benign endothelial cells that are positive for CD31, VEGFR-3, and D2-40.

VENOUS MALFORMATIONS
Common Venous Malformation

Venous malformation (VM) is a slow-flow vascular malformation typically present at birth and exhibits rapid growth secondary to trauma, infection, or hormonal influences.[19] VM is soft and easily compressible, occurs in segmental distribution, and can involve multiple organ sites. It grows in proportion with the child's growth. VM increases in size with Valsalva maneuver and dependency position. Complications of VM include pain, venous thrombosis, and pulmonary embolism.

Unlike infantile hemangioma, VM does not spontaneously regress.

VM typically involves the dermis and subcutis.[7] It consists of abnormally formed blood vessels with irregularly shaped and enlarged lumen lined by thin, flattened endothelial cells and thin basement membrane (**Fig. 5**). The vascular wall has variable thickness of smooth muscles with some areas entirely devoid of smooth muscles, resulting in discontinuous tunica media. Because of vascular congestion in VM, intravascular thrombi and phleboliths are common, with red blood cell extravasation, hemorrhage, and hemosiderin deposition. The presence of phleboliths helps to distinguish VM from other types of vascular malformations. Mucinous changes are often present around adnexal structures, such as sweat glands, in the skin. Malformations involving lymphatic vessels are present as seen on immunostains for the lymphatic marker D2-40. Thus, some VM may have mixed venous and lymphatic components.

Sporadic VM is associated with somatic mutations in *TIE2/TEK2* gene in 50% of the cases.[20,21] *TIE2* (p.L914F) is the most common hot spot mutation in sporadic VM, accounting for more than 70% of patients with *TIE2* mutations. *TIE2* (p.R849W) is the most common mutation in hereditary VM, such as familial mucocutaneous VM. More than 50% of

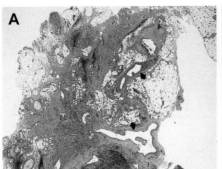
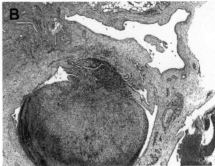

Fig. 5. Venous malformation. (*A*) Irregularly shaped, enlarged blood vessels in fibrous tissue (*arrows*). (*B*) Thrombus formed inside the lumen of a malformed venous channel. H&E stains. (*A*) X20, (*B*) X100.

VMs carry pathogenic somatic mutations in *PIK3CA* gene with hot spot mutations p.E542K, p.E545K, and p.H1047R accounting for more than 90% of *PIK3CA* alterations in VM.[22,23]

Familial Venous Malformation Cutaneomucosal

Familial VM cutaneomucosal is a "slow flow" VM occurring in the skin and oral mucosa that typically appears by puberty.[7] VM cutaneomucosal is associated with activating mutation in *TIE2* gene.[20,21] The lesion involves the deep dermis and subcutis, and consists of large dilated venous vessels lined by thin, flattened endothelial cells. The vascular wall has variable thickness and may have smooth muscles similar to venous channels. Thrombosis and calcification in the vascular wall and lumen are seen.

Blue Rubber Bleb Nevus Syndrome

Blue rubber bleb nevus syndrome (BRBNS) is characterized by multiple "blue rubbery-like" VMs in the skin and gastrointestinal tract.[24] Gastrointestinal bleeding from the lesions is a major morbidity. Lesion consists of large dilated venous channels in the dermis and subcutis of the skin, and submucosa in the gastrointestinal tract (**Fig. 6**). The vessel walls have smooth muscles of variable thickness. Intravascular thrombi, calcification, and intravascular papillary endothelial hyperplasia (Masson tumor) may be present and can cause clinical complications because of bleeding and thrombosis.[25] Even though BRBNS is primarily a VM, it also has a lymphatic component as seen on D2-40 immunostain. Activating mutation in *TIE-2* has been identified in BRBNS.[26]

Glomuvenous Malformation

Glomuvenous malformation (GVM) presents as bluish or violaceous lesion that occurs mainly on the extremities and trunk as solitary or multiple lesions. GVM may have segmental distribution associated with tissue mosaicism nature of the disorder. Familial GVM is linked to loss-of-function mutations in *glomulin* gene.[27] GVM is poorly circumscribed and consists of predominantly irregularly shaped enlarged blood vessels surrounded by small numbers of glomus cells. In some cases, glomus cell component may be limited or inconspicuous. These cells are uniform and cuboidal in size with eosinophilic cytoplasm, and are positive for smooth muscle actin and vimentin.[7] The abnormal vessels have smooth muscles with variable thickness as in other types of VMs. Thrombi may be present. GVM is distinguished from glomus tumor because the latter is a small, well-circumscribed proliferation of sheets of glomus cells without associated vascular malformation.

Verrucous Venous Malformation (Verrucous Hemangioma)

Verrucous venous malformation (VVM) is a congenital vascular malformation that presents at birth or during early childhood and grows in proportion with the child's growth.[28] VVM is single or multiple, and most occur in the extremity. The lesion appears as raised, hyperkeratotic, and warty bluish red papules that coalesce into plaques.

VVM is characterized by papillomatous or verrucous epidermal hyperplasia with hyperkeratosis that overlies markedly dilated blood vessels in the dermis and subcutis (**Fig. 7**).[29] Some vessels are juxtaposed close to the epidermis. The abnormal vasculature is most notable in the papillary dermis, and there is a deep component that extends into the deep dermis and subcutis. Malformed venous channels with irregular smooth muscle wall are present in the deep vascular

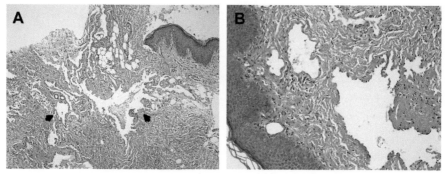

Fig. 6. Blue rubber bleb nevus syndrome. (*A*) Dilated irregular venous channels dissecting through the dermis (*arrows*). (*B*) Venous malformations lined by benign flattened endothelial cells. H&E stains. (*A*) X40, (*B*) X200.

component. VVM is differentiated from angiokeratoma by deep extension into the dermis, whereas angiokeratoma consists of dilated vessels limited to the upper dermis. The superficial portion of the two lesions is almost indistinguishable. VVM is focally positive for GLUT-1, a biomarker uniquely shared with infantile hemangioma. VVM is often negative for the lymphatic marker D2-40, but focal positivity has been observed. It has been suggested that VVM is a vascular malformation with an incomplete lymphatic phenotype. Some cases of VVM show mosaicism for somatic missense mutation in *MAP3K3* (c.1323 C > G; p.Iso441Met).[30]

ARTERIOVENOUS MALFORMATIONS
Sporadic Arteriovenous Malformation

Arteriovenous malformation (AVM) can occur sporadically or in association with inherited disorders, such as capillary malformation-arteriovenous malformation syndrome.[31] AVM presents at birth and grows in proportion with the child's growth. AVM is a fast-flow, compressible lesion with palpable thrill and bounding pulses. It can cause pain with activity and subsequently progress to pain at rest ("vascular steal phenomenon").

AVM is composed of arterial vessels feeding directly into venous vessels without intervening

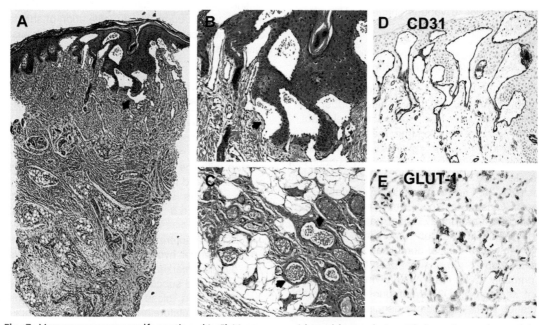

Fig. 7. Verrucous venous malformation. (*A*, *B*) Verrucous epidermal hyperplasia with hyperkeratosis overlying dilated blood vessels (*arrow*). (*C*) Enlarged vessels in the deep dermis (*arrows*). Blood vessels express (*D*) CD31 and (*E*) GLUT-1 focally. Red blood cells also express GLUT-1. H&E stains and immunostains. (*A*) X40, (*B*, *C*, *D*) X200, (*E*) X400.

capillary bed (direct shunting).[7] A distinguishing feature of AVM is blood shunting through a collection of tortuous dysmorphic vessels, known as the "nidus," which is identified *in situ* by radiologic imaging. Arteriovenous shunt is identified on elastin stain of tissue sections. It may require multiple serial sections to obtain the exact section where the shunt is located. Vessels in AVM have irregular thickened vascular wall with variable amounts of elastic fibers and haphazardly oriented smooth muscle fibers (**Fig. 8**). Thrombi may be present in malformed vessels. There are proliferative clusters of capillaries surrounding the periphery of the lesion and numerous branching capillaries in the papillary dermis overlying an AVM. Stain for elastic fibers may be useful in identifying arterial internal elastic lamina present in AVM. AVM may be associated with acroangiodermatitis, a vasoproliferative disorder consisting of proliferation of small, dilated blood vessels, edematous stroma, erythrocyte extravasation, and hemosiderin deposition. Acroangiodermatitis can resemble Kaposi sarcoma, thus requiring careful clinical and histologic evaluation.[32]

Capillary Malformation–Arteriovenous Malformation

This is an autosomal-dominant disorder with capillary malformations that appear as reddish tan, ovoid macules diffusely in the skin and surrounded by pale halo. These are fast-flow lesions with associated AVM in deep soft tissues or muscles elsewhere in the body.[7] In some cases, dermal arteries and veins may be enlarged, and large thin-walled vessels may be found around skin adnexal structures and in the subcutis. AVM in CM-AVM has histologic features similar to common sporadic AVM. CM-AVM shares similar clinical phenotypic characteristics with Parkes Weber syndrome, and both disorders are associated with pathogenic mutations in *RASA1* gene.[33]

VASCULAR MALFORMATIONS ASSOCIATED WITH OTHER ANOMALIES
Klippel-Trénaunay Syndrome

Klippel-Trénaunay syndrome (KTS) is a somatic overgrowth disorder that falls under the umbrella of PIK3CA-related overgrowth spectrum. Classic clinical manifestation of KTS includes diffuse CM (port-wine stain), VM, and LM with varicosities and tissue overgrowth, which is due to hypertrophy of bone and soft tissues, typically localized to the limb.[34] Histologic features of cutaneous CM in KTS are indistinguishable from those seen in lesions without KTS. CMs are dilated thin-walled blood vessels present in the papillary and reticular dermis.[7] As the patient ages, vascular lesions become progressively enlarged with thickened vascular wall and may contain phleboliths, creating nodules and varicosities in the skin.[35] Abnormal lymphatic vessels with enlarged, irregularly-shaped lumen and variable amounts of smooth muscles in the lymphatic walls are present. The presence of thrombi and associated endothelial cell hyperplasia and vascularization (Masson tumor) in VM may lead to diagnostic challenge from a true vascular neoplasm. In longstanding lesions, venous channels may come arterialized with disorganized elastic fibers in the vascular wall, and may lead to misidentification as AVM.

There are secondary skin changes in KTS. These include spongiotic eczematous inflammatory reaction (Meyerson phenomenon) and acroangiodermatitis, which is characterized by small blood vessel proliferation, red blood cell extravasation, and hemosiderin deposition.[36,37]

Parkes Weber Syndrome

Parkes Weber syndrome clinically consists of CM, multiple arteriovenous fistulas, and tissue overgrowth of the affected limb. Large arteries and

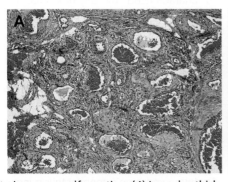
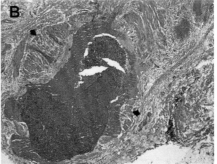

Fig. 8. Arteriovenous malformation. (*A*) Irregular, thick-walled blood vessels in the dermis. (*B*) A thrombus is present in a malformed vessel with variably thickened vascular smooth muscle wall (*arrows*). H&E stains. (*A*) X40, (*B*) X200.

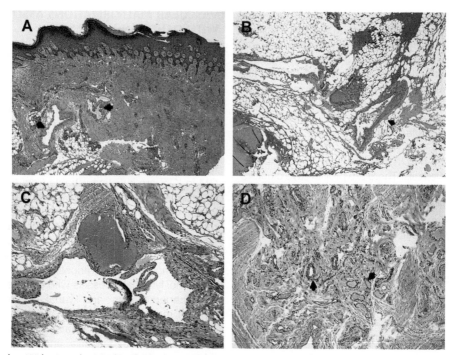

Fig. 9. Parkes Weber syndrome. (*A*, *B*) Abnormal irregularly-shaped blood vessels occupying the dermis and sub-cutis (*arrows*). (*C*) Arteriovenous fistula with valve and variably thickened smooth muscle wall. (*D*) Numerous small vessels in soft tissue (*arrows*). H&E stains. (*A*, *B*) X40, (*C*) X200, (*D*) X100.

veins with wall thickening and a small-vessel component are seen.[7] CMs have a lobular and infiltrative pattern throughout the dermis, and consist of numerous enlarged, dilated small vessels lined by benign, flattened endothelial cells (**Fig. 9**). Arteriovenous fistula component consists of blood vessels with irregularly thickened vascular walls, and is associated with high-flow arteriovenous shunting. Pathogenic mutations in *RASA1* gene have been associated with this syndrome.[38]

Sturge-Weber Syndrome

This syndrome is characterized by diffuse CMs (port-wine stains) with soft tissue overgrowth.[39] Histologic features of CMs associated with Sturge-Weber syndrome (SWS) are indistinguishable from those of sporadic CMs (**Fig. 10**). Some patients with SWS also have pigmented lesions of phakomatosis pigmentovascularis type IIb.[40] Pathogenic mutation in *GNAQ* gene (c.548 G > A, p.R183Q) has been identified in more than 80% of patients with SWS and in those with nonsyndromic port-wine stains.[41]

Maffucci Syndrome

Maffucci syndrome is a nonhereditary disorder of mesodermal dysplasia. Major clinical manifestation of Maffucci syndrome includes vascular

anomalies (spindle cell hemangioma and VM) and enchondroma, which is a benign cartilaginous tumor.[42] Malignant transformation of enchondroma and cutaneous angiosarcoma have been reported in patients with the syndrome.[43] Somatic mosaic mutations in *IDH1* (p.R132C and p.R132H) and *IDH2* (p.R172S) have been reported in more than 70% of patients with Maffucci syndrome.[44,45]

Congenital Lipomatous Overgrowth, Vascular Malformations, Epidermal Nevi, and Skeletal Anomalies (CLOVES) Syndrome

CLOVES is a somatic overgrowth disorder in the PIK3CA-related overgrowth spectrum. CLOVES is characterized by asymmetrical body overgrowth, skeletal anomalies, and vascular malformations, including CM, VM, LM, and AVM, or mixed types.[7] These malformations are usually associated with adipocyte overgrowth and increase in collagenous materials. Small abnormal venous channels often infiltrate fatty tissue. Somatic mosaic mutations in *PIK3CA* were identified in affected tissues of six patients with CLOVES syndrome.[46]

Proteus Syndrome

Proteus syndrome's manifestation includes cerebriform connective tissue nevi, lipomas, ovarian and salivary gland tumors, asymmetrical skeletal

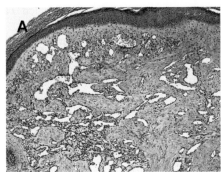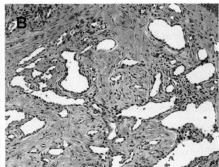

Fig. 10. Capillary malformations in Sturge-Weber syndrome. (*A*) Dilated vascular channels in the dermis. (*B*) Dermal vessels have irregular, enlarged lumen lined by flattened endothelial cells. H&E stains. (*A*) X40, (*B*) X200.

overgrowth as well as eye, lung, and renal abnormalities. Vascular anomalies in Proteus syndrome consist of CM, VM, and LM with development of intravascular thrombi and thromboemboli.[7] Proteus syndrome is caused by somatic mosaic *AKT1* mutation (*AKT1* p.E17K).[47]

CLINICS CARE POINTS

- Correlation between clinical, diagnostic imaging, and histologic features is important in diagnosing vascular malformations.

- H&E tissue stain is the primary modality of histologic diagnosis that can be supplemented with immunostains and molecular studies.

- Vascular malformations can have local or systemic effects that impact overall care of the patient.

- Targeted therapy based on the presence of pathogenic gene mutations is an emerging important treatment modality for vascular malformations.

ACKNOWLEDGMENTS

The author thanks John Larrimore for his excellent assistance with the article preparation.

DISCLOSURE

The author has no conflict of interest to disclose pertaining to this article.

REFERENCES

1. Wassef M, Blei F, Adams D, et al. Vascular anomalies classification: recommendations from the International Society for the Study of Vascular Anomalies. Pediatrics 2015;136(1):e203–14.

2. Phung TL, Wright TS, Pourciau CY, et al. Pediatric dermatopathology. 1st edition. New York: Springer; 2017. p. 427–59.

3. Neumann R, Leonhartsberger H, Knobler R, et al. Immunohistochemistry of port-wine stains and normal skin with endothelium-specific antibodies PAL-E, anti-ICAM-1, anti-ELAM-1, and anti-factor VIIIrAg. Arch Dermatol 1994;130:879–83.

4. Fujita M, Darmstadt GL, Dinulos JG. Cutis marmorata telangiectatica congenita with hemangiomatous histopathologic features. J Am Acad Dermatol 2003;48:950–4.

5. Shoukier M, Teske U, Weise A, et al. Characterization of five novel large deletions causing hereditary haemorrhagic telangiectasia. Clin Genet 2008;73: 320–30.

6. Hashimoto K, Pritzker MS. Hereditary hemorrhagic telangiectasia: an electron microscopic study. Oral Surg Oral Med Oral Pathol 1972;34:751–8.

7. Mulliken JB, Burrows PE, Fishman SJ. Mulliken & Young's vascular anomalies: hemangiomas and malformations. 2nd edition. New York (NY): Oxford University Press; 2013. p. 480–507. Check page number.

8. Castro EC, Galambos C. Prox-1 and VEGFR3 antibodies are superior to D2-40 in identifying endothelial cells of lymphatic malformations: a proposal of a new immunohistochemical panel to differentiate lymphatic from other vascular malformations. Pediatr Dev Pathol 2009;12(3):187–94.

9. Osborn AJ, Dickie P, Neilson DE, et al. Activating PIK3CA alleles and lymphangiogenic phenotype of lymphatic endothelial cells isolated from lymphatic malformations. Hum Mol Genet 2015; 24:926–38.

10. Luks VL, Kamitaki N N, Vivero MP, et al. Lymphatic and other vascular malformative/overgrowth disorders are caused by somatic mutations in PIK3CA. J Pediatr 2015;166(4): 1048–1054 e1041, 1045.

11. Lala S, Mulliken JB, Alomari AI, et al. Gorham-Stout disease and generalized lymphatic

anomaly: clinical, radiologic, and histologic differentiation. Skeletal Radiol 2013;42:917–24.

12. Manevitz-Mendelson E, Leichner GS, Barel O, et al. Somatic NRAS mutation in patient with generalized lymphatic anomaly. Angiogenesis 2018;21(2):287–98.

13. Rodriguez-Laguna L, Agra N, Ibañez K, et al. Somatic activating mutations in PIK3CA cause generalized lymphatic anomaly. J Exp Med 2019;216(2):407.

14. Barclay SF, Inman KW, Luks VL, et al. A somatic activating NRAS variant associated with kaposiform lymphangiomatosis. Genet Med 2019;21(7):1517–24.

15. Foster JB, Li D, March ME, et al. Kaposiform lymphangiomatosis effectively treated with MEK inhibition. EMBO Mol Med 2020;12:e12324.

16. Homayun-Sepehr N, McCarter AL, Helaers R, et al. KRAS-driven model of Gorham-Stout disease effectively treated with trametinib. JCI Insight 2021;9(15):e149831.

17. Nozawa A, Ozeki M, Niihori T, et al. A somatic activating KRAS variant identified in an affected lesion of a patient with Gorham-Stout disease. J Hum Genet 2020;65(11):995–1001.

18. Liu Y, Zhong DR, Zhou PR, et al. Gorham-Stout disease: radiological, histological, and clinical features of 12 cases and review of literature. Clin Rhematol 2016;35(3):813–23.

19. Boon LM, Mulliken JB, Enjolras O, et al. Glomuvenous malformation (glomangioma) and venous malformation: distinct clinicopathologic and genetic entities. Arch Dermatol 2004;140:971–6.

20. Vikkula M, Boon LM, Carraway KL, et al. Vascular dysmorphogenesis caused by an activating mutation in the receptor tyrosine kinase TIE2. Cell 1996;87(7):1181–90.

21. Limaye N, Wouters V, Uebelhoer M, et al. Somatic mutations in angiopoietin receptor gene TEK cause solitary and multiple sporadic venous malformations. Nat Genet 2009;41(1):118–24.

22. Limaye N, Kangas J, Mendola A, et al. Somatic activating PIK3CA mutations cause venous malformation. Am J Hum Genet 2015;97(6):914–21.

23. Castel P, Carmona FJ, Grego-Bessa J, et al. Somatic PIK3CA mutations as a driver of sporadic venous malformations. Sci Transl Med 2016;8(332):332ra342.

24. Agnese M, Cipolletta L, Bianco MA, et al. Blue rubber bleb nevus syndrome. Acta Paediatr 2010;99(4):632–5.

25. Ishii T, Asuwa N, Suzuki S, et al. Blue rubber bleb naevus syndrome. Virchows Arch A Pathol Anat Histopathol 1988;413:485–90.

26. Nobuhara Y, Onoda N, Fukai K, et al. TIE2 gain-of-function mutation in a patient with pancreatic lymphangioma associated with blue rubber-bleb nevus

syndrome: report of a case. Surg Today 2006;36(3):283–6.

27. Brouillard P, Boon LM, Mulliken JB, et al. Mutations in a novel factor, glomulin, are responsible for glomuvenous malformations ("glomangiomas"). Am J Hum Genet 2002;70(4):866–74.

28. Tennant LB, Mulliken JB, Perez-Atayde AR, et al. Verrucous hemangioma revisited. Pediatr Dermatol 2006;23(3):208–15.

29. Wang L, Gao T, Wang G. Verrucous hemangioma: a clinicopathological and immunohistochemical analysis of 74 cases. J Cutan Pathol 2014;41:823–30.

30. Couto JA, Vivero MP, Kozakewich HP, et al. A somatic MAP3K3 mutation is associated with verrucous venous malformation. Am J Hum Genet 2015;96(3):480–6.

31. Whitehead KJ, Smith MC, Li DY. Arteriovenous malformations and other vascular malformation syndromes. Cold Spring Harb Perspect Med 2012;3(2):a006635.

32. Earhart RN, Aeling JA, Nuss DD, et al. Pseudo-Kaposi sarcoma: a patient with arteriovenous malformation and skin lesions simulating Kaposi sarcoma. Arch Dermatol 1974;110:907–10.

33. Eerola I, Boon LM, Mulliken JB, et al. Capillary malformation-arteriovenous malformation, a new clinical and genetic disorder caused by RASA1 mutations. Am J Hum Genet 2003;73:1240–9.

34. Garzon MC, Huang JT, Enjolras O, et al. Vascular malformations: part II: associated syndromes. J Am Acad Dermatol 2007;56:541–64.

35. Klapman MH, Yao JF. Thickening and nodules in port-wine stains. J Am Acad Dermatol 2001;44:300–2.

36. Hofer T. Meyerson phenomenon within a nevus flammeus. The different eczematous reactions within port-wine stains. Dermatology 2002;205(2):180–3.

37. Kofoed ML, Klemp P, Thestrup-Pedersen K. The Klippel-Trenaunay syndrome with acro-angiodermatitis (pseudo-Kaposi's sarcoma). Acta Derm Venereol 1985;65(1):75–7.

38. Daboub AJ, Grimmer JF, Frigerio A, et al. Parkes Weber syndrome associated with two somatic pathogenic variants in RASA1. Cold Spring Harb Mol Case Stud 2020;6(4):a005256.

39. Comi AM. Sturge-Weber syndrome. Handb Clin Neurol 2015;132:157–68.

40. Fernandez-Guarino M, Boixeda P, de Las Heras E, et al. Phakomatosis pigmentovascularis: clinical findings in 15 patients and review of the literature. J Am Acad Dermatol 2008;58(1):88–93.

41. Shirley MD, Tang H, Gallione CJ, et al. Sturge-Weber syndrome and port-wine stains caused by somatic mutation in GNAQ. N Engl J Med 2013;368(21):1971–9.

42. Pellegrini AE, Drake RD, Qualman SJ. Spindle cell hemangioendothelioma: a neoplasm associated

with Maffucci's syndrome. J Cutan Pathol 1995; 22(2):173–6.

43. Davidson TI, Kissin MW, Bradish CF, et al. Angiosarcoma arising in a patient with Maffucci syndrome. Eur J Surg Oncol 1985;11(4):381–4.

44. Amary MF, Damato S, Halai D, et al. Ollier disease and Maffucci syndrome are caused by somatic mosaic mutations of IDH1 and IDH2. Nat Genet 2011;43:1262–5.

45. Pansuriya TC, van Eijk R, d'Adamo P, et al. Somatic mosaic IDH1 and IDH2 mutations are associated with enchondroma and spindle cell hemangioma in Ollier disease and Mafucci syndrome. Nat Genet 2011;43:1256–61.

46. Kurek KC, Luks VL, Ayturk UM, et al. Somatic mosaic activating mutations in PIK3CA cause CLOVES syndrome. Am J Hum Genet 2012;90: 1108–15.

47. Lindhurst MJ, Sapp JC, Teer JK, et al. A mosaic activating mutation in AKT1 associated with the Proteus syndrome. N Engl J Med 2011;365(7):611–9.

Histopathology of Vascular Tumors

Thuy L. Phung, MD, PhD

KEYWORDS

- Vascular anomalies • Histopathology • Vascular tumors • Molecular pathogenesis

KEY POINTS

- Vascular tumors are classified into specific categories based on their biological behavior.
- Clinico-pathologic correlation is important to arrive at the correct diagnosis.
- Identification of key driver mutations leads to better insights into tumor pathogenesis.

INTRODUCTION

Vascular tumors comprise a broad and complex area of vascular anomalies. Correspondingly, classification of vascular tumors is also evolving, reflecting new insights and understanding into the clinical, pathogenesis, and molecular basis of these lesions. This article follows the International Society for the Study of Vascular Anomalies classification,[1] and describes key tissue histopathologic characteristics of these lesions.

BENIGN VASCULAR TUMORS
Infantile Hemangioma

Infantile hemangioma (IH) affects about 5% of all infants, and is more common in females and in infants with prematurity and low birth weight.[2] IH appears shortly after birth as erythematous papules, nodules, or plaques with focal localized distribution or segmental distribution that covers an entire area of skin. IH has a unique course of evolution, which consists of early rapid growth during proliferative phase, followed by gradual stabilization, and spontaneous regression or involution of the lesion over months to years.

Histologic features of IH depends on the natural evolution of the lesion. During proliferative phase, IH is a hypercellular mass that occupies the entire dermis and may extend into the subcutis.[3,4] The tumor is composed of lobules of tightly packed small capillaries with small to nonconspicuous lumen lined by benign endothelial cells and surrounded by pericytes (**Fig. 1**). Intervening stroma consists of fibroblasts, lymphocytes, and mast cells. Proliferating IH is mitotically active with no apparent feature of atypical mitotic figures or endothelial cell atypia. IH undergoes spontaneous involution, a cellular process in which hypercellular endothelial cell component is gradually replaced by fibroadipose tissue. As the lesion involutes, fibrous septae between lobules becomes broader and more conspicuous. There is increase in endothelial cell apoptosis and reduction in cellularity, and a decrease in the number of blood vessels. The remaining vessels have enlarged lumen. At the end of involution, IH remnant consists mainly of fibroadipose tissue with scattered remaining blood vessels. Useful immunostains for IH include endothelial cell marker CD31, and vascular smooth muscle cell marker SMA. A distinguishing biomarker of IH is GLUT-1, which stains IH strongly and is absent in other types of vascular tumors, such as congenital hemangioma.[5] Although GLUT-1 is highly specific for IH, it is also expressed in verrucous venous malformation. Moreover, strong expression of GLUT-1 in red blood cells may lead to misinterpretation of GLUT-1 positivity in cases in which red blood cells are adherent to vascular lumen. IH also expresses unique placenta-related biomarkers, including Lewis Y antigen, merosin, and FcgammaRII.[6] WT-1, a transcription factor encoded by Wilms tumor 1 gene, is a marker

Department of Pathology, University of South Alabama, 2451 University Hospital Drive, Moorer Building, Room 133, Mobile, AL 36617, USA
E-mail address: tphung@health.southalabama.edu

Dermatol Clin 40 (2022) 357–366
https://doi.org/10.1016/j.det.2022.06.009

Abbreviations	
EHE	Epithelioid hemangioendothelioma
HHV-8	Human herpes virus 8
IH	Infantile hemangioma
KHE	Kaposiform hemangioendothelioma
KS	Kaposi sarcoma
NICH	Noninvoluting congenital hemangioma
RICH	Rapidly involuting congenital hemangioma

expressed in hemangiomas but not in vascular malformations.[7]

Rapidly Involuting Congenital Hemangioma

Rapidly involuting congenital hemangioma (RICH) presents as infiltrating violaceous plaques or nodules with surrounding pale halo and large peripheral radiating vessels.[8] Central scar or ulceration may be present. RICH develops in utero and is detectable by prenatal ultrasound by 12 weeks of gestation. RICH is fully developed at birth, which is an important distinguishing clinical feature from IH, which develops after birth. RICH often spontaneously involutes by 12 to 14 months of age.

RICH is characterized by hypercellular lobules of small, well-formed blood vessels with centrally located prominent draining vessels with enlarged lumen (**Fig. 2**).[4,8] The endothelial cells are plump and may have cytoplasmic inclusions. There is minimal mitotic activity and no cytologic atypia. Intravascular thrombi and hemosiderin deposition are seen in some lesions. Consistent with the rapid involution of RICH, there is prominent perilobular fibrous tissue. Involution seems to start in the central portion of the tumor and progresses radially, creating a zonal effect. Unlike IH that stains positively for GLUT-1, RICH does not express GLUT-1. Congenital hemangiomas have been reported to carry somatic activating mutations in *GNAQ* and *GNA11* (p.E209L).[9] The same gene mutation is found in RICH and noninvoluting congenital hemangioma (NICH).

Noninvoluting Congenital Hemangioma

Noninvoluting congenital hemangioma (NICH) appears clinically similar to RICH. It grows in the fetus in utero and is fully developed at birth. The tumor is coarse with overlying telangiectasias and admixed areas of pallor and a pale peripheral halo.[4] NICH grows in proportion to the child, and does not spontaneous involute like RICH.

NICH consists of large lobules of small, tightly packed blood vessels and pericytes (**Fig. 3**). Large, stellate draining vessels may appear in the central portion of the lesions.[3] Endothelial cells may protrude into the vascular lumen, creating

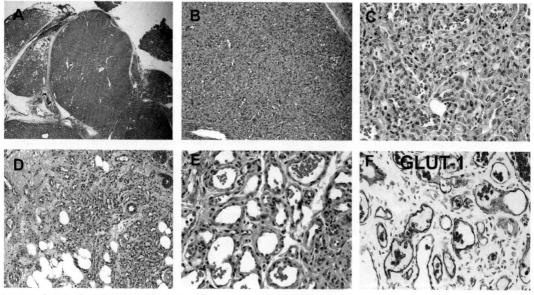

Fig. 1. Infantile hemangioma. (*A–C*) Hemangioma in proliferating phase with well-circumscribed hypercellular lobules of tightly packed endothelial cells and small capillaries. (*D, E*) Hemangioma in involuting phase has increased fibrous stroma and reduced number of blood vessels. Remaining vessels have markedly dilated lumen. (*F*) Vessels express GLUT-1 (*brown immunostain*). Pericytes and stromal cells are GLUT-1 negative. H&E stains. (*A*) X20, (*B*) X40, (*C*) X200, (*D*) X40, (*E, F*) X200.

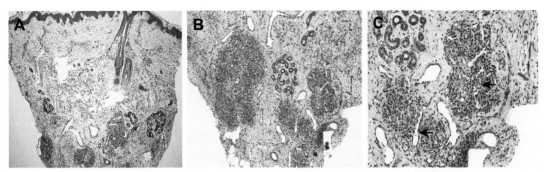

Fig. 2. Rapidly involuting congenital hemangioma. (*A, B*) Presence of hypercellular lobules of small, compact blood vessels in the dermis separated by perilobular fibrous tissue. (*C*) Vascular lobules have prominent centrally located draining vessels with enlarged lumen (*arrows*). H&E stains. (*A*) X20, (*B*) X40, (*C*) X200.

"hobnail" appearance. The lobules are surrounded by dense fibrotic tissue, and hemosiderin and pigment-laden macrophages are present. Extramedullary hematopoiesis may be observed. NICH is negative for GLUT-1 by immunostains, which is a useful tool to distinguish NICH from IH. Somatic activating mutations in *GNAQ* and *GNA11* (p.E209L) has been identified in congenital hemangioma, including NICH.[9]

Tufted Angioma

Tufted angioma is present at birth or appears within the first year of life. It typically occurs as a solitary infiltrative plaque with violaceous and mottled appearance.[10] Lanugo hair and port-wine stain may be seen overlying tufted angioma. The tumor grows over months to years, and can stabilize or regress.[11] It is associated with Kasabach-Merritt phenomenon, a consumptive coagulopathy.

At low scanning magnification, tufted angioma is a diffuse, poorly circumscribed vascular tumor (**Fig. 4**). It has a cannon ball appearance of discreet lobules present in the upper to deep dermis.[3,4] The lobules consist of spindle-shaped endothelial cells, pericytes, and small blood vessels with oval or slit-like lumen. The lobules are surrounded peripherally by crescent-shaped

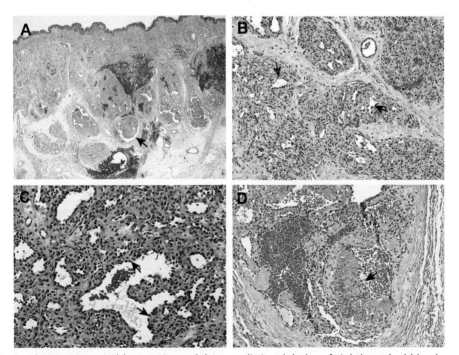

Fig. 3. Noninvoluting congenital hemangioma. (*A*) Large distinct lobules of tightly packed blood vessels with curvilinear channels around the lobules (*arrow*). (*B*) Enlarged central draining vessels in lobules (*arrows*). (*C*) "Hobnail" endothelial cells (*arrows*) protrude into vascular lumen. (*D*) Thrombi in some blood vessels (*arrow*). H&E stains. (*A*) X20, (*B*) X100, (*C*) X200, (*D*) X100.

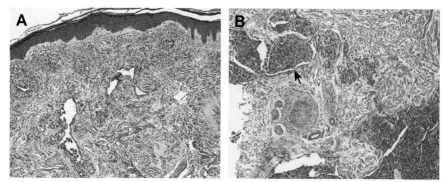

Fig. 4. Tufted angioma. (*A*) The tumor has a cannon ball appearance of distinct hypercellular lobules. (*B*) Lobules are surrounded peripherally by crescent-shaped lymphatic channels (*arrow*). H&E stains. (*A*) X20, (*B*) X100.

lymphatic channels that are positive for the lymphatic marker D2-40.[12] Rare mitotic figures are present and there is no significant cytologic atypia. Endothelial cells are positive for CD31, CD34, and factor VIII–related antigen, and negative for GLUT-1. Tufted angioma is considered to be along the continuum of vascular tumors as kaposiform hemangioendothelioma (KHE). It has tendency for local recurrence and progressive growth, but there are no reported cases of distant metastasis.

Spindle Cell Hemangioma

Spindle cell hemangioma is seen in association with Maffucci syndrome, especially in cases with multifocal lesions. The lesion appears as a bluish and firm nodule, often in the legs. It is based in the dermis and subcutis, and has three major tissue components: (1) a vascular component of markedly dilated thin-walled blood vessels, some of which may contain intravascular thrombi; (2) a solid component of spindle cells with slitlike vascular spaces; and (3) an endothelial component that lines the vascular channels or is present in cellular clusters.[13,14] Endothelial cells are epithelioid with cytoplasmic vacuoles (**Fig. 5**). There are large, malformed vessels and bundles of smooth muscle cells present near enlarged vessels and in solid areas. The spindle cell component appears bland with minimal cytologic atypia. The endothelial cell component is positive for vascular markers CD31, CD34, and factor VIII–related antigen, whereas the solid spindle cell component is negative for these markers.[14] Spindle cell hemangioma is negative for human herpes virus 8 (HHV-8), which is a useful marker to distinguish it from Kaposi sarcoma (KS). Pathogenic mutations in *IDH1* gene have been found in spindle cell hemangioma associated with Maffucci syndrome.[15]

Epithelioid Hemangioma

Epithelioid hemangioma (angiolymphoid hyperplasia with eosinophilia) typically presents as solitary or multiple flesh-to-plum-colored papules or nodules on the head and neck.[16] The lesion has some histologic features of a reactive process. It occupies the dermis and subcutis and consists of well-circumscribed nodular proliferation of thick- and thin-walled blood vessels with

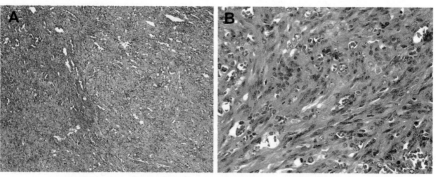

Fig. 5. Spindle cell hemangioma. (*A*) Solid sheet-like proliferation of spindle-shaped cells with slit-like vascular spaces. (*B*) Spindle cells coursing between irregular vascular channels. H&E stains. (*A*) X20, (*B*) X200.

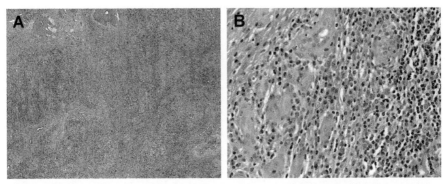

Fig. 6. Epithelioid hemangioma. (A) Dense infiltrates of lymphocytes and lymphoid follicles with inconspicuous blood vessels. (B) Abundant eosinophils and lymphocytes admixed with blood vessels. H&E stains. (A) X20, (B) X200.

prominent "epithelioid" endothelial cells lining the vascular lumen (Fig. 6).[17] Intermixed with endothelial cells and blood vessels is a dense infiltrate of lymphocytes, sometimes with lymphoid follicles, mast cells, and a large number of eosinophils. The inflammatory cell infiltrate may be the dominant component and can even obscure the vascular component. The stroma may be fibrous, edematous, and myxoid. Mitotic figures may be present, but there is no cytologic atypia. The endothelial cells are positive for CD31, CD34, and factor VIII–related antigen.[17]

Pyogenic Granuloma

Pyogenic granuloma (lobular capillary hemangioma) is a common benign vascular tumor that presents as an erythematous and pedunculated mass which tends to bleed repeatedly.[4] The overlying epidermis is often atrophic and ulcerated (Fig. 7). A collarette of elongated rete ridges wraps around multilobular vascular proliferation. A dense proliferation of capillaries and small blood vessels in discreet lobules of variable sizes is present in the dermis.[4] A larger "feeder" vessel

deep to the lobules may be seen. The lobules are larger toward the skin surface, and smaller and more compact in the deep aspect. The intervening stroma may be myxoid, edematous, or fibrotic. Early lesions are hypercellular with increased mitosis, but there is no cytologic atypia. Ulcerated lesions often have a dense inflammatory reaction that resembles granulation tissue. Pyogenic granuloma expresses CD31 and CD34 and is negative for GLUT-1. Bacillary angiomatosis has some histologic features that can mimic pyogenic granuloma.

Hobnail Hemangioma

Hobnail hemangioma (targetoid hemosiderotic hemangioma) presents as a solitary violaceous papule or nodule surrounded by a pale halo and an ecchymotic rim. It is a poorly circumscribed vascular tumor present in the dermis and extends into the subcutis (Fig. 8). There are dilated blood vessels lined by plump endothelial cells that protrude into the vascular lumen (hobnail endothelial cells) and intraluminal papillary projections in the blood vessels.[18] The vessels intercalate between collagen

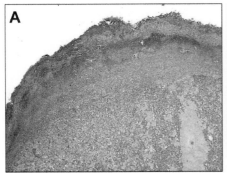
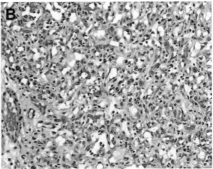

Fig. 7. Pyogenic granuloma. (A) Lobular vascular mass with surface ulceration and inflammation. (B) Dense proliferation of endothelial cells and small blood vessels. H&E stains. (A) X20, (B) X200.

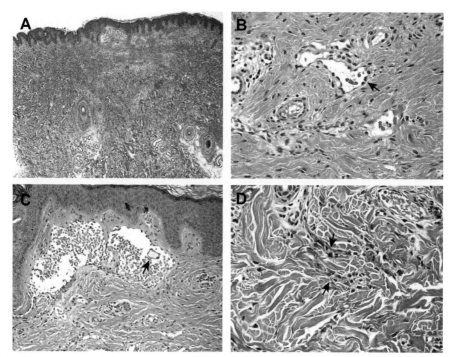

Fig. 8. Hobnail hemangioma. (*A*) Poorly circumscribed vascular tumor in the dermis. (*B*) Hobnail endothelial cells (*arrow*) and (*C*) intravascular papillary processes (*arrow*) are present. (*D*) Narrow vessels intercalate between collagen bundles with hemosiderin deposition (*arrows*). H&E stains. (*A*) X20, (*B*) X200.

bundles with angular, narrow vascular spaces surrounding sweat glands in the deep dermis. There are inflammatory cells, red blood cell extravasation, and hemosiderin deposition. Endothelial cells stain for CD31 and lymphatic markers VEGFR-3 and podoplanin (D2-40 antigen), suggesting lymphatic differentiation of the lesion.[18,19] The lesion is negative for WT-1 expression, which is a biomarker expressed in vascular tumors but not vascular malformations, suggesting that hobnail hemangioma may be a vascular malformation with lymphatic differentiation, and not a true vascular tumor.[20]

Intravascular Papillary Endothelial Hyperplasia

Intravascular papillary endothelial hyperplasia (Masson tumor) is thought to be a reactive vascular proliferative process that occurs within the lumen of a blood vessel, typically a vein. Masses of papillary fronds are observed within the vascular lumen and often associated with intravascular thrombi (**Fig. 9**).[4] Papillary projections are lined by a layer of benign endothelial cells with occasional mitosis but no cytologic atypia. There is upregulation of vascular endothelial

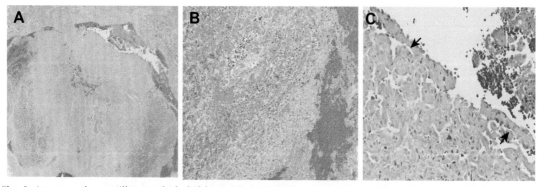

Fig. 9. Intravascular papillary endothelial hyperplasia (Masson tumor). (*A, B*) Thrombus within a large venous vessel and associated vascular proliferative processes. (*C*) Papillary projections are lined by a layer of benign endothelial cells (*arrows*). H&E stains. (*A*) X20, (*B*) X40, (*C*) X200.

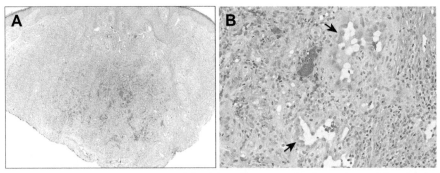

Fig. 10. Cutaneous epithelioid angiomatous nodule. (*A*) Well-circumscribed vascular proliferation in the dermis. (*B*) Numerous blood vessels lined by endothelial cells with abundant eosinophilic cytoplasm (*arrows*). Extravasated red blood cells and inflammatory infiltrates with eosinophils are present. H&E stains. (*A*) X20, (*B*) X200.

growth factor and hypoxia-induced factor 1α expression within thrombi and intravascular endothelial hyperplasia.[21]

Cutaneous Epithelioid Angiomatous Nodule

Cutaneous epithelioid angiomatous nodule is a benign vascular proliferation that often presents as a single red-blue nodule on the trunk, extremities, and head. It is a well-circumscribed proliferation of polygonal endothelial cells with enlarged nuclei in the upper dermis (**Fig. 10**).[22] Endothelial cells may have abundant eosinophilic cytoplasm

and intracytoplasmic vacuoles. Extravasated red blood cells and hemosiderin are often observed. There is an associated mild inflammatory infiltrate, occasionally with eosinophils. The lesional cells are positive for CD31 and focally for CD34.

LOCALLY AGGRESSIVE OR BORDERLINE VASCULAR TUMORS
Kaposiform Hemangioendothelioma

Kaposiform hemangioendothelioma (KHE) is a locally aggressive vascular tumor that can recur

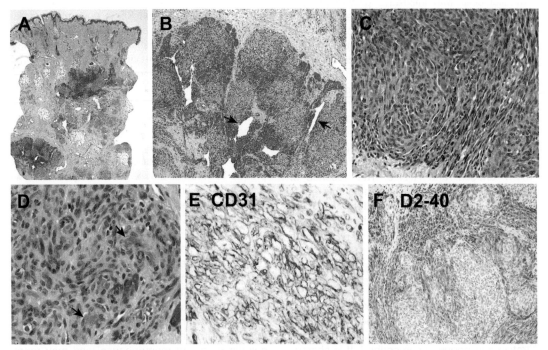

Fig. 11. Kaposiform hemangioendothelioma. (*A*) Lobular proliferation of hypercellular, tightly packed blood vessels with hemorrhage. (*B*) Tumor lobules with paralobular draining vessels (*arrows*). (*C*) Dense hypercellular epithelioid and spindle-shaped cells. (*D*) Microthrombi (*arrows*) are present in vascular lumen. (*E*) Tumor cells are positive for CD31. (*F*) Presence of lymphatic marker D2-40 in the periphery of the lobules. H&E stains. (*A*) X20, (*B*) X40, (*C*) X200, (*D*) X400, (*E*) X100, (*F*) X40.

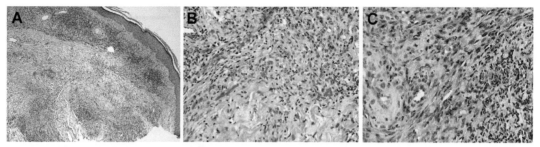

Fig. 12. Kaposi sarcoma. (*A*) Dense proliferation of abnormal blood vessels with hemorrhage in the dermis. (*B*) Infiltrative, irregular slit-like vascular channels dissecting through dermal collagen. (*C*) Interlacing bundles of atypical spindle-shaped cells with lymphocytes and extravasated red blood cells. H&E stains. (*A*) X20, (*B*) X100, (*C*) X200.

but rarely metastasizes.[23,24] The tumor usually presents at birth or within the first year of life, and is characterized as a single infiltrative, deep red, violaceous plaque surrounded by a rim of purpura or ecchymosis. A major complication of KHE is Kasabach-Merritt syndrome, which is a consumptive coagulopathy resulting in thrombocytopenia and disseminated intravascular coagulation.[24] Sirolimus, which inhibits mTOR signaling pathway, is an efficacious and well-tolerated drug for treatment of KHE.[25]

KHE occupies the dermis and extends into the subcutaneous tissue (**Fig. 11**). It consists of lobular proliferations of blood vessels with slit-like or crescent-shaped lumen and spindle-shaped endothelial cells with infiltrative growth pattern, resembling Kaposi sarcoma (KS).[23] Areas of blood vessels, and dense cellularity of endothelial cells and other spindled cells are present. KHE has characteristic features of endothelial cells forming small islands or "glomeruloid" areas in the lobules. There are cytologic atypia and mitoses with intratumoral hemorrhage and hemosiderin. Enlarged and malformed lymphatic vessels are present within and in the periphery of the lobules. Spindled endothelial cells in the lobules are positive for CD31, CD34, and FLI1, but negative for GLUT-1, Lewis Y antigen, and HHV-8. The absence of HHV-8 in KHE aids in distinguishing this entity from KS. KHE has lymphatic differentiation as shown by expression of podoplanin as detected by the antibody D2-40.[12]

Retiform Hemangioendothelioma

Retiform hemangioendothelioma is a locally aggressive, slow-growing vascular tumor that is nodular or plaque-like in appearance, and involving the dermis and subcutis. The tumor is infiltrative and poorly circumscribed. It is characterized by long, thin, arborizing vascular channels that bear resemblance to the rete testis, hence the name.[26] The vessels are lined by hobnail endothelial cells that protrude into the lumen. There is

prominent lymphocytic infiltrate that may obscure the vessels in some cases. There are solid areas with spindle cells arranged in cords with narrow lumen. The tumor expresses von Willebrand factor, CD31, and CD34, but not lymphatic markers D2-40 and VEGFR-3.[27] Spindle cells in the solid areas also express CD31, indicating their endothelial cell differentiation.

Kaposi Sarcoma

Kaposi sarcoma (KS) consists of four clinical variants: (1) classic type, (2) African (endemic) type, (3) immunosuppression-associated type, and (4) HIV-associated type.[4] Classic-type KS affects mainly older men. African-type KS is endemic in areas of Africa, particularly eastern Zaire and western Uganda, affecting mostly males, and it is linked to HHV-8 and Epstein-Barr virus infections.[28] KS associated with immunosuppression often arises in the setting of organ transplantation, cancer chemotherapy, and chronic steroid use. HIV-associated KS is caused mainly by HIV-1 and in some cases HIV-2.[29]

The four clinical variants of KS have similar histologic features. The lesions evolve from patch to plaque to nodular stage. Patch-stage KS shows a dermal proliferation of jagged, irregular vascular channels dissecting through dermal collagen (**Fig. 12**).[4,30] These channels partly surround normal dermal blood vessels in some areas, creating the "promontory sign." Lymphocytes, plasma cells, hemosiderin, and extravasated red blood cells may be present. Plaque-stage and nodular-stage KS show dense dermal proliferation of interlacing bundles of atypical spindle-shaped cells and infiltrative, irregular slit-like vessels. Eosinophilic hyaline globules are present within spindle cells and macrophages, and may represent phagocytosed-red blood cells. The globules are periodic acid Schiff–positive and stain bright red with Mallory trichrome stain.[31] KS expresses CD31 and the lymphatic marker D2-40. Calcitonin

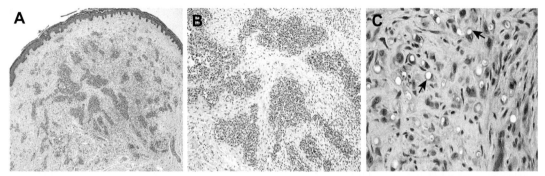

Fig. 13. Epithelioid hemangioendothelioma. (*A, B*) Proliferation of atypical epithelioid and spindle-shaped endothelial cells in nests and cords. (*C*) Atypical endothelial cells have cytoplasmic vacuoles, giving them a "ring cell" appearance (*arrows*). There is characteristic dense hyalinized stroma. H&E stains. (*A*) X20, (*B*) X100, (*C*) X400.

receptor–like receptor is also strongly expressed in KS.[32] HHV-8 in KS may be detected by antibody against HHV-8 latency-associated nuclear antigen LNA-1.[33]

MALIGNANT VASCULAR TUMORS
Epithelioid Hemangioendothelioma

Epithelioid hemangioendothelioma (EHE) is a borderline malignant vascular tumor that occurs in the liver, bone, soft tissue, and skin. EHE is a proliferation of atypical epithelioid and spindle-shaped endothelial cells in nests and cords (**Fig. 13**).[34] Tumor cells may contain cytoplasmic vacuoles, thus giving them a "popcorn" or "ring cell" appearance. Nuclear atypia and mitosis are present. The tumor has a characteristic dense fibromyxoid stroma. Many EHE cases express CD34 and D2-40.[34] ERG, FLI-1, and TFE are also expressed in EHE. *WWTR1-CAMTA1* gene fusion has been identified in many cases of EHE, and *YAP1-TFE3* gene fusion has been found in a small subset of EHE.[35,36] Antibody to the C-terminus of CAMTA1 may be useful in differentiating EHE from other vascular tumors.[37] Loss of expression of YAP1 C-terminus as detected by immunostains may serve as a good ancillary marker for EHE variants with *YAP1-TFE3* gene fusion.[38]

CLINICS CARE POINTS

- Correlation between clinical and histologic features is important in diagnosing vascular tumors.
- H&E tissue stain is the primary modality of histologic diagnosis that can be supplemented with immunostains and molecular studies.
- Vascular tumors can have local or systemic effects that impact overall care of the patient.

ACKNOWLEDGMENTS

The author thanks John Larrimore for his excellent assistance with the article preparation.

DISCLOSURE

The author has no conflict of interest to disclose pertaining to this article.

REFERENCES

1. Wassef M, Blei F, Adams D, et al. Vascular anomalies classification: recommendations from the International Society for the Study of Vascular Anomalies. Pediatrics 2015;136(1):e203–14.
2. Haggstrom AN, Frieden IJ. Hemangiomas: past, present, and future. J Am Acad Dermatol 2004;51: S50–2.
3. Phung TL, Wright TS, Pourciau CY, et al. Pediatric dermatopathology. 1st edition. New York (NY): Springer; 2017. p. 427–59.
4. Mulliken JB, Burrows PE, Fishman SJ. Mulliken & Young's vascular anomalies: hemangiomas and malformations. 2nd edition. New York, NY (NY): Oxford University Press; 2013. p. 43–67 (check page number).
5. North PE, Waner M, Mizeracki A, et al. GLUT1: a newly discovered immunohistochemical marker for juvenile hemangiomas. Hum Pathol 2000;31(1):11–22.
6. North PE, Waner M, Mizeracki A, et al. A unique microvascular phenotype shared by juvenile hemangiomas and human placenta. Arch Dermatol 2001; 137(5):559–70.
7. Lawley LP, Cerimele F, Weiss SW, et al. Expression of Wilms tumor 1 gene distinguishes vascular malformations from proliferative endothelial lesions. Arch Dermatol 2005;141:1297–300.
8. Berenguer B, Mulliken JB, Enjolras O, et al. Rapidly involuting congenital hemangioma: clinical and histopathologic features. Pediatr Dev Pathol 2003; 6(6):495–510.
9. Ayturk UM, Couto JA, Hann S, et al. Somatic activating mutations in GNAQ and GNA11 are

associated with congenital hemangioma. Am J Hum Genet 2016;98(6):1271.

10. Herron MD, Coffin CM, Vanderhooft SL. Tufted angiomas: variability of the clinical morphology. Pediatr Dermatol 2002;19:394–401.

11. Miyamoto T, Mihara M, Mishima E, et al. Acquired tufted angioma showing spontaneous regression. Br J Dermatol 1992;127:645–8.

12. Arai E, Kuramochi A, Tsuchida T, et al. Usefulness of D2-40 immunohistochemistry for differentiation between kaposiform hemangioendothelioma and tufted angioma. J Cutan Pathol 2006;33:492–7.

13. Marušić Z, Billings SD. Histopathology of spindle cell vascular tumors. Surg Pathol Clin 2017;10(2):345–66.

14. Fletcher CD, Beham A, Schmid C. Spindle cell haemangioendothelioma: a clinicopathological and immunohistochemical study indicative of a non-neoplastic lesion. Histopathology 1991;18:291–301.

15. Kurek KC, Pansuriya TC, van Ruler MA, et al. R132C IDH1 mutations are found in spindle cell hemangiomas and not in other vascular tumors or malformations. Am J Pathol 2013;182(5):1494–500.

16. Adler BL, Krausz AE, Minuti A, et al. Epidemiology and treatment of angiolymphoid hyperplasia with eosinophilia (ALHE): a systematic review. J Am Acad Dermatol 2016;74(3):506–12.

17. Guo R, Gavino AC. Angiolymphoid hyperplasia with eosinophilia. Arch Pathol Lab Med 2015;139(5):683–6.

18. Mentzel T, Partanen TA, Kutzner H. Hobnail hemangioma ('targetoid hemosiderotic hemangioma'): clinicopathologic and immunohistochemical analysis of 62 cases. J Cutan Pathol 1999;26:279–86.

19. Al Dhaybi R, Lam C, Hatami A, et al. Targetoid hemosiderotic hemangiomas (hobnail hemangiomas) are vascular lymphatic malformations: a study of 12 pediatric cases. J Am Acad Dermatol 2011;66(1):116–20.

20. Trindade F, Tellechea O, Torrelo A, et al. Wilms tumor 1 expression in vascular neoplasms and vascular malformations. Am J Dermatopathol 2011;33(6):569–72.

21. Kim S, Jun JH, Kim J, et al. HIF-1 alpha and VEGF expression correlates with thrombus remodeling in cases of intravascular papillary endothelial hyperplasia. Int J Clin Exp Pathol 2013;6:2912–8.

22. Brenn T, Fletcher CD. Cutaneous epithelioid angiomatous nodule: a distinct lesion in the morphologic spectrum of epithelioid vascular tumors. Am J Dermatopathol 2004;26:14–21.

23. Lyons LL, North PE, Lai FM, et al. Kaposiform hemangioendothelioma: a study of 33 cases emphasizing its pathologic, immunophenotypic, and biologic uniqueness from juvenile hemangioma. Am J Surg Pathol 2004;28:559–68.

24. Croteau SE, Liang MG, Kozakewich HP, et al. Kaposiform hemangioendothelioma: atypical features and risks of Kasabach-Merritt phenomenon in 107 referrals. J Pediatr 2012;162(1):142–7.

25. Adams DM, Trenor CC, Hammill AM, et al. Efficacy and safety of sirolimus in the treatment of complicated vascular anomalies. Pediatrics 2016;137(2): e20153257.

26. Calonje E, Fletcher CD, Wilson-Jones E, et al. Retiform hemangioendothelioma. A distinctive form of low-grade angiosarcoma delineated in a series of 15 cases. Am J Surg Pathol 1994;18(2):115–25.

27. Parsons A, Sheehan DJ, Sangueza OP. Retiform hemangioendothelioma usually do not express D2-40 and VEGFR-3. Am J Dermatopathol 2008;30:31–3.

28. Chow JW, Lucas SB. Endemic and atypical Kaposi's sarcoma in Africa: histopathological aspects. Clin Exp Dermatol 1990;15:253–9.

29. Barre-Sinoussi F, Chermann JC, Rey F, et al. Isolation of a T-lymphotropic retrovirus from a patient at risk for acquired immune deficiency syndrome (AIDS). Science 1983;220:868–71.

30. Leu HJ, Odermatt B. Multicentric angiosarcoma (Kaposi's sarcoma). Virchows Arch A Pathol Anat Histopathol 1985;408:29–41.

31. Kao GF, Johnson FB, Sulica VI. The nature of hyaline (eosinophilic) globules and vascular slits of Kaposi's sarcoma. Am J Dermatopathol 1990;12:256–67.

32. Hagner S, Stahl U, Grimm T, et al. Expression of calcitonin receptor-like receptor in human vascular tumours. J Clin Pathol 2006;59:1104–7.

33. Hong A, Davies S, Lee CS. Immunohistochemical detection of the human herpes virus 8 (HHV8) latent nuclear antigen-1 in Kaposi's sarcoma. Pathology 2003;35:448–50.

34. Flucke U, Vogels RJ, de Sait Aubain Somerhausen N, et al. Epithelioid hemangioendothelioma: clinicopathologic, immunohistochemical, and molecular genetic analysis of 39 cases. Diagn Pathol 2014;9:131.

35. Tanas MR, Sboner A, Oliveira AM, et al. Identification of a disease-defining gene fusion in epithelioid hemangioendothelioma. Sci Transl Med 2011;3(98):98.

36. Antonescu CR, Loarer FL, Mosquera JM, et al. Novel YAP1-TFE3 fusion defines a distinct subset of epithelioid hemangioendothelioma. Genes Chromosomes Cancer 2013;52(8):775–84.

37. Doyle LA, Fletcher CD, Hornick JL. Nuclear expression of CAMTA1 distinguishes epithelioid hemangioendothelioma from histologic mimics. Am J Surg Pathol 2016;40:94–102.

38. Anderson WJ, Fletcher CD, Hornick JL. Loss of expression of YAP1 C-terminus as an ancillary marker for epithelioid hemangioendothelioma variant with YAP1-TFE3 fusion and other YAP1-related vascular neoplasms. Mod Pathol 2021; 34(11):2036–42.

Diagnostic Imaging

John McAlhany, MD*, Ricardo Yamada, MD

KEYWORDS

- Vascular • Malformations • Anomaly • Imaging

KEY POINTS

- Although typically diagnosed clinically, imaging of vascular anomalies is important in confirming the diagnosis and planning for appropriate treatment.
- Imaging workup of vascular anomalies is performed in a stepwise approach, predominantly using ultrasound and MRI.
- Advanced imaging modalities such as magnetic resonance angiography and computed tomography angiography should not be ordered routinely and be reserved for treatment planning of high-flow lesions only.
- Imaging can identify aggressive features of some vascular tumors and prompt further evaluation with tissue sampling.

OVERVIEW

Vascular tumors and malformations encompass a spectrum of pathology that varies widely in presentation, severity, and treatments. Detection of these lesions are frequently made clinically; capillary malformations (port-wine stains) in the newborn, swelling and skin discoloration in venous and lymphatic malformations (LMs), and high-output heart failure in an arteriovenous malformation (Fig. 1). Although clinically detected, the accurate classification of lesions is often challenging. Imaging plays an integral role in confirming the clinical diagnosis, determining the extent of disease, and planning treatment strategies. Ultrasound (US) and MRI constitute the backbone of diagnostic imaging in vascular anomalies; however, other modalities such as radiography, computed tomography, and conventional angiography can play a role in certain situations.

BACKGROUND

Diagnostic imaging of vascular anomalies (VAs) is used for the confirmation of clinically detected lesions and treatment planning. As mentioned earlier, most instances a clear diagnosis can be made based on history and physical examination alone. Key information to obtain during imaging evaluation includes extent of lesion, hemodynamics, and association with adjacent structures.[1] Imaging is typically obtained in a stepwise approach, from least invasive to more invasive, with consideration for minimizing ionizing radiation and cost. General practitioners should not take the responsibility to order imaging studies, especially advanced imaging modalities. US might be an appropriate initial step, but a specialist can determine that in a more cost-effective way. Ordering cross-sectional images, such as computed tomography and magnetic resonance (MR), should be limited to a specialist.

The American College of Radiology Appropriateness Criteria recommends US and MR as the first step in the evaluation of suspected VAs.[2] US is relatively inexpensive, does not use ionizing radiation, allows dynamic evaluation of the lesion, and can assess flow and velocities with spectral Doppler. The disadvantages include difficulty imaging lesions that are deep or adjacent to air or bone and a narrow field of view.[3–5] MR with and without intravenous contrast provides excellent soft tissue contrast and the ability to image the entire lesion. It is the best study to evaluate the

Medical University of South Carolina, 96 Jonathan Lucas, Suite 210, MSC 323, Charleston, SC 29425, USA
* Corresponding author. Medical University of South Carolina, 25 Courtenay Drive, MSC 226, Charleston, SC 29425.
E-mail address: Mcalhajo@musc.edu

Dermatol Clin 40 (2022) 367–377
https://doi.org/10.1016/j.det.2022.06.010
0733-8635/22/© 2022 Elsevier Inc. All rights reserved.

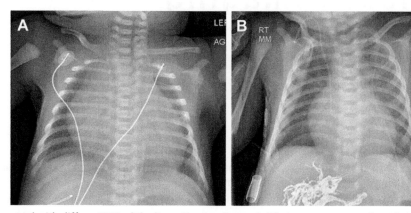

Fig. 1. Neonatal with diffuse AVM of the liver. Chest radiograph (*A*) demonstrates profound cardiomegaly in the setting of high-output heart failure. Following onyx embolization (*B*) of the hepatic AVM that was causing a left to right there is resolution of cardiomegaly.

extension of the lesion and relationship with adjacent structures. Considerations for MRI are the increased time required to acquire images, which may require sedation/anesthesia for young patients and high costs.[4,6]

Hemodynamic assessment of high-flow lesions, including delineation of feeding vessels and drainage veins, is possible with computed tomography angiography (CTA) and magnetic resonance angiography (MRA) (**Fig. 2**). CTA has quick scan times and high spatial resolution, which may afford better evaluation of abdominal/pelvic lesions, where breathing artifact may impose some limitation. CTA is also helpful evaluating lesions involving osseous structures and lungs. However,

CTA lacks the soft tissue contrast of MRA and exposes the patient to ionizing radiation, limiting its clinical use in the workup of VAs.[2] It is important to emphasize that CTA/MRA are mostly reserved for treatment planning of high-flow lesions only. CTA/MRA performed in slow-flow lesions (eg, venous and LMs) do not provide any additional relevant information and will increase overall cost to patient care (see Clinics Care Points).

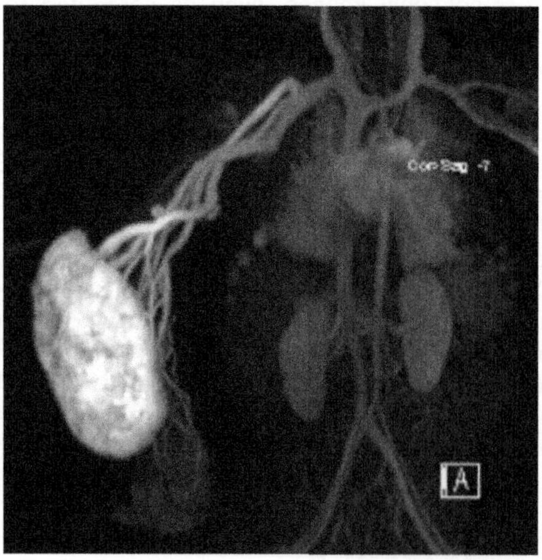

Other imaging modalities, including radiography and conventional angiography, are not part of the initial workup, however, are often used in specific situations. Radiography is frequently obtained in the workup of limb pain or swelling and incidental secondary findings of VAs may be found, such as phleboliths in venous malformations (VMs) (**Fig. 3**). Conventional angiography provides the highest resolution of vessels and allows for the treatment at the same time but is invasive and exposes the patient to ionizing radiation.[2] Therefore, it is usually obtained during endovascular treatment of high-flow lesions.

VASCULAR TUMORS

Vascular tumors are characterized by endothelial cell hyperproliferation and are classified as benign, locally aggressive or borderline, and malignant.[7] Imaging can be particularly useful identifying aggressive/malignant features that would prompt further evaluation with tissue sampling.

BENIGN

Benign tumors include infantile hemangiomas (IHs), congenital hemangiomas (CHs), and less common subtypes such as tufted angiomas, pyogenic granulomas, epithelioid hemangioma, and spindle cell hemangioma.

Fig. 2. MRA of a right upper extremity congenital hemangioma shows a homogenous, hypervascular mass with multiple dilated feeding arteries and draining veins. This image demonstrates the ability of MRA to determine the vascularization pattern of the lesion.

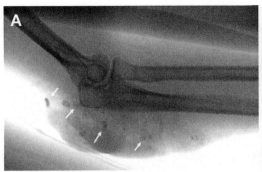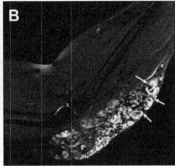

Fig. 3. Radiograph of the elbow (*A*) reveals a soft tissue mass with multiple phleboliths (*arrows*), which are pathognomonic for venous malformations. T2W MRI (*B*) shows hyperintense, dilated, vascular channels with internal low-intensity foci (*arrows*) representing phleboliths.

Infantile Hemangiomas

IHs are the most common vascular tumors of infancy with a prevalence of 2% to 3%. Given the typical clinical evolution and often superficial location, IHs are not commonly imaged. Diagnostic studies are usually reserved for deeper lesions that cannot be fully assessed clinically. The timeline is typically a postnatal presentation, followed by a rapid proliferative phase over the first year, with regression occurring during childhood.[8] Imaging characteristics vary between the proliferative and involuting phase; the former exhibiting well-circumscribed and lobulated margins with internal hypervascularity, whereas the latter shows fatty replacement and decreasing vascularity. Using US, proliferative phase IHs demonstrate a soft tissue mass of variable echogenicity that gradually becomes hyperechoic during involution. Doppler US reveals a high vascular density, and spectral analysis may show arteriovenous shunting.[9] MRI is reserved for determining the extent of involvement of IHs, which are primarily low to intermediate intensity on T1-weighted (T1W) images and high intensity on T2-weighted (T2W) images. Flow voids, which represent high-flow vascular structures, are commonly seen on T2W images. With the addition of contrast, arterial inflow provides early enhancement with persistent enhancement of the mass on delayed images. MRI evaluation of the involutory phase reflects fibrofatty replacement, with foci of increased intensity on T1-weighted imaging and less-avid arterial enhancement.[10]

Congenital Hemangiomas

CHs are much less common than IHs and differ in that they are present at birth. CHs are classified into rapidly involuting CHs, partially involuting CHs (PICHs), and noninvoluting CHs based on whether they fully involute by 1 to 2 years of age (Fig. 4).[8] Imaging findings of CHs are overall similar to IHs with a few differences. On US, the mass component of CHs is heterogenous and the borders are less distinct than in IHs. The characteristic features of CHs include visible vessels, calcifications, and vascular aneurysms.[11]

Less Common Benign Vascular Tumors

Tufted hemangiomas typically present at birth, less than 10% present over the age of 50, as red or violet vascular plaques. Consumptive coagulopathy occurs in 10% of tufted hemangiomas, an association known as Kasabach–Merritt syndrome,[12] and less commonly in intramuscular hemangiomas (Fig. 5). Pyogenic granuloma is a red papule that frequently ulcerates and bleeds, occurs in children, and usually presents on the head and face. These lesions are usually clinical diagnoses and do not require imaging during workup.

LOCALLY AGGRESSIVE OR BORDERLINE

Hemangioendotheliomas represent vascular tumors that fall between benign hemangiomas and malignant angiosarcomas and are classified as kaposiform, retiform, papillary intralymphatic, and composite.[9] US evaluation reveals ill-defined soft tissue masses, frequently with calcifications and necrosis. Degree of vascularity and echogenicity is highly variable. MRI characteristics are similar to those seen in IHs, low to intermediate intensity on T1W imaging and high intensity on T2W imaging with flow voids in highly vascular lesions. Prior hemorrhage and blood products are seen as signal voids on gradient-recalled echo, and post-contrast MRI reveals heterogenous enhancement.[13]

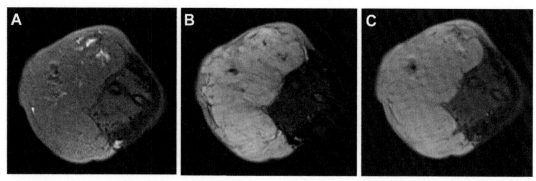

Fig. 4. MRI of a congenital hemangioma of the forearm demonstrates a homogenous T1W (*A*) hypointense and T2W (*B*) hyperintense soft tissue mass. There is homogenous enhancement with contrast administration (*C*), differentiating this congenital hemangioma from the heterogenous enhancement of a venous malformation.

MALIGNANT

Malignant vascular tumors, angiosarcoma and epithelioid hemangioendotheliomas being the two most common, are rare tumors that can present in both pediatric and adult patients. In contrast to previously described lesions, imaging features suggestive of malignancy include ill-defined margins, high-resistive indices on spectral Doppler, and perilesional edema on T2W imaging.[13]

Angiosarcoma

Angiosarcoma is a malignant tumor composed of vascular and lymphatic elements, most commonly within soft tissue of the face and neck in the elderly. Although predominantly sporadic, angiosarcoma may arise from precursor vascular lesions, have associations with toxic exposures, or occur in the setting of chronic lymphedema in Stewart–Treves syndrome.[8,9] Imaging findings are nonspecific and similar to other aggressive vascular tumors with low to intermediate signal

intensity on T1W images and high signal intensity on T2W images. Angiosarcoma is an infiltrative mass with serpentine, predominantly peripheral, avidly enhancing vessels (**Fig. 6**) that will restrict diffusion on diffusion-weighted imaging.[14]

Epithelioid Hemangioendothelioma

Epithelioid hemangioendothelioma most commonly involves the liver in adults. Characteristic imaging findings include multiple peripheral hepatic lesions that are hypoattenuating to hepatic parenchyma on noncontrast CT. Owing to a relative avascular zone surrounding the lesion, a hypoenhancing or T2 hypointense peripheral rim is present and produces a classic targetoid appearance. As peripheral lesions become confluent during disease progression, fibrosis and capsular retraction occur.[15]

VASCULAR MALFORMATIONS

Vascular malformations, in contrast to tumors, are present at birth and grow proportionally with the

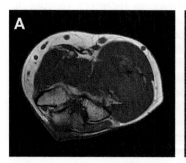
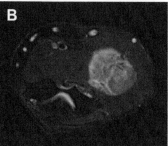
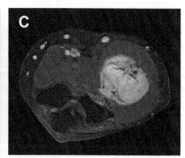

Fig. 5. MRI of a 40-year-old patient with swelling of the left elbow reveals a well-circumscribed, intramuscular hemangioma without invasion of surrounding structures. Similar to other types of hemangiomas, this lesion demonstrates low-intensity T1W (*A*) and high-intensity T2W (*B*) signal with homogenous enhancement on contrast-enhanced sequences (*C*).

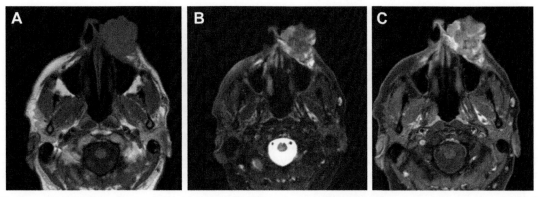

Fig. 6. Axial MRI of the face reveals an irregular, T1W hypointense (*A*) soft tissue mass arising anterior to the left maxillary sinus. The soft tissues surrounding the lesion have high-intensity signal on T2W images (*B*), which represents perilesional edema and is a malignant feature. There is heterogenous contrast enhancement (*C*) and this lesion represents a malignant angiosarcoma.

child, never involuting. Vascular malformations are believed to result from abnormal vessel morphogenesis. They are often not recognized at birth and only become evident secondary to thrombosis, trauma, infections, or periods of hormonal fluctuations, such as puberty and pregnancy.[10] Unlike vascular tumors, vascular malformations tend to defy tissue planes and can involve any tissue, including skin, soft tissue, bone, joints, or viscera.[7] Malformations historically have been characterized as low flow or high flow by the presence of an arterial feeding vessel, as flow rates may affect intervention options. The International Society for the Study of Vascular Anomalies (ISSVA) classification differentiates capillary, venous, lymphatic, arteriovenous fistulas, and arteriovenous malformations (AVMs) into simple malformations or those occurring in combination or associated with other anomalies.[16]

CAPILLARY MALFORMATIONS

The diagnosis of CMs is primarily clinical, as US and MRI evaluation may reveal only nonspecific dermal or subcutaneous thickening and enhancement.[10,17] Although generally isolated, CMs may be associated with underlying anomalies that should be excluded with MRI or other imaging modalities. An example is Sturge–Weber syndrome, which consists of a port-wine stain, neurologic malformations, and ophthalmic abnormalities. Piram and colleagues found that 7% to 28% of patients with port-wine stains in the V1 facial nerve distribution had Sturge–Weber syndrome and require MRI to assess for intracranial vascular malformations.[18] Other associations requiring imaging include CMs overlying the spine associated with

underlying spinal abnormalities and mucosal telangiectasias associated with pulmonary and intracranial telangiectasias in hereditary hemorrhagic telangiectasia syndrome.[16]

LYMPHATIC MALFORMATIONS

LMs arise from abnormal lymphatic development during fetal angiogenesis and result in varying degrees of dilated lymphatic channels that are cystic in nature. LMs are typically diagnosed in the neonatal or early childhood periods and have a propensity to affect the superficial lymphatic rich spaces of the head and neck (70%–80%) and axilla (20%), with a small incidence of deep involvement of the mediastinum, retroperitoneum, pelvis, and extremities.[19] Microcystic and macrocystic LMs are differentiated based on having cystic components less than or greater than 1 to 2 cm, respectively.[16] Defining the predominant cystic component drives treatment, as macrocystic LMs are amenable to percutaneous sclerotherapy rather than surgical or medical management options available for microcystic LMs.

Macrocystic Lymphatic Malformations

Macrocystic LMs have cystic components greater than 1 to 2 cm in size and have smooth cystic spaces underlying normal skin and subcutaneous tissue. Although sporadic cases are the most common, large cervical macrocystic LMs can compromise respiratory or digestive function.[7] Gray scale US reveals noncompressible, anechoic spaces which may contain few thin intervening septa (**Fig. 7**). Fluid–fluid levels may be present in the setting of recent hemorrhage or increased proteinaceous fluid and is not specific to LMs. Doppler

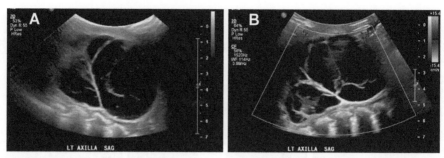

Fig. 7. Gray scale ultrasound (*A*) of a macrocystic LM with anechoic cystic components and thin intervening septations. Doppler ultrasound (*B*) of the same lesion shows no flow within the cystic space, supporting the diagnosis of LM.

US may demonstrate arterial flow within septa, but there should be no flow within the cystic spaces. CT is seldom used in the workup of macrocystic LMs, but when obtained will reveal lobulated cystic structures that are primarily fluid attenuation, although can have increased attenuation in the setting of recent hemorrhage.[20] MRI is the optimal modality to assess macrocystic LMs, which typically feature a low to intermediate intensity on T1W imaging and high intensity on T2W imaging, although variable T1 imaging characteristics can be seen due to degree of proteinaceous contents or hemorrhage within cystic components. On contrast-enhanced MRI, rim and septal enhancement may be present, but there should be no enhancement of the internal cystic spaces (**Fig. 8**).

Microcystic Lymphatic Malformations

Microcystic LMs are composed of diffuse cystic structures with thin intervening septations. Gray scale US will display small anechoic cystic spaces with posterior acoustic enhancement. The background may appear solid, as the combined echogenicity of the septations are all that may be visualized if the cystic spaces are below the resolution of US (**Fig. 9**). The latter pattern can be difficult to differentiate from a vascular tumor on gray scale US; however, on Doppler US, there should be no increased vascularity.[17] MRI of microcystic LMs reveals similar T1 and T2 tissue characteristics to macrocystic LMs; however, on contrast-enhanced MRI, microcystic LMs should not reveal any enhancement (**Fig. 10**). A small subset will show diffuse enhancement due to cumulative enhancement of the walls of the imperceptible cystic components and can be difficult to differentiate from VMs or some vascular tumors with delayed contrast enhancement.[10]

VENOUS MALFORMATIONS

VMs, like other vascular malformations, are present at birth, grow with the child, and do not regress. VMs are the most common, making up to two-thirds of the total cases of vascular malformations.[21] They occur on the extremities (40%) and the head and neck (40%) and can involve any type of tissue including skin, subcutaneous, muscles, joints, and bones. VMs are composed of dilated, thin-walled, postcapillary vascular channels with abnormal smooth muscle, which predisposes to gradual expansion over time.

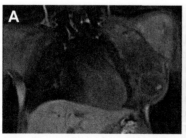
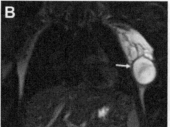
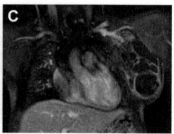

Fig. 8. MRI with coronal views of the same patient reveals a lobulated lesion in the left axilla with macrocystic spaces demonstrating low-intensity T1W (*A*) and high-intensity T2W (*B*) signal with thin low-intensity septations (*arrow*). (*C*) T1W contrast-enhanced image shows septal enhancement without any internal enhancement of cystic spaces, differentiating this lesion from a venous malformation.

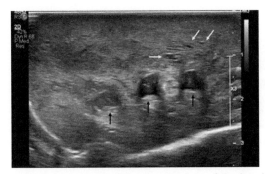

Fig. 9. Gray scale US of the dorsal aspect of the hand reveals diffuse microcystic spaces (*white arrows*) in an echogenic background composed of the walls of cysts that are below the resolution of US. This appearance of microcystic LM can simulate a mass involving the soft tissue layers of the entire hand. Note second to fourth phalanges (*black arrows*).

Drainage occurs through tributaries that connect to normal veins of the superficial or deep venous system.[10]

US is the first line for imaging of VMs as it allows detailed assessment of superficial structures and the ability to perform dynamic maneuvers. VMs are primarily anechoic to hypoechoic, sponge-like vascular channels, separated by hyperechoic septations of variable thickness (**Fig. 11**). VMs are compressible and should exhibit engorgement with application of a tourniquet, dependent on positioning, or removal of compression. Thrombus within the dilated venous spaces may be noncompressible and have a hyperechoic appearance, which can appear solid and mimic a vascular tumor.[20] Small, rounded, hyperechoic foci with posterior shadowing correspond to calcifications or phleboliths and are nearly pathognomonic for VMs; however, these are visualized only 16% of the time (see **Fig. 3**).[22] Fluid–fluid levels occasionally occur secondary to slow flow within the malformations, although this is not specific and is also found in LMs. Flow within VMs is detected 84% of the time, most commonly exhibiting a monophasic waveform. This means that the diagnosis of VM cannot be excluded based only on the absence of flow on Doppler US. Evaluation for turbulent flow and aliasing artifact is important, as this indicates a high-flow arterial component and will change the diagnosis and the treatment approach.[23]

MRI can determine the full extent of VMs, which may cross tissue planes and involve deep structures such as muscles, joints, or bone. VMs are intermediate to low intensity on T1W images, although can have heterogenous signal intensities if significant thrombus burden is present. The most sensitive sequence for evaluating the full extent of VMs is a fat-suppressed T2W sequence, as this allows for nulling of fat signal within septations.[10,20] The absence of flow voids, which indicate high flow, on spin echo sequences is critical to the diagnosis of VMs. Low signal intensity striations, thrombus, and phleboliths can mimic flow voids; however, true flow voids will have high signal intensity on contrast-enhanced and gradient response echo sequences while phleboliths will be low intensity on all sequences. VMs are characterized by slow gradual contrast enhancement that becomes homogenous enhancement on delayed post-contrast T1W imaging.[10] These represent venous "lakes" slowly filled by the contrast agent (**Fig. 12**).

Direct percutaneous phlebography allows for direct contrast injection into the VM to evaluate outflow veins and communication with the deep venous system. This is only performed during sclerotherapy and is a critical step to reduce the risk of extravasation of the sclerosant agent into the normal circulation, as some of those outflow veins need to be compressed/blocked.

ARTERIOVENOUS MALFORMATIONS

AVMs are high-flow lesions with abnormal connections between arteries and veins, bypassing the capillary bed. AVMs shunt blood from at least one feeding artery to the draining system that could be represented by one or multiple veins.

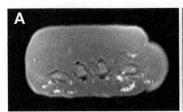
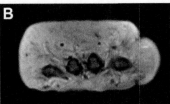
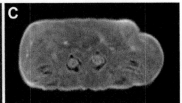

Fig. 10. MRI of the same patient reveals a homogenous low-intensity T1W (*A*) and high-intensity T2W (*B*) lesion without significant contrast enhancement (*C*), differentiating this LM malformation from a venous malformation.

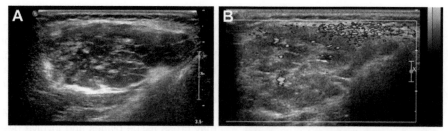

Fig. 11. Gray scale US (*A*) reveals dilated and tortuous hypoechoic vascular channels with thin hyperechoic septations. Power Doppler US (*B*) displays vascular flow within these channels and confirms a VM.

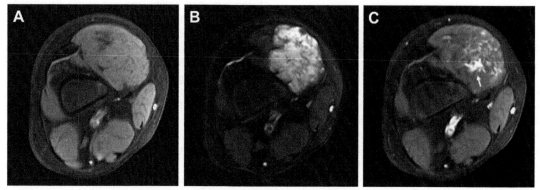

Fig. 12. MRI of the lower extremity reveals a T1W (*A*) isointense and T2W (*B*) hyperintense lesion within the vastus lateralis. Heterogenous enhancement filling venous lakes (*arrow*) within the lesion on the contrast-enhanced image (*C*) in the absence of flow voids is diagnostic of VM.

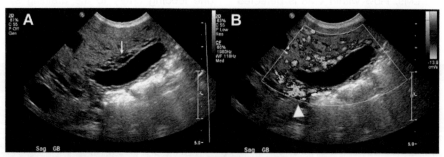

Fig. 13. Gray scale US of the liver (*A*) shows dilated and tortuous anechoic channels (*arrow*) with hyperechoic septations surrounding the gallbladder fossa. Color Doppler (*B*) reveals profound hypervascularity with aliasing (*arrowhead*) representing high flow and confirms a hepatic AVM.

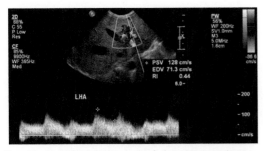

Fig. 14. Doppler ultrasound of the same patient reveals tangle of dysmorphic vessels intimately associated with the left hepatic artery and left portal vein. Spectral waveform analysis displays an arterial waveform with elevated diastolic velocity and a reduced resistive index, consistent with the left to right shunt of an AVM.

The abnormal connection between the arterial and venous system can occur through a tangle of dysmorphic, tortuous vessels known as the nidus, or through a direct single fistulous connection, such as seen in pulmonary AVMs. These malformations are present at birth, although frequently not detected until adolescence or a period of rapid growth, such as following trauma, infection, hormonal fluctuations, or pregnancy.[24]

Initial evaluation with gray scale US will reveal findings similar to those seen in VMs: a nest of hypoechoic, tortuous ducts with intervening hyperechoic septal fat. Doppler US with spectral waveform analysis will differentiate between AVMs and VMs, as AVMs will demonstrate high-flow characteristics such as aliasing, intralesional turbulence, and high diastolic flow and arterialization of the draining vein(s) (**Figs. 13** and **14**). The arterial inflow directly communicating with a low-pressure venous outflow confirms the presence of AVM.[20,25]

After determining the presence of an AVM and before intervention, cross-sectional imaging with CTA or MRA is necessary to determine extent of disease, and better characterize inflow and outflow vessels. The rapid image acquisition of CTA is valuable for evaluation of acute complications of AVM, such as hemorrhage, ischemia, and thrombosis, particularly in osseous or pulmonary AVM, which are less amenable to MRA evaluation.[20]

Characteristic MRI findings are serpentine, dilated inflow, and draining high-flow vessels, which appear as flow voids on T1W and T2W sequences. The intervening nidus appears as a tangle of dysplastic vessels with scattered flow voids (**Fig. 15**). Gradient response echo will demonstrate high signal intensity foci of vessels with no significant mass effect, although there can be adjacent fatty hypertrophy and muscle atrophy.[21,25] On T1W images, hyperintense foci can be seen with thrombosis or hemorrhage and loss of normal high intensity signal within the marrow may indicate intraosseous involvement.[10,25] Gadolinium-enhanced 3D time-resolved dynamic MRA provides high temporal resolution and allows delineation of specific inflow vessels, opacification of the nidus, and characteristic early contrast filling of draining veins.[20]

Angiography is the gold standard for evaluating AVM and should be performed before or in conjunction with every intervention. Findings will include dilated arteries and early opacification of dilated veins (**Fig. 16**), with a more detailed evaluation of the nidus than using MRA.[24]

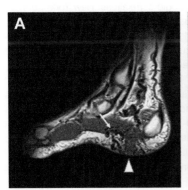
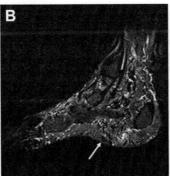
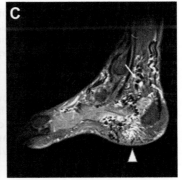

Fig. 15. MRI of the right foot shows dilated, tortuous high-flow vessels that appear as flow voids (*arrows*) on all sequences leading into and within the vascular nidus (*arrowheads*) of the AVM. The nidus appears as a tangle of vessels that are hypointense on T1W images (*A*), hyperintense on T2W images (*B*), and enhance with contrast administration (*C*).

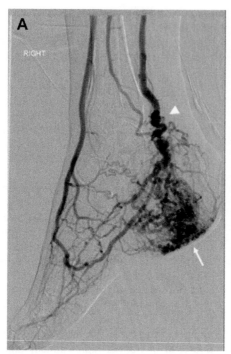
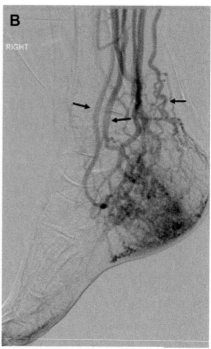

Fig. 16. Digital subtraction angiography of the same patient during arterial phase (*A*) better demonstrates a dilated, tortuous distal posterior tibial artery (*arrowhead*) feeding the nidus (*white arrow*) of the AVM. Venous phase (*B*) shows early venous filling of the veins draining the nidus (*black arrows*).

CLINICS CARE POINTS

- Vascular and lymphatic malformations are typically a clinical diagnosis. US and MRI are most commonly utilized and allow for further lesion classification.

- CTA/MRA are reserved for evaluation of and treatment planning in high-flow lesions only. Use of these modalities in slow-flow lesions will increase cost without improving patient care.

- Vascular tumors can have similar imaging characteristics and definitive diagnosis may not be possible. However, imaging can identify unusual/aggressive findings that can prompt further evaluation with tissue sampling.

- Detecting features of arterial flow in vascular malformations, such as aliasing in US or flow voids in MRI, is critical to differentiating between low-flow (capillary, lymphatic, and venous) and high-flow (AVM/AVF).

DISCLOSURE

None.

REFERENCES

1. Mattassi R, Loose D, Vaghi M. Principles of diagnostics. In: Hemangiomas and vascular malformations an atlas of diagnosis and treatment. Milano: Springer; 2015. p. 187–8.
2. Obara P, McCool J, Kalva S, et al. Clinically suspected vascular malformations of the extremities. Available at: https://acsearch.acr.org/docs/3102393/Narrative/. Accessed February 20, 2022.
3. Peer S, Wortsman X. Hemangiomas and Vascular Malformations. In: Dermatologic ultrasound with clinical and histologic correlations. New York: Springer Science+Business Media; 2013. p. 183–234.
4. Schmidt V, Masthoff M, Czihal M, et al. Imaging of peripheral vascular malformations-current concepts and future perspectives. Mol Cell Pediatr 2021;8(1):19.
5. Hyodoh H, Hori M, Akiba H, et al. Peripharial vascular malformations: imaging, treatment approaches, adn therapeutic issues. Radiographics 2005;25:159–71.
6. Samet J, Restrepo R, Rajeswaran S, et al. Pediatric vascular malformations imaging guidelines and recommendations. Radiol Clin North Am 2021;60: 179–92.
7. Steiner J, Drolet B. Classification of vascular anomalies. An Update 2017;34:225–32.
8. Monroe E. Brief description of ISSVA classification for radiologist. Tech Vasc Interv Radiol 2019;22(4):1–13.

9. Nozaki T, Matsusako M, Mimura H, et al. Imaging of vascular tumors with an emphasis on ISSVA classification. Jpn J Radiol 2013;31:775–85.

10. Flors L, Leiva-Salinas C, Maged I, et al. MR imaging of soft-tissue vascular malformations: diagnosis, classification, and therapy follow-up. RadioGraphics 2011;31:1321–40.

11. Gorincour G, Kokta V, Rypens F, et al. Imaging characteristics of two subtypes of congenital hemangiomas: rapidly involuting congenital hemangiomas and non-involuting congenital hemangiomas. Pediatr Radiol 2005;35:1178–85.

12. Herron M, Coffin C, Vanderhooft S. Tufted angiomas: variability of the clinical morphology. Pediatr Dermatol 2002;19(5):394–401.

13. Dubois J, Rypens F. Diagnostics of Infantile Hemangiomas Including Visceral Hemangioma. In: Hemangiomas and vascular malformations an atlas of diagnosis and treatment. 2nd edition. Milano: Springer; 2015. p. 81–8.

14. Walker E, Salesky J, Fenton M, et al. Magnetic resonance imaging of malignant soft tissue neoplasms in the adult. Radiol Clin North Am 2011;49:1219–34.

15. Chung E, Lattin G, Cube R, et al. Pediatric liver masses: radiologic-pathologic correlation part 2. malignant tumors. RadioGraphics 2011;31:483–507.

16. Merrow A, Gupta A, Patel M, et al. 2014 Revised classification of vascular lesions from the international society for the study of vascular anomalies: radiologic-pathologic update. RadioGraphics 2016; 36:1494–516.

17. Reis J, Koo K, Monroe E, et al. Ultrasound evaluation of pediatric slow-flow vascular malformations:

18. Piram M, Lorette G, Sirinelli D, et al. Sturge-Weber Syndrome in Patients with Facial Port-Wine Stain. Pediatr Dermatol 2012;29(1):32–7.

19. Mulligan P, Prajapati H, Martin L, et al. Vascular anomalies: classification, imaging characteristics and implications for interventional radiology treatment approaches. Br J Radiol 2014;87(1035):1–18.

20. Green J, Resnick S, Restrepo R, et al. Spectrum of imaging mainfestations of vascular malformations and tumors beyond childhood. Radiol Clin North Am 2020;58:583–601.

21. Fayad L, Hazirolan T, Bluemke D, et al. Vascular malformations in the extremities: emphasis on MR imaging features that guide treatment options. Skeletal Radiol 2006;35:127–37.

22. Trop I, Dubois J, Guibaud L, et al. Soft-tissue venous malformations in pediatric and young adult patients: diagnosis with doppler US. Radiology 1999;212(3): 841–5.

23. Abernethy L. Classification and imaging of vascular malformations in children. Eur Radiol 2003;13: 2483–97.

24. Lam K, Pillai A, Reddick M. Peripheral arteriovenous malformations: classification and endovascular treatment. Appl Radiol 2017;46(5):15–21.

25. Madani H, Farrant J, Chhaya N, et al. Peripheral limb vascular malformations: an update of appropriate imaging and treatment options of a challenging condition. Br J Radiol 2015;88(1047):1–16.

practical diagnostic reporting to guide interventional managment. AJR 2020;216:494–506.

Timing and Rationale of Treatment
Achieving the "Best Result"

Marcelo Hochman, MD

KEYWORDS

- Hemangioma • Surgery • Treatment • Timing • Self image

KEY POINTS

- Multi-modality treatment is the norm for vascular anomalies.
- Timing and modality of treatment are dependent on age, stage, location, and size of the lesion.
- Timing of treatment should be in concert with known developmental milestones of the development of self.

INTRODUCTION/BACKGROUND

Various clinical disciplines defend the modality of therapy available to them (eg, medical vs surgery) when, in fact, multi-modality therapy is usually in the best interest of the patient. The aim of any modality of treatment is to obtain the best possible result for a given patient. To successfully achieve that aim for infantile hemangiomas (IH) and all vascular anomalies, defining what is meant by the *best possible result* and by *when to achieve* that, the result needs to be defined. Perhaps more important is to make a determination of what is an *acceptable result*. The impact of a 1-cm IH of the nasal tip is different from that of the same exact lesion on the thigh. The functional import of a 5-mm IH involving the lower eyelid is potentially very different from the same lesion involving the upper eyelid. These examples highlight that variables, such as size and location, are important. What is considered acceptable as a result of treatment of the nasal tip and upper eyelid IH is different from that for the corresponding thigh and lower lid lesions.

To recap what has been enumerated many times in this volume, IHs are true neoplasms that typically appear within the first few weeks of life and undergo the most rapid proliferation in the first 2 months. The rate of endothelial tumor cell hyperplasia slows down by approximately the sixth month and is overcome by the apoptosis and regression of the tumor volume, most rapidly over the first 2 years and then more slowly after that. Though the involution curve is diagrammed as asymptotic in the literature, clinically relevant involution beyond 5 to 6 years is negligible because the tumor is biologically so inactive. The involution is characterized by the slow replacement of the tumor burden by fibro-fatty scar.

Thus, during proliferation, the tissue that the clinician observes is quite different from that in involution and likewise variably responsive to different therapeutic modalities. Thin, superficial, and proliferating tumors may be amenable to laser or topical medical therapy. Thicker, larger, or functionally threatening proliferating lesions may require systemic medical therapy. During involution, the type of IH (as defined by the depth of cutaneous involvement) determines the type of persistent tissue—thin superficial IHs may involute with no significant residuum, whereas a compound IH may have significant anetoderma and a deep IH may present as a mass underlying perfectly normal skin. Each scenario requires different potential medical, laser, and surgical options and combinations, which are discussed throughout this issue. Thus, tumor size, location, and phase of the natural history for which

Oto/HNS and Plastic Surgery, Medical Univ of South Carolina, 526 Johnnie Dodds Blvd, Suite 202, Mt Pleasant, Charleston, SC 29464, USA
E-mail address: drhochman@facialsurgerycenter.com

Dermatol Clin 40 (2022) 379–382
https://doi.org/10.1016/j.det.2022.06.003
0733-8635/22/

the tumor presents for treatment have an impact on treatment options.

DISCUSSION

The choice of treatment options, however, cannot be based exclusively on the tumor qualities. The biology of the tumor clearly plays a role in decision making as just described. Yet, the patient carrying the tumor needs to be taken into account. This may seem an explicit concept when dealing with patients who can speak for themselves and make decisions and value judgments on their own behalf. Because the patients affected by IH and most vascular anomalies are infants and young children, however, the burden of this decision making falls on parents and clinicians. Beyond just relying on the characteristics of the anomaly, the best course of action for a given child can be further determined by considering that child's place on the continuum of psycho-social development, the known data on the development of consciousness of self, and on the societal value of restoration of appearance.

Self-awareness is a fundamental issue in developmental psychology that is germane to the issue of when to strive to obtain the best possible result regardless of the modality of therapy and to which not enough attention is devoted. Humans are a uniquely self-conscious species—caring how they look with others in mind. It is through the gaze of others that humans measure how securely accepted by others they are. Furmark[1] has shown that there is no more dreadful phobia than that of being socially rejected and alienated from others, which explains why people rank public speech as the most common, greatest fear. A review of the entire sequence of development of self-awareness, although fascinating, is beyond the scope of this article. There is a general consensus, however, on a few major landmarks that are pertinent.[2] Infants between 3 months and 12 months old tend to treat their own image in a mirror as a playmate, an "other." They are oblivious to a sticker that has surreptitiously been placed on their forehead and is visible on the image in the mirror. By the end of the first year, children demonstrate enhanced curiosity about the specular image by touching or looking behind the mirror but still do not recognize themselves. It is only by 18 months that infants begin to look for the sticker (or "rouge" in the original experiments) on their own bodies to remove it. This is the literal beginning of identity.

At approximately 2 years of age, children begin to express embarrassment—the first signs of awareness of their public appearance.[3] A stranger pointing at the hemangioma on a two and a half year old's face is recognized by the child as being about "me," that there is something that others see in "me." Over time, this sense of self becomes rooted and by 3 years children begin to grasp the temporal dimension of the self—that their selves endure beyond what can be seen in the mirror or a photo. The cognitive ability to run a simulation of others' minds (what others are thinking of "me") is clearly established by age 3 years to 4 years. The basic fear and embarrassment that the red mark on the cheek that they see on themselves in the mirror persists and is visible to others at all times become ingrained by 4 years to 5 years of age. A psychological profile survey of children with hemangiomas and their families showed that given earlier intervention, affected children did not seem to experience significant emotional trauma from their condition; their families, however, experienced appreciable emotional and psychological distress in dealing with a child with a facial difference.[4] That the presence of facial lesions induces a significant social penalty, specifically which observers are less comfortable communicating with people who have facial defects, has been demonstrated.[5] Other studies have shown that people with facial deformities are perceived as less attractive and are ascribed emotionally negative labels.[6] Another study showed that casual observers perceive that facial defects significantly decrease quality of life, an effect improved by reconstructive surgery.[7] The value of the reconstruction, although highly valued by society, is valued even more so by the affected patient. Patients' perceived improvement in appearance and function is greater than that of objective observers, reiterating humans' concern about how they look.[8]

The reviewed current knowledge of the biology of the IHs, the data on the development of self, and on the value of restoration of appearance can be used to help inform the role of any therapy in the management of these tumors. If the known timelines about the biology of IH are superimposed on developmental milestones in the determination of self-image, important considerations appear (Fig. 1). By the time 85% of tumors have ceased proliferating (6 months), an infant has not met any psychological milestones pertinent to this discussion. The maximum rate of involution occurs between 12 months and 24 months of age.[9] Beyond that, the rate of regression of the tumor slows remarkably, to the point that by 4 years to 5 years it is barely clinically detectable. The replacement by fat and scar may continue at a reduced rate for some time but not in an asymptotic fashion (never crossing the x-axis), as

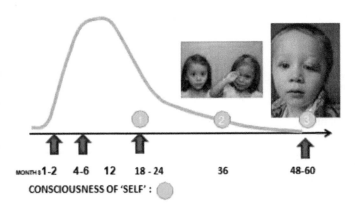

MONTHS **1-2   4-6   12   18 - 24   36   48-60**

CONSCIOUSNESS OF 'SELF' :

Fig. 1. Natural history of IH versus developmental milestones. The figure shows the known natural history of IH (*blue curve*) with proliferation and involution (*size/y-axis*) over time (*months/x-axis*). Most involution curves are shown to be asymptotic to the time axis yet clinically this is not supported so this curve intersects at approximately 5 years of age. The maximum rate of proliferation occurs within the first 2 months (*first red arrow*) and is complete in more than 85% of tumors by 6 months of age (*second arrow*). The maximum rate of involution occurs by 24 months (*third arrow*), coinciding with the infant's recognition of the sticker or rouge in the specular image as being on their own body (development of "self identity," 1st green circle). The rate of apoptosis and involution decreases over time (2nd *green circle*), coinciding with further development of self-consciousness evidenced by embarrassment and avoidance behavior. By 4 to 5 years of age, the rate of involution has decreased to a clinically insignificant level (*fourth arrow*) and coincides with an established sense of "me" (3rd *green circle*).

depicted in most diagrams in the literature. As discussed previously, a child's ability to pass the mirror sticker test occurs at approximately 18 months—during the fastest rate of involution. By 24 months to 36 months, a sense of "me" is established and the realization that "there is something on my face" coincides with the dramatic decrease in the rate of involution.

By late involution, 5 years to 6 years of age, a child's sense of self-image is ingrained. By then, most children are getting ready to enter formal schooling, with its attendant peer pressures from the other children who are comparing their appearances with that of the affected child because they are all on the same developmental timetable of self-recognition. Synthesizing the previous discussions, if an acceptable result for a given IH can be obtained by surgery during involution, for example, but within the timeframe of specified developmental milestones, it is reasonable to propose it as an option. The collective experience of surgery for IH at various locations shows that acceptable results are readily achievable.[10] In addition, these results are achievable with a limited number of procedures by the time a child is aware of the impact of these on his or her-self. Surgery in the proliferative phase of IHs is not usual because the tumor needs to be completely removed lest the remnant continues to proliferate according to its biological "clock." Therefore, topical or systemic medical therapy may be the best option depending on the other physical qualities of the tumor as previously touched upon. Laser therapy while excellent at treating the superficial component of any lesion does nothing for the volume of established tumors. Again, the timing of laser

treatment is affected by the stage, location, type of tumor, and the age (psycho-social and temporal). Surgery during involution has become common when a procedure can achieve a result that is at least as good as waiting for involution to be complete. Focal tumors are more likely to benefit from single-stage, definitive excisions, whereas segmental, diffuse, and/or large lesions can be addressed in a serial fashion. Sequelae of involution and complications, such as scarring, distended skin, and distortion of anatomic features, fall into the surgical realm without much dissent. The key judgment is in the timing of the surgical interventions.[11,12]

SUMMARY

In my opinion, as much as possible, the goal of treatment of IH, in particular, is to obtain the best possible result by the age of 3 years so the child's image of self is not affected. If this is not possible because of the complexity of the excision and reconstruction or timing of presentation to the clinician, then the best effort should be made to finalize the result by the time the affected child is entering formal schooling, at approximately 6 years of age. The concept of intervening by this age for elective otoplasties taking into account the known anatomic variables of cartilage growth and avoiding the stigma of facial difference has been applied for decades. Multi-modality therapy for IH is now commonplace and can achieve excellent results as demonstrated in the clinical literature. It is the timing of the intervention in accord with developmental milestones that need to be kept in focus to give these children the best chance to literally face the world.

CLINICS CARE POINTS

- Multi-modality therapy is typical for the management of vascular anomalies, including infantile hemangioma.
- The tumor location, size, stage in natural history and associated complications are important in determining management.
- The age of the child - in relation to known pyschological stages of the development of 'self' is important in determining best management of the tumor.
- Mapping the natural history of the tumor to the known stages of development of 'self image' helps inform goals for treatment.
- 'Leave it alone, it will go away' is not a universally valid recommendation for all infantile hemangioma.

DISCLOSURE

The author has nothing to disclose.

REFERENCES

1. Furmark T. Social phobia: overview of community surveys. Acta Psychiatr Scand 2002;105(2):84–93.
2. Rochat P. Five levels of self-awareness as they unfold early in life. Conscious Cogn 2013;12:717–31.
3. Amsterdam BK, Levitt M. Consciousness of self and painful self-consciousness. Psychoanal Stud Child 2006;35:67–83.
4. Williams EF, Hochman M, Rodgers BJ, et al. A psychological profile of children with hemangiomas and their families. Arch Facial Plast Surg 2003;5:229–34.
5. Dey JK, Ishii LE, Byrne PJ, et al. The social penalty of facial lesions. New evi- dence supporting high quality reconstruction. JAMA Facial Plast Surg 2015;17(2):90–6.
6. Godoy A, Ishii M, Dey J, et al. How facial lesions impact attractiveness and perception. Laryngoscope 2011;121(12):2542–7.
7. Dey JK, Ishii LE, Joseph AW, et al. The cost of facial deformity. A health utility and valuation study. JAMA Facial Plast Surg 2016;18(4):241–9.
8. Byrne M, Chan JCY, O'Broin E. Perceptions and satisfaction of aesthetic outcome following secondary cleft rhinoplasty: evaluation by patients versus health profes- sionals. J Craniomaxillofac Surg 2014;42:1062–70.
9. Razon MJ, Kra ling BM, Mulliken JB, et al. Increased apoptosis coincides with onset of involution in infantile hemangioma. Microcirculation 1998;5(2–3):189–95.
10. Keller RG, Stevens S, Hochman M. Modern Management of Nasal Hemangiomas. Facial Plast Surg 2017;19(4):327–32.
11. Kulbersh J, Hochman M. Serial excision of facial hemangiomas. Arch Facial Plast Surg 2011;13(3):199–202.
12. Hochman M, Mascareno A. Management of nasal hemangiomas. Arch Facial Plast Surg 2005;7:295–300.

Infantile Hemangiomas

Divina Justina Hasbani, MD[a], Lamiaa Hamie, MD, MS[b],*

KEYWORDS

- Infantile hemangioma • Pediatric dermatology • Propranolol • Timolol • Vascular laser
- Vascular neoplasm

KEY POINTS

- Infantile hemangiomas (IHs) are the most common, benign soft tissue tumors of infancy.
- Although they usually spontaneously regress, they may cause significant parental distress, permanent disfigurement, and functional impairment, which need to be promptly addressed.
- Recognizing high-risk features is important to guide the workup and management of patients with IH.
- Systemic or topical β-blockade has become the first-line treatment in the management of IHs when indicated.

INTRODUCTION

Infantile hemangiomas (IHs) are the most common vascular tumors of childhood, consisting of benign proliferations of endothelial cells.[1] Characterized by onset in the first few weeks after birth, rapid progression and then spontaneous regression, IHs are usually uncomplicated but in some cases may lead to parental distress, permanent disfigurement, and functional impairment.[2] Hence, awareness of the associated risk factors and appropriately addressing an IH early in its course are key factors in approaching this entity.

Studies estimating the incidence of IHs report their presence in about 4% of infants, and rates of up to 12% have been described.[1] Determining the exact incidence, however, can be challenging, given IHs may not appear until after the immediate newborn period and that various names have previously been used for their identification.[2]

IHs are generally more likely to occur in premature or low-birth-weight female neonates, with low birth weight acting as an independent risk factor.[3] The increasing rates of prematurity and low birth weight have been postulated to be driving the higher incidence of IHs over the last few decades.[1]

The incidence is also greater in the setting of multiple gestations, progesterone therapy use, and positive family history.[3] Previous studies have also suggested maternal smoking, older maternal age, in vitro fertilization, White race, prenatal instrumentation with amniocentesis or chorionic villus sampling, and factors associated with placental insufficiency, such as in placenta previa and preeclampsia, to increase the risk of IH development.[1]

Although the pathogenesis of IHs is not well defined, the risk factors associated with their development have provided valuable clues to their underlying pathogenesis.

The main cell of origin of IHs has been postulated to be progenitor endothelial cells arising from the chorionic villi of the placenta; this is supported by their common expression of placenta-associated antigens such as glucose transporter protein-1 (GLUT-1), merosin, FcγRII, and Lewis Y antigen, which are specifically expressed by the chorionic villi.[4] This hypothesis, however, has never been definitively demonstrated. The expression of GLUT-1 throughout all of phases of progression is unique to IHs among other vascular

No funding sources.
[a] Department of Dermatology, American University of Beirut Medical Center, Riad El Solh/ Beirut, P.O. Box 11-0236, Beirut 1107 2020, Lebanon; [b] Department of Dermatology, Division of Pediatric Dermatology, Medical College of Wisconsin, Pediatrics TBRC, 2nd floor, Suite C2010, 8701 Watertown Plank Road, Milwaukee, WI 53226, USA
* Corresponding author.
E-mail address: lhamie@mcw.edu

Dermatol Clin 40 (2022) 383–392
https://doi.org/10.1016/j.det.2022.06.004

tumors and malformations,[4] as is their life cycle mirroring that of the placenta.[5] Another factor associated with IHs is vascular endothelial growth factor A (VEGF-A), which is known for its function in angiogenesis, may be a key driving force of IH proliferation, and may partially justify the response to corticosteroids and propranolol.[2] VEGF-A and GLUT-1, as well as insulin-like growth factor 2, are downstream targets of hypoxia-inducible factor-1alpha;. Therefore, recent studies have shifted their focus to the role of hypoxia in inducing or enhancing the development of IHs[5]; this may explain the increased risk of IHs following chorionic villus sampling during pregnancy.[5] In addition, the renin-angiotensin system seems to be a contributor via angiotensin II, which indirectly promotes angiogenesis and tumor survival.[1] Hence, the physiologically higher levels of renin in infancy and decline thereafter throughout childhood may explain the natural progression of IHs. Serum renin levels are also higher in female, premature, and White neonates, possibly accounting for the greater incidence of IHs in these groups.[1] Another explanation for the association of female gender with IH development is the suggested synergy between estrogen, progesterone, and vascular endothelial growth factors, which may also support the role of progesterone therapy in IH development.[3] Furthermore, genetic factors may participate in the pathogenesis of IHs, although less than other factors.[3] These factors include somatic mutations in VEGF signaling pathway proteins[6] and germline mutations in VEGF receptor-2 and anthrax toxin receptor 1, which encodes an endothelial cell receptor.[5] Specifically, the development of IHs is reportedly linked to genetic factors located on chromosome 5q.[7]

CLINICAL AND HISTOLOGIC FEATURES

IHs usually emerge in the first few weeks erof life, and they may begin as a precursor lesion at birth; this presents subtly in the form of telangiectasias, areas of pallor, erythematous macules, or ecchymosis-like patches. The most common site of involvement is the trunk, followed by the head and neck, especially at positions over the embryonic fusion lines, but they may occur on any cutaneous or mucosal surface. As their natural progression ensues, IHs take on more distinct clinical features, which vary depending on their depth in the soft tissue. IHs located in the superficial dermis are classified "superficial IH" and exhibit a tense bright red, round papule, nodule, or irregular plaque (**Fig.** 1A–C).[2] Those situated in the deep dermis and/or subcutis are denoted "deep IH" and present as a firm and elastic bluish

to flesh-colored nodule or mass. As for IHs with superficial and deep components, or "mixed IH," the presentation combines features of both, often with an erythematous plaque overlying a larger, poorly circumscribed blue-to-violaceous nodule.[2]

The development of an IH from its precursor form occurs in an early proliferative phase, where it rapidly grows in a volumetric manner within its predetermined territory. Most IHs reach their maximal size by the end of this stage, at around 3 months of age on average,[8] with the quickest growth rate between 5 and 8 weeks.[9] Deep hemangiomas tend to have a delayed presentation, but most expansion is completed by 5 months of age.[8] Propagation then proceeds at a slower rate during the late proliferative phase, until 6 to 9 months of age, or an extended period in some cases.[8] Starting around 12 months of age, a change in the IH's color and texture marks the involution phase, where it becomes more violaceous-grey, soft, and compressible.[1] This phase of gradual spontaneous regression usually takes 3 to 9 years, but it is often near-complete by age 4 years.[9] In up to 69% of cases, involution leaves permanent residual skin changes consisting of telangiectasias, fibrofatty tissue, atrophy, anetoderma, erythema, hypopigmentation, or potentially scarring if ulceration occurs.[9]

IH with minimal or arrested growth (IH-MAG) represents an exception to this usual sequence, demonstrating minimal to no development beyond telangiectatic, erythematous, or violaceous patches over a background of vasoconstriction. This variant exhibits a diminished proliferative phase that may only involve a small portion of the tumor's surface area, and it usually occurs on the lower body.[1]

Another mode of IH classification, more commonly adopted than tumor depth, pertains to its pattern of involvement, being focal, multifocal, segmental, or indeterminate.[1] Focal IHs exhibit spatially confined discrete, oval or round lesions, whereas segmental IHs occupy a large territory in a plaque-like manner and are greater than 5 cm in size.[10] The configuration of a segmental hemangioma seems to follow developmental units rather than dermatomes, Blaschko lines, or neural supply.[1] On the other hand, multiple IHs involving discrete locations are termed multifocal and those that are difficult to categorize are referred to as indeterminate.[10]

Histologically in the proliferation phase, IHs show proliferating endothelial cells forming well delineated masses with surrounding pericytes, whereas, in the involution phase, the endothelium flattens and less mitotic activity is noted, with

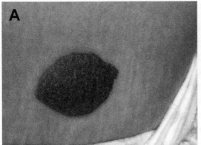 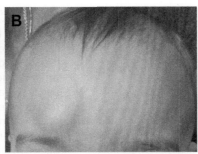 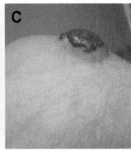

Fig. 1. Types of infantile hemangiomas. (*A*) Superficial IH; exophytic dark red vascular nodule on the lower back. (*B*) Deep IH; skin-colored subcutaneous nodule with a bluish tint on the forehead. (*C*) Mixed IH; exhibiting both superficial and deep features.

fibrous and fatty tissue replacing the vessels.[1] Immunohistochemical analysis shows expression of GLUT-1 by the endothelial cells, and this is a sensitive marker for IHs.[1]

COMPLICATIONS

IHs tend to be small and resolve spontaneously, without the need for intervention. However, in around a quarter of cases,[2] complications may incur, including ulceration, bleeding, associated extracutaneous anomalies, and functional impairment. The risk of developing complications largely depends on factors such as pattern of involvement, size, location, and the patient's age and these are key for the clinician to identify, as they consequently determine the need to intervene and its appropriate timing, as well as the need for further investigations.

Ulceration

Ulceration is the most frequent complication associated with IHs, occurring in around 10% based on recent studies. It can lead to significant impairment in quality of life by causing pain, infection, bleeding, disfigurement, and scarring almost always ensues.[11] Ulceration is attributed to an outgrowth of blood supply during the proliferative phase; hence, it has been observed to occur at a median age of 4 months.[11]

Its risk is generally correlated with increased size and the presence of a superficial component.[10] As for the most common sites, IHs located in the head and neck area, especially the lip, columella, and superior helix of the hear, as well as anogenital and intertriginous sites, are prone to trauma, contamination, and therefore a greater risk of ulcerating and secondary pain and mild bleeding.[9–12] Furthermore, the ulceration of an IH tends to be aggressive (with significant soft tissue destruction, prolonged time to heal, or refractory nature) when it involves a large surface area, is

segmental, or the infant is born to multiple gestations.[11]

Importantly, a sensitive clue to impending ulceration is a change in the IH's color to white-grey (**Fig. 2**) in infants younger than 3 months,[9] so it is crucial for clinicians to be aware of this clinical sign.

Another potentially life-threatening complication arises in the case of intrahepatic hemangiomas, the presence of which should be brought to attention by the clinician when patients present with more than 5 cutaneous IHs (due to significantly higher risk).[13] The liver is the most common site of extracutaneous IH, and when involvement is multifocal and diffuse, macrovascular shunts may result in high-output heart failure.[14] Subsequent complications include consumptive hypothyroidism (in all patients with diffuse HH) and rarely abdominal compartment syndrome due to massive hepatomegaly.[14]

In addition, airway obstruction is a feared complication of IHs occurring over the beard or mandibular area (in an S3 facial distribution) bilaterally, as they are associated with subglottic hemangiomas (**Fig. 3**).[9] These present with hoarse cry, biphasic stridor, and crouplike symptoms, at the age of 4 to 12 weeks.[9,15] Moreover, respiratory distress has been reported as a result of airway obstruction by an IH adjacent to the mainstem bronchus, despite the lack of cutaneous IH.[16] Thus, any patient with an IH involving the bilateral mandibular area must be referred to an otolaryngologist for airway assessment, even if respiratory symptoms are absent.[9]

Visceral Involvement

Segmental hemangiomas occurring over specific sites may indicate the presence of underlying congenital structural anomalies. PHACES (posterior fossa, hemangioma, arterial anomalies of cervical and cerebral vessels, cardiac defects

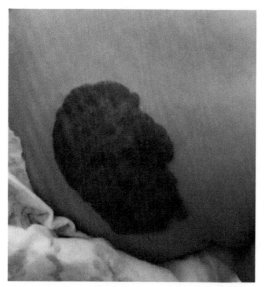

Fig. 2. White gray discoloration of an IH as a clue to impending ulceration.

[especially coarctation of the aorta], eye anomalies, and sternal defects and supraumbilical raphe) syndrome is of concern when an infant presents with a segmental hemangioma over the face, scalp, and/or neck, especially the S1 segment.[17] This syndrome has been observed to occur in around 30% to 58% of patients with this risk factor, and the chance increases with increasing size and number of facial segments involved by the IH.[1,17] As for segmental IHs over the lumbosacral or perineal area, they should raise alarm to LUMBAR (lower body/lumbosacral hemangioma and lipomas or other cutaneous anomalies, urogenital anomalies, myelopathy [spinal dysraphism], bony deformities, anorectal and arterial anomalies, renal anomalies) syndrome. These hemangiomas often are of the IH-MAG type, extend to one lower extremity, and ulcerate.[1] Specifically, those IH located in the midline may indicate spinal dysraphism.[10]

Hypothyroidism

Hypothyroidism due to the inactivation of thyroxine and triiodothyronine (T3) by type 3 iodothyronine deiodinase, which is overexpressed by the endothelium of IHs, is usually seen in cases of diffuse hepatic hemangiomas but also with large cutaneous IH.[18] This complication is refractory to thyroid replacement due to its nature but requires beta-blockade until it is overcome by involution of the IH.[1] Testing for TSH, T3, and T4 should be performed to rule out peripheral hypothyroidism in patients with infantile hepatic hemangiomas or large IH.[1]

Functional Impairment

Functional impairment most often results from IHs on the head and neck and around natural body orifices. Periocular hemangiomas pose a significant threat to the infant's visual development. Although usually small, mass effect on the cornea can cause refractive errors such as astigmatism in around one-third of affected patients, as well as visual axis obstruction, strabismus, and ptosis. Amblyopia, which could progress to permanent visual impairment if not promptly addressed, may result from any interference in an infant's formation of images, as in the presence of periocular hemangiomas.[19] Its occurrence is 20 times more likely when the upper eyelid is involved, and large IH diameter (greater than 1 cm) and a deep component are other associated traits.[19]

When perioral, IHs may lead to impaired feeding and swallowing, especially if ulcerated; this is more significant with upper lip hemangiomas when focal, as well as with segmental his and large size, which are independent factors.[20] In addition, IHs could obstruct the nostrils or auditory channels leading to conductive hearing loss, on rare occasions, and large IH on the neck may lead to positional torticollis.[21]

Permanent Disfigurement

The risk for an IH leading to alteration in anatomic landmarks and/or disfigurement is greater than that of obstruction or functional impairment, yet it can significantly impair the patient's and parents' quality of life.[10] For example, IHs on the nasal tip (**Fig. 4**) might leave behind residual skin alterations and occasionally cause local deformation of nasal tip support structures.[10,12] The lip is another cosmetically sensitive site, especially when the vermillion border is involved.[20] As for relatively large IHs (at least 2 cm in size during infancy), the potential for scarring and other permanent sequelae becomes relevant when occurring anywhere on the face.[10] Moreover, scalp IHs can lead to alopecia and breast IH to breast asymmetry or altered nipple contour in female patients.[10] These cosmetic consequences increase in likelihood when the IH exhibits a thick superficial component.[9]

EVALUATION

Knowing the various complications that can emerge from one or more IHs, it is important for the clinician to recognize high-risk features to refer the patient to a hemangioma specialist and/or proceed with the appropriate workup and management, as highlighted in the following section.

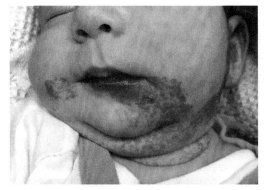

Fig. 3. Segmental infantile hemangioma in an S3 facial distribution. The patient was found to have asymptomatic laryngeal hemangiomas over the arytenoids and false vocal cords.

- Doppler ultrasound of the abdomen to detect hepatic IH if 5 or more cutaneous IHs exist. If detected, thyroid function screening should be performed and hepatic IH should be monitored with serial ultrasounds thereafter until hemangioma resolution is noted radiographically.[14,21]
- MRI and MR angiography of the head and neck when PHACES syndrome suspected, as in the case of segmental scalp or facial IH. Echocardiography may also be performed for cardiac evaluation.[10]
- Doppler ultrasound of abdomen, pelvis, and spine for infants younger than 6 months to screen for LUMBAR syndrome, when lumbosacral/perineal segmental IH present. However, MRI is a more sensitive modality that may be needed to exclude the diagnosis.[10]
- Referral of patients with segmental IH in the beard area to an otolaryngologist for endoscopic airway examination to rule out subglottic hemangioma.[21]

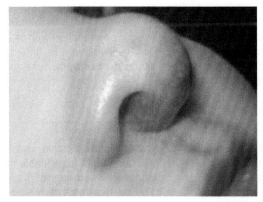

Fig. 4. Deep infantile hemangioma over the nasal tip and columella.

- Referral of patients with periocular IH to an ophthalmologist for early evaluation and follow-up.[19]

DISCUSSION OF THERAPEUTIC OPTIONS

Although most infantile hemangiomas resolve spontaneously with minimal consequence, certain cases warrant specific attention and management, which includes hemangiomas that are ulcerated/or at risk for ulceration, are located in areas with possible functional impairment or permanent disfigurement, and are associated with PHACES/LUMBAR or infantile hepatic hemangiomas.[22] When necessary, referral to a hemangioma specialist and/or initiation of therapy should be considered at 1 month of age,[21] and the younger the patient starts therapy, the better the cosmetic result.[23] Therapy aims to impede growth and accelerate involution while limiting permanent sequelae.

In order to clarify the indications for referrals, the Infantile Hemangioma Referral Score has been recently developed as a screening tool that may guide primary care clinicians to appropriately refer IH patients to expert centers; this would allow early intervention and minimize the possibility of complications in those hemangiomas requiring active medical therapy.[21]

Systemic Therapy

Oral propranolol

Oral propranolol, a nonselective beta-adrenergic receptor antagonist, is the first-line and only treatment approved by the US Food and Drug Administration (FDA) and European Medicines Agency (EMA) for complicated IHs.[10,21] Its precise mechanism of action has not been determined, but several theories have been postulated. Available evidence points to a role in vasoconstriction, inhibition of angiogenesis, regulation of the renin-angiotensin system, inhibition of nitric oxide, and induction of apoptosis in hemangioma-derived endothelial cells.[10] Propranolol has also recently been shown to exert its effects by directly regulating the transcription factor SOX18, independently of the beta-adrenergic receptor, thereby interfering with the differentiation of hemangioma stem cells into hemangioma endothelial cells.[24]

It is a significantly effective medication resulting in complete resolution in most of the cases and response rates of up to 100%, with improvement even in quality of life of their parents.[10,25] Plus, response to therapy may be more advanced when the IH exhibits increased vascularity on ultrasound, whereas those with pronounced fat component on MRI are less likely to respond.[26]

Before initiation, a thorough history and physical examination should be undertaken, including family history of arrhythmia or maternal connective tissue disease.[21] Furthermore, findings suggesting potential compromise of cardiovascular and/or respiratory function may be addressed by requesting further workup such as an electrocardiogram and echocardiography and possibly consulting a pediatrician or pediatric cardiologist.[21,22]

The recommended propranolol hydrochloride dosing varies between 2 and 3 mg/kg daily according to different practice guidelines. Propranolol may be initiated at a dose of 1 mg/kg daily and increased after 1 day to a target of 2 mg/kg/d or 3 mg/kg/d, if needed.[20] Nonetheless, dosing should be continuously adjusted to weight throughout the treatment.[21] Also, the dosing frequency (twice vs three times daily) is not well established, yet the FDA and EMA labeling indicate twice daily dosing.[10] Despite previous recommendations for vital signs monitoring, propranolol has been deemed safe for initiation at home, unless the infant is younger than 5 weeks of age, born preterm, or has feeding difficulties or significant comorbidities.[20,21] Nevertheless, it is fundamental that caregivers be educated about drug administration and advised to interrupt therapy when the patient is inadequately feeding to avoid hypoglycemia,[21] the risk of which increases with the concomitant use of systemic corticosteroids.[27] The dose escalation may also be slower in outpatient settings, starting at 0.5 mg/kg/d and increasing by 0.5 mg/kg increments to reach the target.[21]

As for the duration of treatment, 6 months seem to be superior to 3 months according to a recent large trial, but a consensus has not been reached.[10] Evidence has shown that rebound growth can occur in around 10% to 25% of cases, even after 6 months of propranolol, especially if discontinued before 12 months of age.[10] Tapering propranolol before discontinuation has also been suggested to decrease the risk of rebound tachycardia and hypertension, as well as that of potential rebound growth.[21]

Contraindications to propranolol therapy include second- and third-degree heart block and hypersensitivity, and individualized treatment initiation planning could be considered in cases of uncontrolled heart failure, frequent wheezing, PHACES syndrome, hypoglycemic episodes, and hemodynamic abnormalities.[1,21] Propranolol is a safe medication, but potential side effects are sleep disturbances, cold extremities, diarrhea, and less commonly bronchospasm, hypotension, hypoglycemia, and bradycardia.[1,21,28] Hyperkalemia, coma, and generalized hypertrichosis have also been reported.[25,28,29] Despite its lipophilic nature and penetration of the blood-brain barrier (BBB), evidence shows that neurodevelopmental consequences need not be of concern.[10]

Other β-blockers

Alternatively, atenolol and nadolol are β-blockers that theoretically cannot cross the BBB, offering a reduced risk of sleep disturbance and cognitive effects.[21,30] When atenolol (1 mg/kg/d) was compared with propranolol (2 mg/kg/d) in a recent randomized controlled trial, atenolol showed similar efficacy with fewer complications but no difference in severe adverse events.[31] Moreover, the noninferiority of nadolol (2 mg/kg/d) to propranolol (2 mg/kg/d) and similar safety were illustrated in a recent prospective study.[32]

One should keep in mind that the occurrence of neurologic side effects is not eliminated with the use of these β-blockers independent of their ability to cross the BBB, as they amend the release of nitric oxide and hydrogen peroxide in the hypothalamus and could lead to central toxicity.[21] Nevertheless, atenolol is a cardioselective β-blocker with a reduced risk of bronchospasm and hypoglycemia.[22] Also, its long half-life allows once daily dosing.[31] On the other hand, nadolol has been associated with a case of death in an infant with IH who had not been passing bowel movements for 10 days prior, whereas feces are the primary route of elimination of nadolol.[21]

Acebutolol is another cardioselective β-blocker with the potential for efficacy on IH involution and a better side-effect profile than propranolol, although further investigations are needed to explore its efficacy.[33]

Systemic corticosteroids

In the event of contraindications to propranolol or an unsatisfactory outcome to propranolol therapy, oral prednisolone or prednisone may be considered. Dosing ranges between 2 and 5 mg/kg/d, administered either for long durations of up to 12 months or at multiple short intervals.[10] Corticosteroids may also be used in combination with oral propranolol to accelerate involution in urgent cases.[22] Several other treatments may be suitable, as highlighted in **Table 1**.

Topical Therapy

Topical timolol

Timolol maleate is another nonselective beta-adrenergic receptor antagonist that is available in gel or liquid formulation for the treatment of glaucoma. It may be useful for the treatment of thin, superficial IHs, having shown similar efficacy to oral propranolol with fewer side effects.[10,21] The

Table 1
Systemic treatments for infantile hemangiomas aside from β-blockers and corticosteroids[21,22,34,35]

Medication	Mode of Action	Comments
Sirolimus (rapamycin)	mTOR inhibitor; prevents the differentiation of IH stem cells and hinders vasculogenesis	Combination with propranolol may be beneficial in cases refractory to propranolol and corticosteroids
Vincristine	Chemotherapeutic agent that impedes microtubule formation during mitosis	May be used for life-threatening or functionally impairing IHs Unfavorable safety profile
Interferon-α (2a and 2b)	Inhibits angiogenesis	May be considered for severe recalcitrant IHs (short-term use) Unfavorable safety profile
Itraconazole	Inhibits cellular proliferation	Satisfactory results in reported cases Relatively safe
Captopril	Angiotensin-converting enzyme inhibitor	Less effective than propranolol

0.5% solution or gel is applied twice daily, and most studies have demonstrated significant response rates to reduce IH color and size when compared with laser, placebo, or observation.[22] Nevertheless, a recent trial did not find a significant effect in the treatment of IH compared with placebo when initiated during the early proliferative phase.[21] Side effects consist mainly of local reactions such as irritation and rarely events similar to propranolol. Thus, caution should be exercised when it is used on ulcerated IHs and preterm infants due to potential for significant systemic absorption.[10]

Other local therapies
Topical and intralesional corticosteroids, topical imiquimod, and other intralesional therapies may prove beneficial on further investigation (**Table 2**).

Table 2
Local treatments for infantile hemangiomas aside from timolol[10,21,22,25]

Medication	Efficacy	Comments
Topical corticosteroids	Outcomes significantly better with topical timolol vs corticosteroids	Potent corticosteroids usually
Topical β-blockers propranolol and carteolol	Evidence for efficacy in a prospective study of 2% carteolol twice daily	Less evidence than other modalities
Topical imiquimod	No significant difference between topical imiquimod and topical timolol	5% ointment formulation More side effects than timolol
Intralesional corticosteroids	Triamcinolone exhibits an average expected clearance of 58%	Triamcinolone or betamethasone For focal, bulky IHs during proliferation or in sensitive anatomic sites As an adjunct to β-blockade or for nonresponders
Intralesional bleomycin	Inferior efficacy to oral propranolol	May be considered as an adjunct to oral propranolol in cases of propranolol nonresponse Significant risk of toxicity
Intralesional bevacizumab	Less effective than intralesional triamcinolone	Anti-VEGF-A Could be considered as an adjuvant therapy

Laser Therapy

The use of the 595 nm pulsed dye laser (PDL) or the long-pulse Nd:YAG has been addressed over the past several years, although the outcomes evaluated have been heterogeneous.[10] PDL has been well established for the treatment of the residual telangiectasias of IHs, but it has also shown benefit in speeding the involution of superficial IHs.[22,36] The 1095 nm Nd:YAG, on the other hand, may be used to target deep IHs due to its longer wavelength.[22] The pertinent benefit of laser therapy, especially PDL, appears with its use in conjunction with oral β-blockers.[37] In addition, PDL used at low fluences has been reported to accelerate healing in ulcerated IH and assist in pain control.[9] Ablative lasers have also been tried to help transdermal delivery of timolol for deep IH.[22]

Surgical Options

Despite the multitude of medical options available, procedures may be warranted for the satisfactory treatment of IHs or their sequelae. Moreover, surgical excision and reconstruction may be considered during infancy, for life-threatening cases, or when the risks of pharmacologic options supersede those of surgery, although usually deferred until after involution to excise residual fibrofatty tissue or correct deformity.[21] In addition, embolization may be necessary in life-threatening IH that is refractory to medical management, especially cases of visceral IH.[21]

MANAGEMENT OF COMPLICATIONS

Ulceration is the most common complication arising from IH, and the first step in addressing this issue is local wound care with barrier creams and nonadhesive dressings, plus pain control. In addtion, propranolol is pivotal in the treatment of ulcerated IHs, resulting in improved healing specifically at doses less than or equal to 1 mg/kg/d.[11] However, β-blocker therapy may induce or worsen ulceration due to their vasoconstrictive properties.[21] Furthermore, topical timolol and PDL to the bed of the ulcer may improve healing, with caution as to the potentially enhanced systemic absorption of timolol with topical application to ulcers.[21,38] Although the rate of secondary infection of ulcerated IHs is elevated, routine antibiotics are not recommended, and infections may be treated with bacterial sensitivity-guided topical or systemic antibiotics.[21,22] As for the management of the cutaneous sequelae of IHs, various surgical interventions may be performed, as outlined in **Table 3**.

Table 3
Interventions for the cutaneous sequalae of infantile hemangiomas

Complication	Intervention
Telangiectasia	Vascular lasers such as PDL or 532 nm KTP laser
Fibrofatty tissue	Surgery Liposuction Intralesional deoxycholic acid
Scarring or textural changes such as atrophy and anetoderma	Ablative fractional laser resurfacing Surgery
Structural deformity	Reconstructive surgery

Data from Sebaratnam DF, Rodríguez Bandera AL, Wong LF, Wargon O. Infantile hemangioma. Part 2: Management. J Am Acad Dermatol. 2021 Dec;85(6):1395-1404.

SUMMARY

In conclusion, IHs are benign tumors with a peculiar natural progression that ultimately spontaneously resolve. However, in order to maximize the chance of the best possible result for each individual patient, accurate early recognition, diagnosis and treatment is important.

CLINICS CARE POINTS

- Infantile hemangiomas can present as superficial bright red papules or plaques, deep skin-colored masses, or with features of the two.
- The classic presentation of an IH may be preceded by a telangiectatic precursor with surrounding rim of vasoconstriction, from birth.
- Parents should be educated about the natural course of IHs.
- Clinical features and patterns of involvement serve as clues to the risks of developing complications and the need for further evaluation.
- The optimal window for intervention or referral to a hemangioma specialist is at around 1 month of age.
- The most common complication is ulceration, and a sensitive clue to its occurrence is a change in color to white gray in infants younger than 3 months.
- Oral propranolol is the first-line therapeutic option, whereas vascular lasers (PDL), topical

timolol, and systemic or topical corticosteroids may serve as alternative or adjuvant therapies.

- The appropriate management of a patient with IH should be determined on a case-by-case basis.

DISCLOSURE

No commercial or financial conflicts of interest to disclose.

REFERENCES

1. Rodríguez Bandera AI, Sebaratnam DF, Wargon O, et al. Infantile hemangioma. Part 1: Epidemiology, pathogenesis, clinical presentation and assessment. J Am Acad Dermatol 2021;85(6):1379–92.
2. Holland KE, Drolet BA. Approach to the Patient with an Infantile Hemangioma. Dermatol Clin 2013;31(2):289–301.
3. Ding Y, Zhang J-Z, Yu S-R, et al. Risk factors for infantile hemangioma: a meta-analysis. World J Pediatr 2020;16(4):377–84.
4. North PE, Waner M, Mizeracki A, et al. A unique microvascular phenotype shared by juvenile hemangiomas and human placenta. Arch Dermatol 2001;137(5):559–70.
5. Munden A, Butschek R, Tom WL, et al. Prospective study of infantile haemangiomas: incidence, clinical characteristics and association with placental anomalies. Br J Dermatol 2014;170(4):907–13.
6. Pramanik K, Chun CZ, Garnaas MK, et al. Dusp-5 and Snrk-1 coordinately function during vascular development and disease. Blood 2009;113(5):1184–91.
7. Berg JN, Walter JW, Thisanagayam U, et al. Evidence for loss of heterozygosity of 5q in sporadic haemangiomas: are somatic mutations involved in haemangioma formation? J Clin Pathol 2001;54(3):249.
8. Chang LC, Haggstrom AN, Drolet BA, et al. Growth Characteristics of Infantile Hemangiomas: Implications for Management. Pediatrics 2008;122(2):360–7.
9. Luu M, Frieden IJ. Haemangioma: clinical course, complications and management. Br J Dermatol 2013;169(1):20–30.
10. Krowchuk DP, Frieden IJ, Mancini AJ, et al. Clinical Practice Guideline for the Management of Infantile Hemangiomas. Pediatrics 2019;143(1):e20183475.
11. Faith EF, Shah S, Witman PM, et al. Clinical features, prognostic factors, and treatment interventions for ulceration in patients with infantile hemangioma. JAMA Dermatol 2021;157(5):566–72.
12. Mariani LG, Ferreira LM, Rovaris DL, et al. Infantile hemangiomas: risk factors for complications, recurrence and unaesthetic sequelae. Anais brasileiros de dermatologia 2022;97(1):37–44.
13. Horii KA, Drolet BA, Frieden IJ, et al. Prospective Study of the Frequency of Hepatic Hemangiomas in Infants with Multiple Cutaneous Infantile Hemangiomas. Pediatr Dermatol 2011;28(3):245–53.
14. Kulungowski AM, Alomari AI, Chawla A, et al. Lessons from a liver hemangioma registry: subtype classification. J Pediatr Surg 2012;47(1):165–70.
15. Darrow DH. Management of Infantile Hemangiomas of the Airway. Otolaryngol Clin North America 2018;51(1):133–46.
16. Sacco O, Moscatelli A, Nozza P, et al. Respiratory Distress in a 3-Month-Old Infant with a Mass Obstructing the Right Main-Stem Bronchus: An Unusual Localization of Infantile Hemangioma. J Pediatr 2017;182:397. e391.
17. Haggstrom AN, Garzon MC, Baselga E, et al. Risk for PHACE Syndrome in Infants With Large Facial Hemangiomas. Pediatrics 2010;126(2):e418–26.
18. Igarashi A, Hata I, Yuasa M, et al. A case of an infant with extremely low birth weight and hypothyroidism associated with massive cutaneous infantile hemangioma. J Pediatr Endocrinol Metab 2018;31(12):1377–80.
19. Zhao J, Huang AH, Rainer BM, et al. Periocular infantile hemangiomas: Characteristics, ocular sequelae, and outcomes. Pediatr Dermatol 2019;36(6):830–4.
20. Solman L, Glover M, Beattie PE, et al. Oral propranolol in the treatment of proliferating infantile haemangiomas: British Society for Paediatric Dermatology consensus guidelines. Br J Dermatol 2018;179(3):582–9.
21. Colmant C, Powell J. Medical Management of Infantile Hemangiomas: An Update. Pediatr Drugs 2021;1–15.
22. Sebaratnam DF, Rodríguez Bandera AI, Wong L-CF, et al. Infantile hemangioma. Part 2: Management. J Am Acad Dermatol 2021;85(6):1395–404.
23. Vivcharuk V, Vy Davydenko. Influence of age and morphological features on the clinical manifestations and treatment efficacy of hemangiomas in children. Inter Collegas 2021;8(1):22–9.
24. Schrenk S, Boscolo E. A transcription factor is the target of propranolol treatment in infantile hemangioma. J Clin Invest 2022;132(3):e156863.
25. Leung AKC, Lam JM, Leong KF, et al. Infantile hemangioma: an updated review. Curr Pediatr Rev 2021;17(1):55–69.
26. Park HJ, Lee S-Y, Rho MH, et al. Ultrasound and MRI findings as predictors of propranolol therapy response in patients with infantile hemangioma. PLoS One 2021;16(3):e0247505.

27. de Graaf M, Breur J, Raphaël MF, et al. Adverse effects of propranolol when used in the treatment of hemangiomas: a case series of 28 infants. J Am Acad Dermatol 2011;1097–6787 (Electronic)).

28. Babiak-Choroszczak L, Giżewska-Kacprzak K, Dawid G, et al. Safety assessment during initiation and maintenance of propranolol therapy for infantile hemangiomas. Adv Clin Exp Med Official Organ Wroclaw Med Univ 2019;28(3):375–84.

29. Mendez-Gallart R, García-Palacios M, Cortizo-Vazquez J, et al. Generalized hypertrichosis in an infant after treatment with propranolol for infantile hemangioma. Indian J Dermatol Venereol Leprol 2020;86(3):311–3.

30. Bayart CB, Tamburro JE, Vidimos AT, et al. Atenolol Versus Propranolol for Treatment of Infantile Hemangiomas During the Proliferative Phase: A Retrospective Noninferiority Study. Pediatr Dermatol 2017; 34(4):413–21.

31. Ji Y, Chen S, Yang K, et al. Efficacy and Safety of Propranolol vs Atenolol in Infants With Problematic Infantile Hemangiomas: A Randomized Clinical Trial. JAMA otolaryngology– head neck Surg 2021;147(7): 599–607.

32. Pope E, Lara-Corrales I, Sibbald C, et al. Noninferiority and Safety of Nadolol vs Propranolol in Infants With Infantile Hemangioma: A Randomized Clinical Trial. JAMA Pediatr 2022;176(1):34–41.

33. Koh SP, Leadbitter P, Smithers F, et al. β-blocker therapy for infantile hemangioma. Expert Rev Clin Pharmacol 2020;13(8):899–915.

34. Zhang L, Zheng JW, Yuan WE. Treatment of alarming head and neck infantile hemangiomas with interferon-α2a: a clinical study in eleven consecutive patients. Drug Des Devel Ther 2015;9:723–7.

35. Liu Z, Lv S, Wang S, et al. Itraconazole therapy for infant hemangioma: Two case reports. World J Clin cases 2021;9(28):8579.

36. Shen L, Zhou G, Zhao J, et al. Pulsed dye laser therapy for infantile hemangiomas: a systemic review and meta-analysis. QJM: An Int J Med 2015; 108(6):473–80.

37. Fei Q, Lin Y, Chen X. Treatments for infantile Hemangioma: A systematic review and network meta-analysis. EClinicalMedicine 2020;26:100506.

38. Wang JY, Ighani A, Ayala AP, et al. Medical, Surgical, and Wound Care Management of Ulcerated Infantile Hemangiomas: A Systematic Review. J Cutan Med Surg 2018;22(5):495–504.

Hemangioma Genetics and Associated Syndromes

Julie Luu, BS[a], Colleen H. Cotton, MD[b],*

KEYWORDS

- Infantile hemangioma • PHACE • LUMBAR • Hemangiomatosis • Arterial anomalies

KEY POINTS

- Any potential underlying genetic cause of IH remains unknown.
- Evaluation for PHACE and LUMBAR syndromes is necessary for large segmental IH, including the imaging of appropriate anatomic areas.
- Five or more cutaneous IH should prompt evaluation for extracutaneous IH with liver ultrasound.

INTRODUCTION

While infantile hemangiomas (IH) are the most common benign vascular tumor of infancy, their genetics have largely remained elusive. Syndromes associated with other vascular anomalies are the result of the same somatic mutation at different times in different tissue types. Additionally, identifying syndromes truly associated with IH is confusing as the term "hemangioma" is often used to refer to different vascular lesions in the literature. The specific mechanisms of IH-associated syndromes are unknown but are related to patterns of anomalies determined by IH location and characteristics. We briefly discuss what is known regarding IH genetics, how to identify patients with IH who need screening for associated syndromes/anomalies, and how to manage these patients.

DISCUSSION

Hemangioma Genetics

The pathogenesis of IH is not yet understood. Repeated studies have failed to identify a specific gene that is responsible for the formation of IH. While a genetic mechanism is likely important, it is highly unlikely to be solely responsible for IH pathogenesis.

Several genes important for angiogenesis, cell growth, transcriptional control, and cell signaling are deregulated in IH (**Table 1**).[1–4] The role of microRNAs (miRNA), circular RNAs (circRNA), and long-noncoding RNAs (lnRNA) have also been the subject of more recent IH research to investigate the pathogenesis and identify potential therapeutic targets.[5–8]

The expression of several genes is also altered by the beta-blocker treatment of IH (see **Table 1**).[4,9] A recent study identified SOX18, a transcription factor, as being the direct target of propranolol. The R enantiomer of propranolol inhibits the dimerization of SOX18 with other key proteins, thereby preventing selective binding to DNA. This may be the mechanism by which propranolol treats IH.[9]

Neonatal Hemangiomatosis

Nature of the problem

It is not uncommon to see more than one cutaneous IH in a single infant. However, multiple cutaneous IH can signify the presence of extracutaneous IH (**Fig. 1**). These can arise in any organ, but the most common extracutaneous site is the liver. These lesions, such as cutaneous IH, are GLUT-1 positive.[10] There is no association between the number of cutaneous IH and the

[a] University of the Incarnate Word School of Osteopathic Medicine, 7615 Kennedy Hill Dr, San Antonio, TX 78235, USA; [b] Department of Dermatology and Dermatologic Surgery, Medical University of South Carolina, 135 Rutledge Avenue, MSC 578, Charleston, SC 29425, USA
* Corresponding author. Department of Dermatology and Dermatologic Surgery, Medical University of South Carolina, 135 Rutledge Avenue, MSC 578, Charleston, SC 29425.
E-mail address: cotton.colleen@gmail.com

Dermatol Clin 40 (2022) 393–400
https://doi.org/10.1016/j.det.2022.07.001

Table 1
Genes relevant for IH pathogenesis and treatment. This list is not exhaustive

Relationship to IH	Relevant Genes
Upregulated in IH[1–3]	6-phosphofructo-2-kinase 3 (PFKFB3) Angiopoietin 2 (ANGPT2) Vascular endothelial growth factors (VEGF, VEGFA, VEGF2) NDRG1 Glucose transporter-1 (GLUT1) Stromal cell-derived factor-1a (SDF1α) Matrix metalloproteinase 9 (MMP9) Insulin-like growth factor 2 (IGF2) MALAT1 Tumor endothelial marker-8 (TEM-8) Kirsten RAt Sarcoma viral oncogene homolog (KRAS) Fibroblast growth factor 2 (FGF2)
Downregulated in IH[3]	KiSS1 metastasis suppressor (KISS1) Forkhead Box O1 (FOXO1) Cyclin-dependent kinase inhibitor 2A (CDKN2A or p16)
Downregulated in involution phase[2,4]	Collagen type IV alpha 2 chain (COL4A2) Integrin subunit alpha 1 (ITGA1) Platelet-derived growth factor receptor-beta (PDGFRB) RNA binding Fox-1 homolog 2 (RBFOX2) Matrix-remodeling-associated protein 5 (MXRA5) Vasohibin 1 (VASH1) Peroxidasin (PXDN)
Upregulated in involution phase[4]	ATPase Na+/K+ transporting subunit beta 1 (ATP1B1) Fibulin 1 (FBLN1) N-Myc downstream regulated 1 (NDRG1) Secreted frizzled-related protein (SRFP1) Cluster of differentiation 9 (CD9)
Expression altered by propranolol treatment[4]	Aldehyde dehydrogenase 1A1 (ALDH1A1) Endothelial PAS domain protein 1 (EPAS1) LIM and SH3 domain protein 1 (LASP1) Solute carrier member family 25 member 23 (SLC25A23) Myosin-binding protein 1 (MYOB1)
Directly targeted by propranolol treatment[9]	SOX18

number of hepatic IH; however, the more cutaneous IH, the higher the likelihood of having hepatic IH.[11]

Neonatal hemangiomatosis is split into 2 categories: diffuse neonatal hemangiomatosis (DNH) with extracutaneous involvement, and benign neonatal hemangiomatosis (BNH) with skin-limited disease. Some have also proposed the term "multifocal IH with or without extracutaneous disease" to separate it from other multifocal vascular anomalies previously included in neonatal hemangiomatosis.[12]

Umbilical cord tumors and chorioangiomas (the most common benign tumor of the placenta) have been reported in cases of BNH and DNH.[13,14] Multifocal IH are more common in premature and low birth weight infants.[11]

Both cutaneous and extracutaneous IH in these conditions follow the classic time course of non-syndromic IH. However, several cases of BNH have been reported with cutaneous IH fully formed at birth, and/or with unusually rapid involution.[15]

Evaluation
Patients with ≥5 cutaneous IH should have a liver ultrasound to evaluate for extracutaneous IH.[16] This cutoff was validated in a prospective study comparing the rate of liver IH in patients with 1 to 4 cutaneous IH (0%) versus patients with ≥5 cutaneous IH (16%).[11] This recommendation only applies to infants younger than 6 months, as the development of clinically relevant liver disease after this age is extremely unlikely. Patients should also be monitored for signs of IH at less common

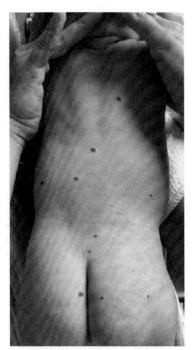

Fig. 1. Neonatal hemangiomatosis. This patient had greater than 50 cutaneous IH and innumerable hepatic IH.

extracutaneous sites, including the gastrointestinal (GI) tract (blood in the stool) and airway (biphasic stridor).

As hepatic IH can follow the classic pattern of rapid growth, a negative liver ultrasound in the early neonatal period should be repeated at 2 to 3 months of age to ensure that new or enlarging liver IH has not developed. Current guidelines recommend complete blood counts and liver function tests at diagnosis and then as needed.[17] Patients with hepatic IH require serial ultrasounds until involution, though specific intervals may vary.[17] An echocardiogram is considered when symptoms of heart failure occur (eg, abdominal distension, failure to thrive, breathing difficulties) or enlarged hepatic veins are seen.

Complications

Complications associated with isolated cutaneous IH can apply to BNH lesions, including ulceration, cosmetic deformity, and functional impairment. However, several life-threatening complications can result from DNH. In the proliferative stage, hepatic IH can be associated with significant arteriovenous shunting, leading to high output cardiac failure.[17] This may present as failure to thrive, respiratory distress, or abdominal distension. Abdominal compartment syndrome and liver

failure are also possible with diffuse hepatic IH replacing the liver parenchyma.

Diffuse hepatic IH can also lead to consumptive hypothyroidism (Fig. 2). This will not be present congenitally and therefore not detected on newborn screening, as it is related to proliferation. These lesions express very high levels of type 3 iodothyronine deiodinase, which converts T4 into biologically inactive reverse T3.[18] Both enzyme activity level and burden of hepatic IH play a role in whether and when patients have clinically relevant hypothyroidism. If unrecognized, this can cause poor growth, lethargy, and feeding difficulties. Thyroid function tests should be performed at diagnosis for all patients with hepatic IH. They should be repeated monthly until 6 months of age for patients with diffuse disease.[17]

GI tract involvement is less common than hepatic IH, and clinically significant bleeding from these lesions is even rarer. Most cases of "hemangiomatosis" with GI bleeding are actually different types of vascular anomalies.[12] Airway hemangiomas have also been reported in DNH.

Treatment

Like isolated cutaneous IH, beta-blockers are the treatment of choice to manage hepatic IH, improving lesion size and ameliorating complications.[19,20] Active nonintervention is reasonable for BNH, with topical timolol in reserve if only a few of the lesions are likely to result in complications. Associated hypothyroidism in DNH should be treated with levothyroxine concomitantly with the underlying hepatic IH. Given its consumptive nature, higher doses are often required.[21]

PHACE Syndrome

Nature of the problem

PHACE(S) syndrome is a neurocutaneous disorder describing a characteristic group of developmental irregularities: posterior fossa malformations, segmental IH, arterial anomalies, cardiac defects, eye abnormalities, and sternal or abdominal ventral midline defects (Table 2).[22–25] The complete spectrum of symptoms encompassed by the PHACE acronym is only seen in a minority of patients. With more than 300 cases reported, PHACE is considered one of the most common neurocutaneous vascular disorders occurring in childhood with a poorly understood underlying pathogenesis.[24,26] During embryogenesis, the migration of neural crest cells and mesoderm-derived endothelial precursors contribute to the vascular formation and midline structural development of the head, heart, and trunk, providing a common pathway for the anomalies seen in PHACE to occur.[25,27] Several hypotheses have

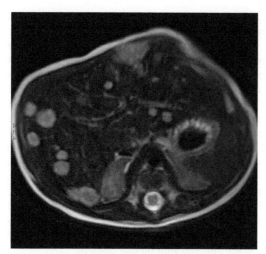

Fig. 2. Numerous T2 hyperintense lesions on abdominal MRI showing diffuse hepatic IH. This patient had consumptive hypothyroidism requiring levothyroxine.

been proposed to explain the development of PHACE including somatic mutations early in development, X-linked inactivation, structural variants, imprinted loci, and a complex combination of these.[27–30] The exact cause remains unknown.

Evaluation/guidelines Segmental cervicofacial IH ≥ 5 cm in diameter should raise suspicion for PHACE.[26,31,32] Between 31% and 58% of patients with large cervicofacial IH will have PHACE.[33–35] Full-body skin examination is necessary to evaluate for ventral midline fusion defects (sternal pit or tag, supraumbilical raphe, congenital scarring). In addition, workup for associated cerebrovascular, ophthalmologic, cardiac, auditory, dental, speech, endocrine, and neurologic deficits is required.[30,31]

Identifying the facial segments involved in facial IH may guide screening decisions. These are based on developmental fusion planes during embryogenesis.[25,36] Patients with IH involving 3 or more facial segments or area ≥25 cm² are at higher risk of having PHACE, whereas patients with parotid gland or maxillary facial segment involvement are at lower risk.[33]

Cerebrovascular anomalies are the most common extracutaneous finding in PHACE leading to the potential for thromboembolism and increased risk of acute ischemic stroke (AIS).[37] Risk stratification is assessed by brain magnetic resonance angiography (MRA) to determine the potential risk of AIS and guide further management.[24,31,37] Patients at intermediate risk should see pediatric neurology, and those with high-risk anomalies

should start prophylactic aspirin therapy and ongoing surveillance with vascular neurology.[31]

Consensus-based diagnostic criteria were most recently revised in 2016.[31] Each category of extracutaneous anomaly (arterial, structural brain, cardiovascular, ocular, and ventral midline) is divided into major and minor criteria. Definite PHACE is diagnosed with a facial IH > 5 cm in diameter with 1 major or 2 minor criteria, or large IH on the upper body with 2 major criteria.[31]

Imaging Magnetic resonance imaging (MRI) and MRA of the head and neck as well as an echocardiogram including the aortic arch must be performed to evaluate for congenital heart disorders, cerebral abnormalities, and arterial anomalies.[24,31,37] A comprehensive eye examination with retinal visualization is also required.

Complications Coarctation of the aorta, aberrant arteries, aplasia, or occlusion of a major cerebral artery is risk factors for AIS in children with PHACE.[37] Although IH is often the initial presenting sign of PHACE, poor prognosis and morbidity result from cerebrovascular changes in anomalous cervical and cerebral arteries leading to neurovascular complications. Adolescents and adults with PHACE may suffer from arteriopathy with debilitating migraine-like headaches, AIS, and moyamoya-type vasculopathy.[37] Further complications that may not present on initial screening include congenital or acquired hypothyroidism, symptoms of dysphagia or speech delay, and dental anomalies.[31,38] Patients should be followed for these throughout their development. While the more severe disease is typically associated with neurodevelopmental deficits (particularly speech delay), no single feature is predictive.[39] Clinicians should have a low threshold to refer for early intervention services.

Lumbar Syndrome

Nature of the problem

LUMBAR syndrome (sometimes called PELVIS or SACRAL syndromes) is the counterpart to PHACE with large segmental IH on the lower extremities or perineal and lumbosacral areas. Distinct underlying congenital anomalies are seen: lower body hemangioma and other cutaneous abnormalities, urogenital defects, ulceration, myelopathy, bone deformities, anorectal malformations, arterial and renal anomalies.[30,40–42] Similar to PHACE, few patients present with the full spectrum summarized by the LUMBAR acronym. The exact pathogenesis is also unknown.

Table 2 Anomalies associated with PHACE syndrome. This list is not exhaustive	
Category	**Anomalies**

Arterial	• Anomalies of the large cerebral or cervical arteries
	  ○ Absence
	  ○ Aberrant origin or course
	  ○ Moyamoya collaterals
	  ○ Significant hypoplasia
	  ○ Stenosis or occlusion
	• Cerebral arterial aneurysm
	• Persistent carotid-vertebrobasilar anastomosis
	  ○ Proatlantal segmental artery
	  ○ Hypoglossal artery
	  ○ Otic artery
	  ○ Trigeminal artery

Structural Brain	Abnormal septum pellucidum
	Arachnoid cyst
	A/dysgenesis of corpus callosum
	Brainstem hypoplasia
	Dural ectasia of Meckel's cave
	Intracranial IH
	Malformations of cortical development
	  ○ Cortical dysplasia
	  ○ Gray matter heterotopia
	  ○ Polymicrogyria
	Optic nerve/chiasm hypoplasia (may also be seen on eye examination)
	Pituitary abnormalities
	Posterior fossa defects
	  ○ Cerebellar hypoplasia
	  ○ Dandy–Walker spectrum
	  ○ Fourth ventricle abnormalities

Cardiovascular	Right aortic arch/double arch Coarctation of aorta Aneurysm of aortic arch Aberrant origin of subclavian artery Vascular rings Ventricular septal defect Systemic venous anomalies Aortic tortuosity or other dysplasia
Ocular	Staphyloma Persistent hyperplastic primary vitreous Persistent fetal vasculature Retinal vascular anomalies Optic nerve hypoplasia (may also be seen on MRI) Morning glory disc anomaly

(continued on next page)

Table 2 (continued)	
Category	**Anomalies**
	Microphthalmia Sclerocornea Coloboma Cataracts Horner syndrome
Ventral Midline	• Sternal pit • Sternal cleft • Supraumbilical raphe • Ectopic thyroid • Hypopituitarism • Midline sternal papule/hamartoma
Other	• Dental root abnormalities • Dental enamel hypoplasia

Evaluation

Children at risk for LUMBAR require a thorough physical examination of the abdomen, pelvis, and lower extremities with a focus on the genital and paraspinal regions.[40] Segmental IH in the lumbosacral region warrants further evaluation for underlying regional congenital abnormalities (abnormal genitalia, imperforate anus, and sacral bony defects), disruptions in vascular formation (aberrant, stenosed, occluded, and tortuous vessels), spinal dysraphism, and organ dysfunction.[30,40] Unlike PHACE, there are currently no defined diagnostic criteria for LUMBAR.

Imaging

MRI is the gold standard to detect occult spinal changes.[42] Current imaging recommendations for a child less than 3 months of age with lumbosacral or perineal segmental IH are ultrasound of the spine, abdomen, and pelvis with color Doppler. For children with normal ultrasound and segmental IH or other cutaneous manifestations spanning across the midline or lower back, MRI of the spine is recommended at 3 to 6 months of age due to the high risk of spinal cord anomalies.[40,42] Spinal ultrasound has a 50% false-negative rate compared with MRI in high-risk patients.[40,42] MRA and magnetic resonance venography (MRV) help evaluate the severity of associated vascular anomalies including the extent of internal IH and blood vessel structure. With extensive involvement of the lower limbs, MRI/MRA/MRV evaluation of the abdominal aorta down to the pedal vessels is optimal.[40] X-ray of the lower limbs during preschool years is also recommended to detect leg length discrepancy.[40]

Table 3
Indications for IH-related syndrome screening and associated work-up

Syndrome	Indications for Screening	Screening Recommended
PHACE syndrome	• Large (>5 cm diameter) cervicofacial IH • Large IH on the trunk or upper extremity	• MRI/MRA of the head and neck • Echocardiogram • Complete eye examination • Careful physical examination for midline anomalies

LUMBAR syndrome	• Large segmental IH on the lower body	• Ultrasound of abdomen and pelvis
		• Careful physical examination for midline and genital anomalies
		• Spinal imaging
		  ○ If < 3 month old, start with spinal ultrasound
		  ○ If > 3 month old or high-risk IH location over midline or other midline anomalies, MRI of the spine
		• If extensive involvement of lower limbs, MRI/MRA/MRV from aorta to pedal vessels
		• X-ray of lower limbs at preschool age

Diffuse neonatal hemangiomatosis	• Five or more cutaneous IH
	• Fewer than 5 cutaneous IH with clinical symptoms of heart failure
		• Ultrasound of liver
		• If liver IH:
		  ○ Complete blood count
		  ○ Liver function tests
		  ○ Thyroid function tests
		  ○ Consider echocardiogram

Complications

Segmental IH is more likely to ulcerate, and this is particularly true of IH in the diaper area, making patients with LUMBAR especially prone to this complication. Life-threatening internal IH, hypotension, and hypoperfusion through stenosed or tortuous vessels may require consultation with vascular specialists.[40] Myelopathy may result in bilateral upper or lower extremity weakness. Abnormal limb development, tissue atrophy, renal artery stenosis, and acute ischemic stroke may also occur.[40,42]

SUMMARY

Many candidate genes have been identified as playing an important role in the pathogenesis and treatment of IH. Ongoing research hopes to better characterize the genetics and epigenetics of IH.

It is important to recognize when additional evaluation may be required for IH with particular characteristics, including PHACE syndrome, LUMBAR syndrome, and neonatal hemangiomatosis. Recommended evaluations are summarized in **Table 3**.

CLINICS CARE POINTS

- There is no role for genetic testing in patients with IH, as true IH is not associated with any genetic syndromes
- Infants less than 6 months of age with ≥5 cutaneous IH should have a liver ultrasound for hepatic IH
- When checking for liver IH, if ultrasound in the first month of life is normal, still need to recheck at 2 to 3 months of age as hepatic IH may have been too small to detect.
- Patients with hepatic IH require laboratory evaluation for consumptive hypothyroidism (TSH, free T4, and reverse T3), complete blood count, and liver function tests.
- Consider echocardiogram in patients with IH that have abdominal distension, failure to thrive, or enlarged hepatic veins during imaging
- Patients with hepatic IH require serial ultrasounds until the IH has involuted

- Patients with large IH of the head or neck >5 cm in diameter should receive a PHACE workup with MRI/MRA of the head and neck, echocardiogram, and eye examination.

- Make sure in a PHACE workup that the arteries of the head and neck are included in imaging to fully evaluate the carotid arteries for anomalies

- The entire aortic arch should be evaluated during a PHACE workup, whether on MRI or echocardiogram

- Patients with large IH of the lower extremities or lumbosacral regions should receive a LUMBAR workup with spinal ultrasound/MRI, MRI/MRV/MRA of underlying vasculature, and abdominal and pelvic ultrasound.

DISCLOSURE

Dr Cotton received honoraria as a consultant for Pierre-Fabre pharmaceuticals. Ms Luu has no relevant disclosures.

REFERENCES

1. Kleinman ME, Greives MR, Churgin SS, et al. Hypoxia-induced mediators of stem/progenitor cell trafficking are increased in children with hemangioma. Arterioscler Thromb Vasc Biol 2007;27(12):2664–70.

2. Luca AC, Miron IC, Trandafir LM, et al. Morphological, genetic and clinical correlations in infantile hemangiomas and their mimics. Rom J Morphol Emryol 2020;61(3):687–95.

3. de Leye H, Saerens J, Janmohamed SR. News on infantile haemangioma. Part 1: clinical course and pathomechanism. Clin Exp Dermatol 2021;46(3): 473–9.

4. Gomez-Acevedo H, Dai Y, Strub G, et al. Identification of putative biomarkers for infantile hemangiomas and propranolol treatment via data integration. Sci Rep 2020;10(1):3261.

5. Bertoni N, Pereira LMS, Severino FE, et al. Integrative meta-analysis identifies microRNA-regulated networks in infantile hemangioma. BMC Med Genet 2016;17:4.

6. Fu C, Lv R, Xu G, et al. Circular RNA profile of infantile hemangioma by microarray analysis. PLoS One 2017;12(11):e0187581.

7. Li J, Li Q, Chen L, et al. Expression profile of circular RNAs in infantile hemangioma detected by RNA-Seq. Medicine (Baltimore) 2018;97(21):e10882.

8. Zhou L, Jia X, Yang X. LncRNA-TUG1 promotes the progression of infantile hemangioma by regulating miR-137/IGFBP5 axis. Hum Genomics 2021;15(1): 50.

9. Schrenk S, Boscolo E. A transcription factor is the target of propranolol treatment in infantile hemangioma. J Clin Invest 2022;132(3):e156863.

10. Mo JQ, Dimashkieh HH, Bove KE. GLUT1 endothelial reactivity distinguishes hepatic infantile hemangioma from congenital hepatic vascular malformation with associated capillary proliferation. Hum Pathol 2004;35(2):200–9.

11. Horii KA, Drolet BA, Frieden IJ, et al. Prospective study of the frequency of hepatic hemangiomas in infants with multiple cutaneous infantile hemangiomas. Pediatr Dermatol 2011;28(3):245–53.

12. Glick ZR, Frieden IJ, Garzon MC, et al. Diffuse neonatal hemangiomatosis: an evidence-based review of case reports in the literature. J Am Acad Dermatol 2012;67(5):898–903.

13. Schwickert A, Seeger K-H, Rancourt RC, et al. Prenatally detected umbilical cord tumor as a sign of diffuse neonatal hemangiomatosis. J Clin Ultrasound 2019;47(6):366–8.

14. Hamouda S, Soussan J, Haumonte J-B, et al. In utero embolization for placental chorioangioma and neonatal multifocal hemangiomatosis. J Gynecol Obstet Hum Reprod 2019;48(8):689–94.

15. Korekawa A, Nakajima K, Nakano H, et al. Benign neonatal hemangiomatosis with early regression of skin lesions: A case report and review of the published work. J Dermatol 2020;47(8):911–6.

16. Dickie B, Dasgupta R, Nair R, et al. Spectrum of hepatic hemangiomas: management and outcome. J Pediatr Surg 2009;44(1):125–33.

17. Iacobas I, Phung TL, Adams DM, et al. Guidance Document for Hepatic Hemangioma (Infantile and Congenital) Evaluation and Monitoring. J Pediatr 2018;203:294–300. e2.

18. Huang SA, Tu HM, Harney JW, et al. Severe hypothyroidism caused by type 3 iodothyronine deiodinase in infantile hemangiomas. N Engl J Med 2000;343(3):185–9.

19. Mazereeuw-Hautier J, Hoeger PH, Benlahrech S, et al. Efficacy of propranolol in hepatic infantile hemangiomas with diffuse neonatal hemangiomatosis. J Pediatr 2010;157(2):340–2.

20. Ishikawa T, Seki K, Uchiyama H. Efficacy of intravenous propranolol for life-threatening diffuse neonatal hemangiomatosis. Pediatr Dermatol 2022. Online ahead of print.

21. Campbell V, Beckett R, Abid N, et al. Resolution of Consumptive Hypothyroidism Secondary to Infantile Hepatic Hemangiomatosis with a Combination of Propranolol and Levothyroxine. J Clin Res Pediatr Endocrinol 2018;10(3):294–8.

22. Frieden IJ, Reese V, Cohen D. PHACE syndrome. The association of posterior fossa brain malformations, hemangiomas, arterial anomalies, coarctation of the aorta and cardiac defects, and eye abnormalities. Arch Dermatol 1996;132(3):307–11.

23. Metry D, Heyer G, Hess C, et al. Consensus State-ment on Diagnostic Criteria for PHACE Syndrome. Pediatrics 2009;124(5):1447–56.

24. Rotter A, Samorano LP, Rivitti-Machado MC, et al. PHACE syndrome: clinical manifestations, diag-nostic criteria, and management. An Bras Dermatol 2018;93(3):405–11.

25. Haggstrom AN, Lammer EJ, Schneider RA, et al. Patterns of infantile hemangiomas: new clues to hemangioma pathogenesis and embryonic facial development. Pediatrics 2006;117(3):698–703.

26. Metry DW, Haggstrom AN, Drolet BA, et al. A Prospective Study of PHACE Syndrome in Infantile Hemangiomas: Demographic Features, Clinical Findings, and Complications. Am J Med Genet A 2006;140(9):975–86.

27. Etchevers HC, Vincent C, Le Douarin NM, et al. The cephalic neural crest provides pericytes and smooth muscle cells to all blood vessels of the face and forebrain. Development 2001;128(7):1059–68.

28. Metry DW, Siegel DH, Cordisco MR, et al. A comparison of disease severity among affected male versus female patients with PHACE syndrome. J Am Acad Dermatol 2008;58(1):81–7.

29. Siegel DH. PHACE syndrome: Infantile hemangi-omas associated with multiple congenital anoma-lies: Clues to the cause. Am J Med Genet C Semin Med Genet 2018;178(4):407–13.

30. Stefanko NS, Davies OMT, Beato MJ, et al. Hamarto-mas and midline anomalies in association with infan-tile hemangiomas, PHACE, and LUMBAR syndromes. Pediatr Dermatol 2020;37(1):78–85.

31. Garzon MC, Epstein LG, Heyer GL, et al. PHACE Syndrome: Consensus-Derived Diagnosis and Care Recommendations. J Pediatr 2016;178: 24–33.e2.

32. Schmid F, Reipschlaeger M, Leenen A, et al. Risk of associated cerebrovascular anomalies in children with segmental facial haemangiomas. Br J Dermatol 2019;181(6):1334–5.

33. Cotton CH, Ahluwalia J, Balkin DM, et al. Association of Demographic Factors and Infantile Hemangioma Characteristics With Risk of PHACE Syndrome. JAMA Dermatol 2021;157(8):1–8.

34. Forde KM, Glover MT, Chong WK, et al. Segmental hemangioma of the head and neck: High prevalence of PHACE syndrome. J Am Acad Dermatol 2017; 76(2):356–8.

35. Haggstrom AN, Garzon MC, Baselga E, et al. Risk for PHACE Syndrome in Infants With Large Facial Hemangiomas. Pediatrics 2010;126(2):e418–26.

36. Endicott AA, Chamlin SL, Drolet BA, et al. Mapping of Segmental and Partial Segmental Infantile Hem-angiomas of the Face and Scalp. JAMA Dermatol 2021;157(11):1328–34.

37. Eisenmenger LB, Rivera-Rivera LA, Johnson KM, et al. Utilisation of advanced MRI techniques to un-derstand neurovascular complications of PHACE syndrome: a case of arterial stenosis and dissection. BMJ Case Rep 2020;13(9):e235992.

38. Youssef MJ, Siegel DH, Chiu YE, et al. Dental root abnormalities in four children with PHACE syn-drome. Pediatr Dermatol 2019;36(4):505–8.

39. Brosig CL, Siegel DH, Haggstrom AN, et al. Neuro-developmental outcomes in children with PHACE syndrome. Pediatr Dermatol 2016;33(4):415–23.

40. Iacobas I, Burrows PE, Frieden IJ, et al. LUMBAR: association between cutaneous infantile hemangi-omas of the lower body and regional congenital anomalies. J Pediatr 2010;157(5):795–801.e8017.

41. Golabi M, An AC, Lopez C, et al. A new case of a LUMBAR syndrome. Am J Med Genet A 2014; 164A(1):204–7.

42. Drolet BA, Chamlin SL, Garzon MC, et al. Prospec-tive study of spinal anomalies in children with infan-tile hemangiomas of the lumbosacral skin. J Pediatr 2010;157(5):789–94.

Vascular Anomalies
Other Vascular Tumors

Kelly Atherton, MSCR[a], Harriet Hinen, MD[b],*

KEYWORDS

- Vascular tumors • Cutaneous • Pediatric • Congenital hemangioma • Pyogenic granuloma
- Kaposiform hemangioendothelioma • Angiosarcoma

KEY POINTS

- Vascular tumors are divided into three categories: benign, locally aggressive/borderline, and malignant.
- Several benign and locally aggressive/borderline tumors are newly identified and characterized and remain rare in the literature.
- Differentiating benign lesions from locally aggressive or malignant tumors is of utmost importance due to differences in treatment and prognosis.
- Diagnosis should be made based on a combination of clinical presentation, anatomic location, histology, immunohistochemistry, and imaging (if applicable).

BENIGN VASCULAR TUMORS

Infantile hemangioma (IH), the most common form of benign vascular tumor, is discussed in Divina Justina Hasbani and Lamiaa Hamie's article, "Infantile Hemangiomas," in this issue.

Congenital Hemangiomas

Congenital hemangiomas (CHs) are present and fully developed at the time of birth and may be diagnosed in utero. CHs were once believed to be a congenital form of IHs, until it was found that that CH does not display GLUT-1 expression, a hallmark of IH.[1,2] Clinical presentation, histology, and immunohistochemistry (IHC) are important for differentiating CH from IH.[1,3]

CHs follow a variable clinical course and exist on a spectrum defined by three main forms: rapidly involuting CH (RICH), partially involuting CH (PICH), and non-involuting CH (NICH).[3,4] RICHs are defined by lesion involution within the first year of life,[2,5] whereas NICHs do not involute. PICHs are a recently defined entity that exists on the spectrum between these other forms,

displaying incomplete involution and appearance and histology similar to NICH.[2,6]

CH occurs equally in both sexes.[6] Clinically, RICH typically presents as an exophytic mass occurring on the head and neck or extremities (Fig. 1).[2,3,7] Following involution, residual atrophy and scaring is common.[3] RICH may be associated with transient mild to moderate thrombocytopenia due to a localized intravascular consumptive coagulopathy,[2,3,8] which is milder than the severe thrombocytopenia of Kasabach–Merritt phenomenon (KMP) seen in tufted angiomas (TAs) and kaposiform hemangioendotheliomas (KHEs).[2,3,8]

NICHs present as solitary pink to violaceous plaques with overlying coarse dark red telangiectasias with possible areas of bluish discoloration and a blanching, halo-like area surrounding the lesion.[2,3,7,9] They are typically found on the trunk and extremities.[9]

PICHs present as red to violaceous patches, plaques, or masses with telangiectasias and surrounding pallor most commonly on the head and neck, trunk, and extremities, similar to NICHs. They also demonstrate subcutaneous draining channels and may develop central ulceration and

a College of Medicine, Medical University of South Carolina, 135 Rutledge Avenue, 11th Floor, Charleston, SC 29425-5780, USA; b Department of Dermatology and Dermatologic Surgery, Medical University of South Carolina, 135 Rutledge Avenue, 11th Floor, Charleston, SC 29425-5780, USA
* Corresponding author.
E-mail addresses: atherton@musc.edu (K.A.); bagnal@musc.edu (H.H.)

Dermatol Clin 40 (2022) 401–423
https://doi.org/10.1016/j.det.2022.06.011

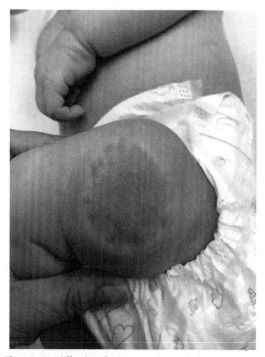

Fig. 1. Rapidly involuting congenital hemangioma located on the lateral thigh of an infant.

composed of large, well-defined lobules of capillary proliferations, separated by a dense fibrotic stroma of collagen, with prominent, thick-walled draining channels.[2,3,6,9,13] The fibrotic stroma may contain arteries, dysplastic veins, and arteriovenous fistulae and are confined to the subcutaneous tissue inferiorly.[9] Overlying epidermis is atrophic with a loss of dermal adnexal structures.[1,3]

Somatic activating missense mutations of exon Glu209 in GNAQ and GNA11 have been identified in many CHs[6,10,14,15] as well as one instance of a de novo germline mutation in MYH9.[16]

Treatment of CH depends on the type, size, location, and associated morbidity. Observation is often first-line management, and biopsy may be necessary if clinical diagnosis is uncertain.[3]

Surgical excision, especially in RICH, is indicated if associated with persistent or severe ulceration, life-threatening hemorrhage and hemodynamic instability, and thrombocytopenia.[3,6] Excision can also be considered for the removal of persistent atrophic tissue following involution[3,6] or may be indicated for functional impairment. **Fig. 2** demonstrates a CH with classical appearance, which was excised due to large size and subsequent functional impairment of the arm. Surgical excision is considered a standard treatment of NICH, which may involve preoperative embolization[6,7] as well as liver CHs causing a high-output cardiac state.[3] The pulse dye laser is sometimes used to treat associated telangiectases.[3,17]

overlying epidermal atrophy.[3,6] Similar to RICHs, PICHs begin to involute shortly after birth, but stabilize without complete involution, and continue to grow proportionately in size with the patient.[3,6]

Proliferation of CHs after birth, termed tardive expansion, is rare but has been described in a subset of NICHs, including one case series of 11 neonates demonstrating proportionate growth for 12 months, followed by spontaneous and rapid expansion within 12 to 61 months of age,[10] and another series describing 9 cases of atypical postnatal growth of NICHs from ages 2 to 10 years.[9] Another case described a rapid growth of a CH between 4 and 5 weeks of age, ultimately involuting by 4 months of age.[4] Tardive expansion CHs, as these lesions have come to be known, may represent a separate type of CH altogether and constitute an area of active research.

Of note, CH may also somewhat commonly involve the viscera, including the liver.[11,12] Large CH may be associated with high cardiac output and subsequent heart failure[2,13] and rarely hemorrhage, so echocardiography and coagulation studies at the time of presentation may be an important component of diagnostic assessment, particularly in very large lesions.[6] Imaging can also be helpful in diagnostic confirmation, particularly MRI and Doppler ultrasound.[2,4,6,10]

Histologically, RICH, NICH, and PICH share nearly indistinguishable morphology. All are

Tufted Angioma

TAs, sometimes referred to as angioblastoma of Nakagawa, are considered benign vascular tumors but must be differentiated from other benign tumors due to the potential complication of KMP, which occurs in 19% to 38% of TA cases.[18,19]

Approximately 15% of TAs are present at birth, the remaining majority developing within the first 5 years of life,[3,20] though there are reports of TA developing in adulthood.[3,21,22]

Clinically, TA presents as a solitary slow-growing, erythematous to violaceous indurated macule or plaque on the head and neck or upper trunk, often poorly demarcated or with a vascular halo.[3,19,20] A few cases of multifocal or disseminated TA have been reported.[23] Some TAs are associated with hypertrichosis and hyperhidrosis.[3,24,25]

Three clinical patterns of TA have been identified: uncomplicated, complicated by KMP, and complicated by chronic coagulopathy without thrombocytopenia.[19] KMP is characterized by a consumptive coagulopathy of microangiopathic hemolytic anemia, profound thrombocytopenia

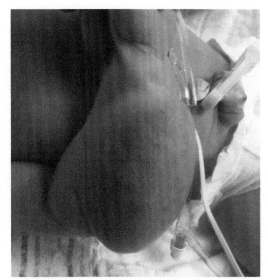

Fig. 2. Large congenital hemangioma causing functional impairment.

with severe hypofibrinogenemia, elevated D-dimer, increased fibrin degradation products and rapidly enlarging vascular tumor.[8,19] Aggressive and prompt treatment is needed. Because of their shared clinicopathologically similar features and association with KMP, some consider TA and KHE to lie on one spectrum.[3,20]

Histologically, TA demonstrates closely packed tufts and lobules of proliferating capillaries in a cannonball distribution within the dermis and subcutis.[3,19,20,26]

IHC of TA reveals positive staining for D2-40, CD31, CD34, WT-1, Prox-1, and LYVE-1,[19,27] of which D2-40, Prox-1, and LYVE-1 are also expressed in KHE.[19]

Somatic activating mutations of GNA14 have been identified in TA associated with KMP,[28] whereas others have found hotspot mutations in NRAS (neuroblastoma RAS viral oncogene homolog).[29] In addition, TA and KHE have been found to share a common methylation pattern, providing further evidence of their spectrum relationship.[29]

Mainstay treatment of TA involves systemic high-dose glucocorticoids. Other attempted treatments include vincristine, interferon, radiation, embolization, oral propranolol, aspirin and sirolimus,[19,22] pulsed-dye laser, intense pulsed light, and surgical excision, though no evidence-based consensus exists.[19,22,30] Some also suggest the use of dermoscopy for close clinical monitoring.[19]

Spindle Cell Hemangioma

Spindle cell hemangiomas (SCHs), formerly known as spindle cell hemangioendotheliomas, were first described in 1986[31] and later renamed to reflect

their benign nature.[32] SCH have an indolent clinical course, yet there is some debate regarding their pathophysiology as a reactive process rather than a true neoplasm.[32] They are currently classified as benign vascular tumors by the ISSVA.[8]

SCH occurs equally in males and females and most commonly affects adolescents and young adults.[32] It presents as a solitary lesion, which usually progresses to form multiple bluish nodules localized to one anatomic region, typically involving the extremities, but can also involve in the head and neck and other locations.[31–35] SCH has been described as both solitary and multifocal lesions, termed spindle cell hemangiomatosis.[36] Multifocal SCH has been associated with Maffucci syndrome, Klippel–Trenaunay syndrome, Ollier disease, Milroy disease, von Willebrand disease, acute myelomonocytic leukemia, early-onset varicose veins, and epithelioid hemangioendothelioma (EHE).[35]

Histologically, SCH is characterized by multiple well-circumscribed, nonencapsulated nodules within the dermis and subcutis and dilated, thin-walled veins sometimes containing thrombi or phleboliths.[32] Fascicles of spindle cells and a second type of round cell in aggregate with vacuolated cytoplasm are also seen.[32]

IHC is positive for CD31, CD34[33] von Willebrand factor (vWF), vimentin,[35] and variably positive for factor VIII, smooth muscle actin, and CD69.[32,35]

Heterozygous mutations in IDH1 and IDH2 have been identified,[37,38] such as somatic mosaic R132 C IDH1 hotspot mutations, among others.[39–41] IDH1 mutations are especially prevalent in association with Maffucci syndrome.[38]

Treatment is simple excision, though local recurrence is common and has been reported in up to 60% of cases. No regional or distant metastases have been reported.[32]

Epithelioid Hemangioma

Epithelioid hemangioma (EH), first recognized in 1969,[42] is classified by the ISSVA as a benign vascular tumor, but is regarded by some as locally aggressive,[8,43,44] and reports of local recurrence and distant metastasis do exist.[45]

EH is better known as angiolymphoid hyperplasia with eosinophilia but may also be referred to as inflammatory angiomatous nodule and histiocytoid hemangioma.[43,46] It is believed to exist on a spectrum of vascular proliferations alongside EHE, epithelioid angiosarcoma, and pseudomyogenic epithelioid sarcoma-like hemangioendothelioma.[47]

EH presents cutaneously as solitary or multiple pink to red-brown papules, nodules, or mass primarily of the head and neck or extremities in young or middle-aged adults, though can form within osseous tissue.[43,48] EH may be asymptomatic or present with pruritis, pain, or bleeding.[48] The pathogenesis of EH is unclear.

Histologically, EH is characterized by proliferations of blood vessels lined by hobnail endothelial cells protruding into vascular lumina and a dense inflammatory infiltrate of lymphocytes, eosinophils, and mast cells, with eosinophilia occurring in 20% of cases.[46]

EH has been associated with TEK gene mutation, TCR rearrangement,[46] and FOS and FOSB gene rearrangements,[49,50] with FOS rearrangements primarily identified in skeletal and soft tissue EH.[49,51]

Surgical treatment options include excision, Mohs micrographic surgery, pulsed dye laser, carbon-dioxide laser or argon laser.[46,48] Medical management options include imiquimod, tacrolimus, isotretinoin, and interferon.[46] Spontaneous resolution has been observed.[48]

Pyogenic Granuloma

Pyogenic granulomas (PGs), also known as lobular capillary hemangiomas (LCHs), are a common acquired benign vascular tumor that is considered a type of inflammatory hyperplasia.[52] PG can develop at any age, though it is unknown whether congenital PGs represent a separate entity.[53]

Clinically, PG presents as an exophytic, red to brown papule on a pedunculated or sessile base which may display overlying ulceration and friability (**Fig. 3**), a collarette of scale, and bleeding spontaneously or with minimal trauma.[3,20,52] PGs are usually less than 2.5 cm in diameter, may develop over weeks to months, and tend not to involute spontaneously.[20,52] They are usually solitary, but may be multiple or disseminated,[53,54] and can be associated with preexisting capillary malformations.[3,55]

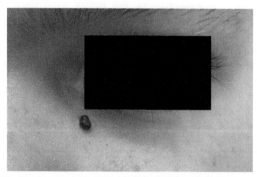

Fig. 3. Pyogenic granuloma occurring on the infraorbital region of a child.

Lesions may occur anywhere but most commonly develop on skin in sites of trauma including the cheek, forehead, hands, or mucous membranes.[3,48,52,56] PGs may be reactive after eczema, infection, insect bite, or burn. They are also found at an increased prevalence during pregnancy or in association with certain medications,[56–58] indicating a multifaceted pathophysiology.

Histologically, PG can be divided into LCH and non-LCH type but generally is characterized as a pedunculated lesion with many small capillaries, composed of bland endothelial cells and filled with red blood cells, in a loose edematous, collagenous matrix, sometimes seen with acute or chronic inflammation.[20]

IHC for PG is positive for CD31, CD34, variably positive for WT-1, and negative for D2-40.[20]

Genetic mutations in PGs are widely believed to upregulate the MAPK/ERK (mitogen-activated protein kinase/extracellular signal regulated kinase) pathway. Somatic activating BRAF (v-raf murine sarcoma viral oncogene homolog B1) and RAS (rat sarcoma) (NRAS, KRAS [Kirsten rat sarcoma viral oncogene homolog], and HRAS [Harvey rat sarcoma viral oncogene homolog]) mutations have been identified in primary PGs. GNAQ mutations are strongly associated with secondary PGs arising from port wine stains.[59,60] GNA11 and GNA14 mutations have demonstrated in vitro upregulation,[60] whereas still other MAPK-activating mechanisms in PGs remain unknown.[61] These mutations are localized to endothelial cells, suggesting some PGs may be benign neoplasms of capillary endothelium or may lie on a spectrum with cherry (senile) angiomas given shared RAS mutations.[59] In addition, paradoxic activation of BRAF has been observed as a side effect of vemurafenib and encorafenib, resulting in PG formation.[62]

Surgical excision with or without electrodessication or curettage of the lesion base is a common treatment as well as removal of traumatic stimulus, use of pulse dye laser, Neodymium-doped Yttrium Aluminum Garnet (Nd:YAG) laser, and continuous-wave/pulsed CO_2 laser.[3,52,63,64] Topical imiquimod, topical or oral beta-blockers, and sodium tetradecyl sulfate sclerotherapy are also options, though lesion recurrence occurs in up to 16% of lesions regardless of method.[52]

Other Benign Vascular Tumors

In addition to the most common benign tumors described above, several rarer benign lesions exist,

Table 1
Differential diagnosis of benign cutaneous vascular lesions

	Hobnail Hemangioma (HH)	Microvenular Hemangioma (MV)	Glomeruloid Hemangioma (GH)	Papillary Hemangioma (PH)	Intravascular Papillary Endothelial Hyperplasia (IPEH)	Cutaneous Epithelioid Angiomatous Nodule (CEAN)	Acquired Elastic Hemangioma (AEH)
General information	Also known as targetoid hemosiderotic hemangioma (THH), primarily cutaneous tumor first described in 1988.[65]	Rare, <100 cases reported in the literature.[66] First described in 1989,[67] name MV coined 2 years later in 1991.[68]	Eruptive cutaneous process strongly associated with systemic conditions. Regarded as a pathopneumonic marker for POEMS syndrome,[69,70] also commonly been reported in TAFRO syndrome,[71,72] Castleman's disease,[70,73] immune thrombocytopenic purpura, and Sjogren's syndrome.[70] One reported case of oral GH unrelated to TAFRO or POEMS.[74]	Very rare, fewer than 20 cases reported in the literature. First described in 2007.[75]	Also known as Masson's tumor. First described in 1923,[76] name IPEH coined in 1976.[77] May be associated with minor trauma or the influence of hormones or growth factor stimulation.[78,79]	Rare, <100 cases described in the literature. First described in 2004.[80] There is debate on whether CEAN represents a distinct entity or a variant of epithelioid hemangioma or pyogenic granuloma.[81,82]	Very rare, <60 cases reported in the literature.[83] First described in 2002.[84] Often mistaken for basal cell carcinoma, squamous cell carcinoma, or other solar damage-associated lesion.[83] May be associated with lichen sclerosis[85] or lichen simplex chronicus.[86,87]
Clinical presentation	Single, soft, compressible reddish to blackish nodule or papule measuring 3–12 mm in diameter,[88] surrounded by an annular, targetoid-appearing, purpuric ring with pale areas.[88,89] Occurs at any age, most commonly second and third decades of life.[90]	Asymptomatic, non-tender, non-blanchable, firm, reddish to violaceous papule, nodule, or plaque.[66] May arise suddenly and exhibit rapid growth before stabilizing.[66] Presentation most common in young to middle-aged adults in the second or third decade of life. Slight female predominance (1.3–1.5:1).[66,91]	Multiple firm, purple-red, papulonodular lesions, ranging from 2 mm to 2 cm in diameter. Sometimes associated with elevated VEGF levels.[70]	Single bluish papule or nodule.[92] Reported in otherwise healthy individuals 2–86 year old, approximately 2:1 male: female predilection.[92,93]	Cutaneous lesions present as asymptomatic, slow-growing, reddish-blue, firm nodules or masses with slight elevation.[94,95]	Rapidly growing, reddish-blue nodule or papule 0.3–1.5 cm in diameter. Typically a single lesion or rarely, multiple lesions.[96,97] Occurs mostly in young adults, no sex predominance.	Elevated erythematous to violaceous angiomatous papule, plaque, or patch with well-demarcated borders.[83,84] Ranging from 4–20 mm in diameter. Typically asymptomatic.[83] Occurs commonly in mid-to-late adulthood, no gender predominance.

(continued on next page)

Table 1
(continued)

	Hobnail Hemangioma (HH)	Microvenular Hemangioma (MV)	Glomeruloid Hemangioma (GH)	Papillary Hemangioma (PH)	Intravascular Papillary Endothelial Hyperplasia (IPEH)	Cutaneous Epithelioid Angiomatous Nodule (CEAN)	Acquired Elastic Hemangioma (AEH)
Anatomic location	Trunk, extremities, head and neck, and less commonly, naso-oral mucous membranes.[98,99] At least one case of orbital HH reported.[100]	Any cutaneous site,[66] most commonly trunk, extremities, and less commonly, head and neck.[66,91]	Trunk and proximal extremities.[101–103]	Head and neck, often involving the face.[92]	Skin and subcutaneous tissues of the trunk, hands, and extremities.[104] May also involve head and neck, favoring the lips, oral mucosa, tongue, gingiva, buccal mucosa, orbit, parotid, masseter, nose, sinus, mandible, pharynx, thyroid, and vocal cords.[94,105,106]	Head and neck, trunk, or extremities.[96,107] Also reported in breast, vulva, penis, and mucosal surfaces.[82,97]	Sun-damaged skin of the forearms, face, legs, or chest.[83,84]
Dermoscopy	Reddish-violaceous or ecchymotic and brownish, with red or dark lacunae. May exhibit vascular structures, delicate pigment network and white structures, including chrysalis.[89]	—	—	—	—	—	Reddish or violaceous appearance with rim of thin, branching vessels at periphery. May be pulsatile.[86] Variable presence of shiny, white structures throughout lesion when viewed under polarized light.[108]
Histology	Non-circumscribed, superficial, ectatic vascular proliferations with intraluminal papillary projections (characteristic "hobnail" morphology), with lesion extension into subcutaneous tissue.[88] Usual stromal hemosiderin	Poorly circumscribed, infiltrative lesion of reticular dermis and subcutaneous tissue. Characterized by central thin-walled, branching vessels, surrounded concentrically by perivascular spindle cells (pericytes).[66,91] Vessels dissect through collagen bundles in the dermis and have sometimes been	Coiled capillary aggregates localized to the dermis, resembling renal glomeruli.[71,72] Appearance comparable to cherry (senile) angiomas, containing multiple branching, randomly arranged vessels lined by flat	Dermal location. Ectatic, branching, papillary, intravascular proliferations which project into the lumen of thin-walled vessels. Endothelial cells contain PAS-positive eosinophilic hyaline	Excessive endothelial proliferation.[76] Three distinct recognized patterns: 1. Arising within the lumen of dilated vessel. 2. Developing within a preexisting vascular lesion such as a hemangioma, PG or arteriovenous malformation. 3. Papillary hyperplasia of an extravascular origin.[94,109,110]	Solid and sheet-like proliferations of large, polygonal epithelioid cells, with similar appearance to EH.[80]	Proliferation of bland-appearing, thin-walled capillaries lined by endothelial cells, arranged in horizontal, band-like pattern parallel to the skin surface. Localized to the upper reticular dermis.[83,86] Intermingled with elastotic fibers, and typically accompanied

	deposition caused by vascular hemorrhage[88] (hence alternative name THH). Biphasic pattern: superficial vessels are dilated; deeper, smaller vessels form slit-like spaces with occasional dissecting collagen fibers.[88] Endothelial cells of superficial portion demonstrate hobnail morphology, whereas deeper endothelial cells are flat.[88]	observed to track along adnexal structures.[91] Presentation and histology can be similar to hobnail hemangioma.[91]	endothelial cells.[101-103] Endothelial and stromal cells contain eosinophilic granules which stain positive for period acid-Schiff (PAS), and kappa and lambda light chains, which are therefore thought to contain immunoglobulins.[71,72,101]	globules.[75,92,93] Numerous pericytes found within the papillary structure as well as a basement membrane-type collagen substance and occasional normal-appearing capillaries.[75,92]	Rarer compared with first two.[94]
					by notable prominence of solar elastosis.[83,84]
Immunohisto-chemistry	Positive for CD31, CD34, von Willebrand factor (VWF), Ki67, BCL-2. Variably positive for CD105 and D2-40 antibodies,[98,111] pericytes variably actin-positive.[112] Endothelial cells negative for GLUT-1, but variably positive for VEGF-3, creating some debate over HHs vascular vs lymphatic origin.[111,112]	Positive for CD31, CD34, SMA,[91,113] WT-1,[91] and more recently, one case of progesterone receptor positivity described, suggesting possible hormonal influence for development of MH.[66] Usually negative for GLUT-1 and D2-40.[91,113]	—	Endothelial lining of papillary projections positive for CD31, CD34 and ERG (ETS-related gene). Intermingled pericytes positive for α-SMA (alpha-smooth muscle actin).[92]	Positive for CD31, CD34. Variably positive for D2-40.[86]

(continued on next page)

Table 1
(continued)

	Hobnail Hemangioma (HH)	Microvenular Hemangioma (MV)	Glomeruloid Hemangioma (GH)	Papillary Hemangioma (PH)	Intravascular Papillary Endothelial Hyperplasia (IPEH)	Cutaneous Epithelioid Angiomatous Nodule (CEAN)	Acquired Elastic Hemangioma (AEH)
Treatment	Simple excision.	Simple excision.[66]	Correct underlying disorder.	Simple excision.[93]	Complete surgical excision.[106]	Simple excision.[96]	Excision, historically (before benign nature established). Currently, usually observation, dual-wavelength laser, pulsed dye laser, or Nd:YAG laser.[83]
Prognosis	No reports of invasion, dissemination, or post-excision recurrence.[111,114] Important to differentiate from more worrisome lesions such as Kaposi sarcoma (KS)[65,98] and well-differentiated angiosarcoma.[88]	No reports of post-excision recurrence.[66] Important to differentiate from KS and angiosarcoma. Unlike KS, MH is HHV-8 negative. Unlike MH, angiosarcoma exhibits cytologic atypia and absence of a pericyte layer.	Almost always associated with systemic illness or manifestations, requiring further care.	One reported case of post-excision local recurrence.[75,93] PH can closely resemble GH; important to differentiate. PH is an exclusively cutaneous process, in contrast systemic illness-associated GH.	Very low post-excision recurrence rate.[95,115]	No reports of dissemination or post-excision recurrence.[96]	No reports of invasion, dissemination, or post-excision recurrence.[83]

which may be cutaneous or non-cutaneous. **Table 1** contains the differential diagnosis of a benign cutaneous vascular tumor, describing seven benign cutaneous tumor types not already discussed.

Related Lesions

Eccrine angiomatous hamartoma

Eccrine angiomatous hamartoma (EAH) is a rare cutaneous tumor characterized by flesh-colored, blue-brown or reddish nodules, plaques or macules which are frequently solitary, but may be multiple, and appear most commonly on the extremities, especially the lower or distal extremities.[116,117] EAH may present with associated hyperhidrosis, hypertrichosis, or pain.[116–118] EAH is often congenital or presents in childhood but rarely may appear in adulthood.[117,118] Histologically, EAH is characterized by vascular proliferation of the dermal capillaries with well-differentiated eccrine secretor and ductal elements.[116,118] Excision is curative and can be considered for symptomatic lesions.[116,118,119]

Reactive angioendotheliomatosis

Reactive angioendotheliomatosis (RAE) is an extremely rare entity first characterized in 1958,[120] though it is currently classified within the broader category of cutaneous reactive angiomatosis.[121]

RAE is characterized by multiple red to blue, variably sized patches, nodules, and indurated plaques with focal purpura, typically distributed over the trunk, limbs, face, or earlobes.[120,122] Ulceration or blisters may develop.[122] RAE can occur at any age, with no predilection for gender.[122]

Histology is characterized by intravascular proliferation of endothelial and myoepithelial cells, which can fill vascular lumens in the papillary and reticular dermis, causing luminal occlusion and variably, intraluminal fibrin thrombi, which can cause secondary necrosis and infarction of the surrounding skin.[122]

This vascular proliferation often occurs in the setting of other systemic disorders such as subacute bacterial endocarditis, tuberculosis, and antiphospholipid syndrome and has been suggested to represent a hypersensitivity reaction.[121,123] RAE may also be associated with elevated erythrocyte sedimentation rate.[122]

Treatment should address the underlying systemic cause, but recently, pulsed dye laser, topical timolol, and lenalidomide have been used with variable success on RAE lesions.[121,124,125]

Bacillary angiomatosis

Bacillary angiomatosis (BA) is a systemic disease caused by *Bartonella henselae* or *Bartonella quintana* infection, which is also the pathogenic organism associated with cat-scratch disease. BA was first identified in the setting of AIDS with very low CD4 count. Today, BA is typically regarded as an opportunistic infection of immunocompromised individuals, including solid organ transplant recipients.[126,127]

BA classically presents with cutaneous vascular proliferations characterized by single or multiple erythematous to violaceous skin papules or nodules, ranging from 1 to 10 cm in diameter, which are firm, rubbery, and freely-mobile on examination.[126,128] Lesions are usually painful, bleed easily with minor trauma, and may ulcerate.[128] BA may additionally involve the mucous membranes.[126] Systemic symptoms include fever, fatigue, myalgia, night sweats, splenomegaly, and lymphadenopathy and have been reported with associated hemophagocytic lymphohistiocytosis.[129]

Histology is generally characterized by ectatic, lobular proliferation of capillaries, neutrophilic infiltration and interstitial bacillary deposition.[127,128] BA further involves four recognized distinct histologic patterns, two of which share resemblance with PG and Kaposi sarcoma (KS).

Treatment includes macrolides, doxycycline, or quinolones.[129]

LOCALLY AGGRESSIVE OR BORDERLINE VASCULAR TUMORS
Kaposiform Hemangioendothelioma

KHEs are rare vascular neoplasms that present in infancy or early childhood; they are classified as locally aggressive or borderline vascular tumors.[8] KHE was first differentiated from IH in 1993 based on its "focal Kaposi-like" appearance and aggressive course[130] and is characterized by progressive angiogenesis and lymphangiogenesis.[131]

It is generally accepted that KHE lies on a spectrum with TAs, given their similar clinicopathology and association with KMP. Some even argue a relationship between KHE and kaposiform lymphangiomatosis for similar reasons.[29,131]

Ninety percent of KHE develop within the first year of life, and 50% of cutaneous KHE are present at birth, though true incidence and prevalence are unknown.[131]

Clinical presentation of KHE is highly variable but most commonly presents as a soft tissue mass with a cutaneous appearance of an erythematous papule, nodule, or plaque to a firm, indurated, violaceous plaque or tumor (**Fig. 4**).[3,131] Lesions often rapidly enlarge, but a small subset of KHEs remain stable.[131] When KMP occurs, KHE lesions are painful, purpuric, swollen, and warm. KHE with KMP can exhibit progressive

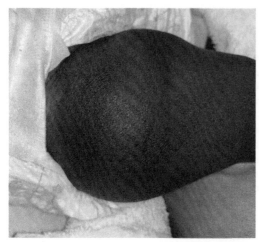

Fig. 4. Intraarticular kaposiform hemangioendothelioma of the knee of an infant.

enlargement, purpura, pain, and hemorrhage. KHE may occur in the retroperitoneum as well as visceral locations, and 12% of cases lack cutaneous involvement.[131]

KMP complicates 42% to 71% of KHEs; these cases have a propensity to occur in large congenital lesions located in the retroperitoneum or intrathoracic region.[3,132,133]

Poor prognosis is associated with local invasion, visceral disease, compression of vital structures such as the trachea and life-threatening KMP, characterized by a profound consumptive coagulopathy and discussed further in the section of TAs.[3,131]

The diagnosis of KHE is difficult, especially when visceral organs or deep soft tissues are involved. Imaging may be helpful, including ultrasound (US) for small, superficial KHE, and MRI with and without contrast for deep or infiltrating lesions. Biopsy is confirmatory[131] but may be contraindicated in the setting of KMP.

Histologically, KHE share features with TA but are distinguished by their Kaposi's sarcoma-like architecture and lymphangiomatosis. Lesions are marked by rounded but irregular, confluent, and infiltrating nodules of spindle-shaped endothelial cells, aligned in abnormal lymphatic and slit-like vascular channels,[131] surrounded by desmoplastic stroma.[29] Platelet thrombi, eosinophilic hyaline granules, and hemosiderin deposition can also be observed.[131]

IHC is positive for vascular endothelial markers CD31 and CD34, and lymphatic endothelial markers VEGFR-2 (vascular endothelial growth factor receptor 2), D2-40, Prox-1, and lymphatic endothelial hyaluronan receptor 1 and negative for Glut-1 and HHV-8.[131]

Genetically, somatic activating GNA14 mutations have been found in KHE and TA,[28] whereas chromosome 13,16 translocation has also been identified.[131,134] One case of RAD50 mutation in KHE has been reported.[29]

Treatment of both KHE and TA is difficult, but management is primarily medical. Historically, interventions have included systemic corticosteroids, cyclophosphamide, vincristine, and oral sirolimus, though these were based on expert opinion and case reports.[135]

Vincristine has been proven effective in steroid-resistant KHE with KMP.[136] Recently, one prospective randomized control trial of KHE and TA associated with KMP found IV vincristine to be superior to IV methylprednisolone for improvement of thrombocytopenia and tumor texture, but overall effectiveness was not significantly different.[137]

In a retrospective study assessing the use of oral sirolimus for treatment of KHE, sirolimus demonstrated significant reduction in tumor size and platelet count normalization with only one possible case of severe side effect when evaluated with long-term follow-up.[138] In a more recent randomized control trial of KHE associated with KMP, prednisolone plus oral sirolimus showed a significant clinical improvement and reduction in mortality compared with prednisolone alone, with significantly lower disease sequelae at 24-month follow-up in the prednisolone plus sirolimus group.[135]

Propranolol, interferon-α, and ticlopidine have been used with variable results and are not recommended as monotherapy[131,134,135,138] Medical management of KHE predominates, but surgery may be considered in small, localized cases, and for resection of fibrofatty residue or adjacent damaged tissue.[131] Supportive treatment of KMP, such as cryoprecipitate, is necessary, and KHE with KMP should be managed by a multidisciplinary care team.

Retiform Hemangioendothelioma

Retiform hemangioendothelioma (RA), first described in 1994,[139] is classified as an intermediate vascular neoplasm which rarely metastasizes.[8]

Clinically, RA presents in the skin or subcutaneous tissues of the lower extremities, or less commonly, head and neck, trunk, penis, vulva,[140] pleura, or mandible,[141] and may occur at any age, but is more common in children and young adults.[142] Local recurrence is common (up to 60%), whereas distant metastasis is rare and has been reported in the lymph nodes and liver.[142]

Cutaneous RA lesions may appear as firm, indurated plaques.[142] RA may be asymptomatic or present with symptoms related to tumor location, such as cough and shortness of breath with mediastinal involvement,[142] and may be visualized on computed tomography (CT) or magnetic resonance imaging (MRI).

RA may occur in association with complex vascular lesions and maybe found alongside composite hemangioendotheliomas (CHEs) or papillary intralymphatic angioendothelioma (PILA), the latter of which may sometimes be indistinguishable from RA.[142] PILA, and relevant differences, will be discussed later in this article.

Histologically, RA is composed of vascular structures with an appearance similar to the rete testis, for which RA is named.[142] The anastomosing vessels are composed of single-layer endothelial cells with hobnail morphology, are variably dilated, and may show intraluminal papillary projections with fibrovascular cores. Nuclear atypia is absent. Mild stromal lymphocytic infiltrate or aggregates are possible.[142] The absence of eosinophils is helpful for differentiating RA from EH.[142]

IHC staining is positive for CD31, CD34, ERG, and claudin-5 and negative for D2-40 and HHV-8.[142]

YAP1 gene rearrangements and YAP1-MAML2 gene fusion have been documented in RA as well as CHE, providing evidence that they lie on a spectrum with each other.[143]

Simple surgical resection or in cutaneous RA, Mohs micrographic surgery,[144] is commonly used.[142] Multifocal and unresectable RA has been treated with chemotherapy and radiation.[145]

Papillary Intralymphatic Angioendotheliomas/Dabska Tumor

PILA, also known as endovascular papillary angioendothelioma or Dabska tumor, was first described in 1969[146] and renamed to PILA in 1999.[147]

PILA is a rare vascular tumor most commonly found in children but can occur at any age.[148] Its original description reported lymph node and lung metastasis, but subsequent cases have demonstrated less aggressive behavior.[147] Lesions may be asymptomatic or present with pain, ulceration, or bleeding.[148] No anatomic or sex predilection is known.

Clinically variable, PILA presents as a slow-growing, erythematous to violaceous or bluish nodule, plaque, or poorly defined mass with palpable projections and atrophic dermis.[3,148]

Histologically, PILA is characterized by intravascular proliferations of hobnail endothelial cells forming papillary intraluminal projections, with intravascular or perivascular lymphocytic inflammatory infiltrate.[3,148]

IHC is positive for CD31, CD34, vimentin, VEGF3, and factor VIII-related antigen, and D2-40, suggesting a lymphatic origin of PILA as opposed to hemangioma.[149]

Treatment of these lesions is surgical excision with wide margins and close follow-up, given the potential for metastasis.[148] Given the rarity of this tumor, no treatment has been developed for unresectable or multifocal disease.

Other Hemangioendotheliomas

In recent decades, several new types of hemangioendothelioma, all classified as borderline or locally aggressive,[8] have been identified and described (**Table 2**). These include CHE,[150] pseudomyogenic hemangioendothelioma,[151] and polymorphous hemangioendothelioma (PHE).[152] These entities were previously categorized as hemangioendothelioma, not otherwise classified,[8] and remain extremely rare, with a relative paucity of literature. It is, however, of utmost importance to differentiate these lesions from other borderline and malignant mimickers and other benign tumors whenever possible due to potential differences in prognosis and treatment.

Kaposi Sarcoma

KS, first described in 1872,[162] is classified as an angioproliferative neoplasm caused by human herpes virus 8 (HHV8) infection, though there is some debate whether KS instead represents a reactive process.[163,164]

Four epidemiologic subtypes exist: classic, African endemic, immunosuppression-related, and AIDS (aquired immuno-deficiency syndrome)-related.[165]

Classic KS is indolent and seen in the lower extremities in men of Mediterranean, eastern European, or Middle Eastern descent.[166] African endemic KS is more aggressive and seen in human immunodeficiency virus (HIV)-negative individuals in sub-Saharan Africa.[167] Immunosuppression-related KS occurs in individuals who are immunosuppressed for reasons other than HIV/AIDS, most commonly recipients of solid organ[168] or stem cell transplant,[169] but also in those receiving corticosteroids and biologic therapy.[165,170] AIDS-related KS typically occurs in HIV-infected men with AIDS and very low CD4 counts, though can occur with nondetectable HIV viral load and normal CD4 count.[171] A fifth,

Table 2
Other hemangioendotheliomas

	Composite Hemangioendothelioma (CHE)	Pseudomyogenic Hemangioendothelioma	Polymorphous Hemangioendothelioma (PHE)
General information	First described in 2000.[150] May be cutaneous or non-cutaneous.	First described in 2011.[63] Also known as epithelioid sarcoma-like hemangioendothelioma.[32]	First described in 1992[152] rare primary, "nodal" neoplasm.
Clinical presentation	Single or multiple erythematous to violaceous papules or nodules.[150,153] May be asymptomatic or present with symptoms related to tumor location such as abdominal distension or back pain.[153] Female > male predominance.[153]	Grouped nodules, may be painful or asymptomatic[3,32] Commonly occurs between second and fifth decades of life.[32] Male predominance.[32]	Frequently indolent. May be asymptomatic or present with symptoms related to tumor location such as pain, mass effect, elevated liver enzymes, and so forth. Occurs primarily in adults[154], at least one reported pediatric case in the setting of immunosuppression.[155]
Anatomic location	Extremities, head and neck, liver, spleen, kidney.[153]	Lower extremities; less commonly, upper extremities, trunk, or head.[3,32]	Primarily lymph nodes. Extranodal locations include liver, paravertebral soft tissue, mediastinum, thoracic spinal cord, and neck.[154]
Histology	Spectrum of vascular components, often with a retiform morphology similar to rete testis, with infiltrative margins.[150,156]	Infiltrative, poorly circumscribed malignant-appearing architecture composed of sheets and cords of spindled cells with eosinophilic cytoplasm.[3,32] Lesions have a fascicular pattern, myxoid stroma, and scattered neutrophils. May involve subcutaneous tissue or skeletal muscle.[32]	Solid, primitive vascular and angiomatous components. Mimics angiosarcoma, but lacks nuclear atypia, infiltrative growth, frequent mitoses, vascular invasion, or necrosis.[152,154]

Imaging (if applicable)	US, CT, MRI for non-cutaneous CHE[150]; lacks specificity.	—	CT, MRI.
Immunohistochemistry	Positive for CD31, CD34, factor VIII, FLI-1, ERG. Variably positive for Ki67[153]	Positive for AE1, AE3, FL1, CD31, CAM 5.2, SMA, EMA, and pancytokeratin MNF-116. Negative for CD34, desmin and S-100 protein.[32]	Positive for CD31 and factor VIII. Variably positive for CD34. May mimic Kaposi sarcoma, but negative for HHV-8.[154]
Genetics	—	Chromosome 7,19 translocation.[157] Gene fusion between FOSB and SERPINE1, ACTB, or WWTR1, resulting in overexpression of FOSB.[158]	
Treatment	Options include surgical excision, limb amputation, chemotherapy, or radiation (Li).[153] Interferon (IFN)-α2b and thalidomide use have been reported.[153,159]	Simple excision with or without radiotherapy is treatment of choice; difficult in multifocal or metastatic disease.[32] Medical management options include gemcitabine, sirolimus, and everolimus.[3]	Radical or aggressive surgical excision is considered to prevent local recurrence.[154,160]
Prognosis	Local recurrence is common. Metastasis is rare and most common to the liver.[150]	Post-excision recurrence is common (>50%).[32]	Clinical behavior not fully characterized due to few cases of PHE recognized in the literature. Local recurrence in lymph nodes and surrounding soft tissue possible. Metastasis to the lungs causing death has been reported.[154,160,161]

"nonepidemic KS" has been reported and resembles classic KS at a younger age, with exclusive cutaneous involvement and good prognosis.[172]

HHV8 exists in a latent and lytic phase, with KS occurring in the lytic phase. Contributing factors for phase transformation include hypoxia, oxidative stress, viral coinfection, epigenetic modification, immune suppression, and hyperglycemia.[173,174]

KS increases risk for solid-organ malignancy, Hodgkin lymphoma, and acute lymphocytic lymphoma.[175]

Clinically, KS is variable and may present as multifocal, scattered pink to purple papules and patches, or as rapidly progressive, ulcerated nodules, and plaques and may disseminate to the visceral organs.[165] Visceral involvement is more common in AIDS-related KS, and oral mucosal KS in this setting portends a poor prognosis.[165,176] Pediatric KS is associated with lymph node involvement, rare cutaneous lesions, fulminant progression, cytopenias, and normal CD4 count.[177]

KS histology evolves with lesion progression. In patch stage, KS is characterized by perivascular dermal and lymphocytic infiltrate.[165] Patch and plaque stage is characterized by the promontory sign, proliferation of dilated, thin-walled vessels lined by endothelial cells with bland endothelial cells, forming around preexisting normal vessels so that the normal vessels seem to protrude into the neoplastic channels.[163,178] In plaque stage, spindle cell proliferations appear in the dermis.[165] Nodular KS lesions exhibit dermal proliferations of spindle cells and slit-like vessels.[165]

IHC staining is positive for HHV8 latent nuclear antigen-1,[165,179] and it is uncertain whether KS has a vascular, lymphatic, or combined origin.

Treatment of KS depends on epidemiologic subtype, tumor size, location, and immune status. Restoration to immunocompetency is ideal, but not always possible and irrelevant in KS unaccompanied by immunosuppression.[180] Local treatment, when appropriate, includes surgical excision, cryotherapy, radiotherapy, intralesional chemotherapy, and alitretinoin gel.[165,180]

Systemic treatment includes single-agent cytotoxic chemotherapy, immunotherapy with IFN-α, anti-PD1 immune checkpoint inhibitors, antiretroviral therapy (in AIDS-related KS), trans-retinoic acid,[165,180] and numerous others.

MALIGNANT VASCULAR TUMORS
Angiosarcoma

Angiosarcoma, a subtype of soft tissue sarcoma, is an uncommon, highly aggressive vascular tumor of endothelial origin which commonly occurs in the skin and soft tissue of the head and neck but can affect any visceral organ.[3,181] Angiosarcomas can be divided into the following subtypes: cutaneous angiosarcoma, lymphoedema-associated angiosarcoma, radiation-induced angiosarcoma, primary breast angiosarcoma, and soft-tissue angiosarcoma.[181]

Angiosarcoma occurs equally in both sexes and can occur at any age, though more commonly in older adults. They are rarely reported in children and account for 0.3% of pediatric sarcomas.[3,182] Cutaneous angiosarcoma mostly commonly occurs in elderly white men.[181,183,184]

Most angiosarcomas develop spontaneously,[181] though known risk factors for developing angiosarcoma include long-standing lymphedema, chronic infections, various toxin exposures including vinyl chloride, prior radiation (with a peak incidence of 5–10 years post-radiation),[185] and inherited familial syndromes including Neurofibromatosis Type I, Klippel–Trenaunay syndrome, and Maffucci syndrome,[3,181,182] and there are reports of angiosarcoma occurring via transformation of preexisting benign vascular lesions.[181]

Angiosarcomas are aggressive and portent a poor prognosis. They most often metastasize hematogenously to the lungs.[3,181] Five-year survival is 35%.[181]

Clinically, angiosarcoma can present as an expanding bruise-like lesion or as an erythematous to violaceous papule, nodule, or plaque, which is commonly multifocal and which may develop rapid growth, infiltration, fungation, ulceration, and hemorrhage (Fig. 5).[3,181] Visceral and deep soft tissue angiosarcomas often present as an expanding mass with or without associated pain.[3,181]

Angiosarcoma has a variable histologic appearance and can be difficult to distinguish from benign or inflammatory lesions on light microscopy.[181,186] Pleomorphic malignant cells may be polygonal, rounded, fusiform, or epithelioid in morphology.[181]

The well-differentiated, low-grade angiosarcomas or tumor portions contain abnormal endothelial cells organized into sinusoids which anastomose with surrounding normal vasculature, with low-grade cytology.[186] These sinusoids can be seen to dissect collagen bundles and may display associated monocytic infiltration.[181] The less well-differentiated areas display abnormal endothelial cell architecture, organized into multilayered papillary structures which may project into the vascular lumen.[181] The poorly differentiated, high-grade areas display sheets of abnormal endothelial cells, hemorrhage, and necrosis with a high mitotic rate.[181]

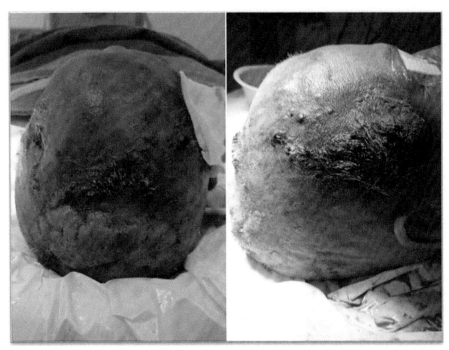

Fig. 5. Angiosarcoma on the scalp of an adult man. (*From* Oley MC, Oley MH, Durry MF, Kepel REM, Faruk M. Cutaneous angiosarcoma: A case report. Int J Surg Case Rep. 2021 Nov;88:106506.)

IHC is typically positive for the endothelial markers CD31, CD34, Ulex europaeus agglutinin I, vWF, and VEGF.[181]

Angiosarcoma demonstrates a wide variety of associated molecular and genetic irregularities, though the causality of these remains unclear. Some case reports have noted a role of BRCA1 and BRCA2 mutations in predisposing affected patients to angiosarcoma following breast cancer treatment.[187] Other mutations include TP53, overexpression of Wilms' tumor-1 and galectin-3, HRAS activation, KRAS mutations, upregulation of KIT (KIT Proto-Oncogene, Receptor Tyrosine Kinase), RET (Ret Proto-Oncogene), and numerous others.[181,188] More recently, amplification and overexpression of MYC on chromosome 8 has been recognized in cutaneous, breast, and postradiation sarcoma.[189–192]

Evidence-based treatment recommendations for angiosarcoma are lacking, and recurrence is common.[181] Localized disease is managed with complete surgical resection with wide margins and adjuvant radiation.[193] Metastatic disease is considered incurable but may be treated with multi-agent cytotoxic chemotherapy.[3,193] Other current and emerging therapies may include immunotherapy, VEGF-A monoclonal antibodies, tyrosine kinase inhibitors, and propranolol.[3,193]

Epithelioid Hemangioendothelioma

EHE, first described in 1975[194] and coined in 1982,[195] is a very rare vascular tumor of intermediate malignancy that has overlapping features of epithelioid angiosarcoma and EH and may undergo high-grade malignant transformation.[3,196] EHE may present at any age, but most often occurs in middle age, and exhibits a sex ratio of 4:1 female: male.[3,196]

Clinically, EHE has a variable presentation and has been reported to affect a variety of tissues including liver, lung, and bone.[3,196,197] EHE may be asymptomatic and is commonly found incidentally on imaging,[196] though imaging findings are similarly variable and lack specificity.[198]

Symptomatic patients may experience weight loss, fatigue, fever, chest pain, hemoptysis, and pleural effusion and anemia.[194,196,199,200] Metastases have an affinity for cortical bone and can cause pathologic fractures or spinal cord compression.[196]

Prognosis is variable depending on tumor behavior, with 5-year survival rates ranging from 49% to 100%.[197] Indolent tumor behavior portends better prognosis, whereas poorer outcomes are associated with lung primary, systemic symptoms, metastases at time of diagnosis, and increased mitoses on pathology.[3,196,197,200,201]

EHE arises from endothelial or pre-endothelial cells and histologically demonstrates endothelial cells arranged in nests or cords, with possible arrangement into vascular channels.[196] Tumors are characterized by pleomorphic nuclei, desmoplastic reaction, and the presence of spindle-shaped or signet-ring appearing cells.[196,202] Compared with epithelioid angiosarcoma, EHE demonstrates intranuclear inclusion, intracytoplasmic vacuoles, and stromal change.[196,202]

Management of EHE is variable given limited data and the rarity of this tumor. Treatment options may include chemotherapeutic agents, immunotherapy, and targeted therapies such as mTOR inhibitor sirolimus, tyrosine kinase inhibitor apatinib targeting VEGFR-2, and immune checkpoint blockade with anti-PD1 antibodies.[3,196,203,204] Surgical resection may be performed for localized disease, and watchful waiting can be considered for asymptomatic disease due to reports of spontaneous regression.[3,200] Successful liver transplant has been reported for liver primary EHE.[3,205]

IHC is positive for CD31, CD34, and friend leukemia integration 1 transcription factor (FLI-1).[194,196]

Genetically, EHE demonstrates a chromosome 1,3 translocation with resulting WWTR1-CAMTA1 fusion protein in 90% of cases.[3,206] A YAP1-TEF3 fusion protein has also been discovered in both WWTR1-CAMTA1 positive and negative tumors.[51,197,206,207] Paired clinical characteristics, some now define two clinical EHE subgroups: TFE3-positive and TFE3-negative.[207]

CLINICS CARE POINTS

- Pyogenic granulomas (PGs) are painless, fleshy nodule often with rapid growth over the course of weeks.

- PGs may be medication-related.

- If pregnancy-related, they may spontaneously regress.

- Treatment warranted for ulceration, bleeding, cosmetic concern, or functional impairment.

- Always counsel about risk of recurrence.

- For cosmetically sensitive areas, consider shave excision or curettage and electrodesiccation, but in the case of recurrent PGs, treatment may be multimodal.

DISCLOSURE

The authors have nothing to disclose.

REFERENCES

1. North PE, Waner M, James CA, et al. Congenital nonprogressive hemangioma: a distinct clinico-pathologic entity unlike infantile hemangioma. Arch Dermatol 2001;137(12):1607–20.
2. Browning JC, Metry DW. Rapidly involuting congenital hemangioma: case report and review of the literature. Dermatol Online J 2008;14(4):11.
3. Hinen HB, Trenor CC 3rd, Wine Lee L. Childhood Vascular Tumors. Front Pediatr 2020;8:573023.
4. Matarneh B, Lillis AP, Fernandez Faith E. Early postnatal proliferation of rapidly involuting congenital hemangioma. Pediatr Dermatol 2022;39(1):137–8.
5. Berenguer B, Mulliken JB, Enjolras O, et al. Rapidly involuting congenital hemangioma: clinical and histopathologic features. Pediatr Dev Pathol 2003;6(6):495–510.
6. Nasseri E, Piram M, McCuaig CC, et al. Partially involuting congenital hemangiomas: a report of 8 cases and review of the literature. J Am Acad Dermatol 2014;70(1):75–9.
7. Krol A, MacArthur CJ. Congenital hemangiomas: rapidly involuting and noninvoluting congenital hemangiomas. Arch Facial Plast Surg 2005;7(5):307–11.
8. Anomalies ISftSoV. ISSVA Classification of Vascular Anomalies. International society for the study of vascular Anomalies. 2022. Available at: issva.org/classification.
9. Cossio ML, Dubois J, McCuaig CC, et al. Non-involuting congenital hemangiomas (NICH) with postnatal atypical growth: A case series. Pediatr Dermatol 2019;36(4):466–70.
10. Hua C, Wang L, Jin Y, et al. A case series of tardive expansion congenital hemangioma: A variation of noninvoluting congenital hemangioma or a new hemangiomatous entity? J Am Acad Dermatol 2021;84(5):1371–7.
11. Lewis D, Vaidya R. Hepatic Hemangioma. 2022 Jun 21. In: StatPearls [Internet]. Treasure Island (FL): StatPearls Publishing; 2022 Jan–. PMID: 30085530.
12. Gasparella P, Singer G, Arneitz C, et al. Rapidly involuting congenital hemangioma of the liver in a newborn with incomplete Pentalogy of Cantrell: description of a new association. J Surg Case Rep 2021;2021(3):rjab047.
13. Mulliken JB, Bischoff J, Kozakewich HP. Multifocal rapidly involuting congenital hemangioma: a link to chorangioma. Am J Med Genet A 2007;143A(24):3038–46.

14. Funk T, Lim Y, Kulungowski AM, et al. Symptomatic Congenital Hemangioma and Congenital Hemangiomatosis Associated With a Somatic Activating Mutation in GNA11. JAMA Dermatol 2016;152(9):1015–20.

15. Ayturk UM, Couto JA, Hann S, et al. Somatic Activating Mutations in GNAQ and GNA11 Are Associated with Congenital Hemangioma. Am J Hum Genet 2016;98(4):789–95.

16. Fomchenko EI, Duran D, Jin SC, et al. De novo MYH9 mutation in congenital scalp hemangioma. Cold Spring Harb Mol Case Stud 2018;4(4).

17. Liang MG, Frieden IJ. Infantile and congenital hemangiomas. Semin Pediatr Surg 2014;23(4):162–7.

18. Osio A, Fraitag S, Hadj-Rabia S, et al. Clinical spectrum of tufted angiomas in childhood: a report of 13 cases and a review of the literature. Arch Dermatol 2010;146(7):758–63.

19. Mehrotra K, Khunger N, Sharma S, et al. Tufted angioma with coagulopathy: a dermoscopic evaluation and successful treatment. Int J Dermatol 2021;60(9):e379–81.

20. Johnson EF, Davis DM, Tollefson MM, et al. Vascular Tumors in Infants: Case Report and Review of Clinical, Histopathologic, and Immunohistochemical Characteristics of Infantile Hemangioma, Pyogenic Granuloma, Noninvoluting Congenital Hemangioma, Tufted Angioma, and Kaposiform Hemangioendothelioma. Am J Dermatopathol 2018;40(4):231–9.

21. Sabharwal A, Aguirre A, Zahid TM, et al. Acquired tufted angioma of upper lip: case report and review of the literature. Head Neck Pathol 2013;7(3):291–4.

22. Fabbri N, Quarantotto F, Caruso A, et al. Surgical excision of a tufted angioma of the hand in an adult-a rare case report with a review of literature. AME Case Rep 2019;3:7.

23. Wang L, Liu L, Wang G, et al. Congenital disseminated tufted angioma. J Cutan Pathol 2013;40(4):405–8.

24. Saito Y, Shimomura Y, Abe R. Tufted angioma associated with hyperplasia of eccrine sweat glands. Clin Exp Dermatol 2017;42(5):548–50.

25. Jakhar D, Singal A, Kaur I, et al. Indurated Dusky Red Swelling on the Forearm of an Infant: Tufted Angioma. Indian J Dermatol 2019;64(2):146–8.

26. Herron MD, Coffin CM, Vanderhooft SL. Tufted angiomas: variability of the clinical morphology. Pediatr Dermatol 2002;19(5):394–401.

27. Su X, Liu Y, Liu Y, et al. A retrospective study: Clinicopathological and immunohistochemical analysis of 54 cases of tufted angioma. Indian J Dermatol Venereol Leprol 2020;86(1):24–32.

28. Lim YH, Bacchiocchi A, Qiu J, et al. GNA14 Somatic Mutation Causes Congenital and Sporadic Vascular Tumors by MAPK Activation. Am J Hum Genet 2016;99(2):443–50.

29. Ten Broek RW, Koelsche C, Eijkelenboom A, et al. Kaposiform hemangioendothelioma and tufted angioma - (epi)genetic analysis including genome-wide methylation profiling. Ann Diagn Pathol 2020;44:151434.

30. Javvaji S, Frieden IJ. Response of tufted angiomas to low-dose aspirin. Pediatr Dermatol 2013;30(1):124–7.

31. Weiss SW, Enzinger FM. Spindle cell hemangioendothelioma. A low-grade angiosarcoma resembling a cavernous hemangioma and Kaposi's sarcoma. Am J Surg Pathol 1986;10(8):521–30.

32. Requena L, Kutzner H. Hemangioendothelioma Semin Diagn Pathol 2013;30(1):29–44.

33. Oukessou Y, Lyoubi M, Hammouda Y, et al. Spindle cell hemangioma in the infratemporal fossa: A unique case report. Int J Surg Case Rep 2021;78:38–41.

34. Degala SMK, Hiriyanna N. Spindle cell haemangioma in head and neck: Report of an uncommon vascular lesion and review of treatment modalities till present. Case Study. Oral Maxillofacial Surg Cases 2020;6(2):100149.

35. Tosios KI, Gouveris I, Sklavounou A, et al. Spindle cell hemangioma (hemangioendothelioma) of the head and neck: case report of an unusual (or underdiagnosed) tumor. Oral Surg Oral Med Oral Pathol Oral Radiol Endod 2008;105(2):216–21.

36. Perkins P, Weiss SW. Spindle cell hemangioendothelioma. An analysis of 78 cases with reassessment of its pathogenesis and biologic behavior. Am J Surg Pathol 1996;20(10):1196–204.

37. Ten Broek RW, Bekers EM, de Leng WWJ, et al. Mutational analysis using Sanger and next generation sequencing in sporadic spindle cell hemangiomas: A study of 19 cases. Genes Chromosomes Cancer 2017;56(12):855–60.

38. Pansuriya TC, van Eijk R, d'Adamo P, et al. Somatic mosaic IDH1 and IDH2 mutations are associated with enchondroma and spindle cell hemangioma in Ollier disease and Maffucci syndrome. Nat Genet 2011;43(12):1256–61.

39. Kurek KC, Pansuriya TC, van Ruler MA, et al. R132C IDH1 mutations are found in spindle cell hemangiomas and not in other vascular tumors or malformations. Am J Pathol 2013;182(5):1494–500.

40. Brown NJ, Ye Z, Stutterd C, et al. Somatic IDH1 variant (p.R132C) in an adult male with Maffucci syndrome. Cold Spring Harb Mol Case Stud 2021;7(6).

41. Sun Y, Fan X, Rao Y, et al. Cell-free DNA from plasma as a promising alternative for detection of gene mutations in patients with Maffucci syndrome. Hereditas 2022;159(1):4.

42. Wells GC, Whimster IW. Subcutaneous angiolymphoid hyperplasia with eosinophilia. Br J Dermatol 1969;81(1):1–14.

43. Okada EMD, Matsumoto MMD, Nishida M, et al. Epithelioid Hemangioma of the Thoracic Spine: A Case Report and Review of the Literature. J Spinal Cord Med 2019;42(6):800–5.

44. Goldblum JR, Weiss S, Folpe AL. Benign vascular tumors. In: Goldblum JR, Weiss S, Folpe AL, editors. Enzinger and Weiss'ssoft tissue tumors. 6th edition. Philadelphia, PA, USA: Elsevier Saunders; 2014. p. 639–80. chap Benign vascular tumors.

45. Nielsen GP, Srivastava A, Kattapuram S, et al. Epithelioid hemangioma of bone revisited: a study of 50 cases. Am J Surg Pathol 2009;33(2):270–7.

46. Guo R, Gavino AC. Angiolymphoid hyperplasia with eosinophilia. Arch Pathol Lab Med 2015; 139(5):683–6.

47. Llamas-Velasco M, Kempf W, Cota C, et al. Multiple Eruptive Epithelioid Hemangiomas: A Subset of Cutaneous Cellular Epithelioid Hemangioma With Expression of FOS-B. Am J Surg Pathol 2019; 43(1):26–34.

48. Adler BL, Krausz AE, Minuti A, et al. Epidemiology and treatment of angiolymphoid hyperplasia with eosinophilia (ALHE): A systematic review. J Am Acad Dermatol 2016;74(3):506–512 e11.

49. Huang SC, Zhang L, Sung YS, et al. Frequent FOS Gene Rearrangements in Epithelioid Hemangioma: A Molecular Study of 58 Cases With Morphologic Reappraisal. Am J Surg Pathol 2015;39(10): 1313–21.

50. Tsuda Y, Suurmeijer AJH, Sung YS, et al. Epithelioid hemangioma of bone harboring FOS and FOSB gene rearrangements: A clinicopathologic and molecular study. Genes Chromosomes Cancer 2021;60(1):17–25.

51. Antonescu CR, Huang SC, Sung YS, et al. Novel GATA6-FOXO1 fusions in a subset of epithelioid hemangioma. Mod Pathol 2021;34(5):934–41.

52. Jafarzadeh H, Sanatkhani M, Mohtasham N. Oral pyogenic granuloma: a review. J Oral Sci 2006; 48(4):167–75.

53. Schneider MH, Garcia CFV, Aleixo PB, et al. Congenital cutaneous pyogenic granuloma: Report of two cases and review of the literature. J Cutan Pathol 2019;46(9):691–7.

54. Alomari MH, Kozakewich HPW, Kerr CL, et al. Congenital Disseminated Pyogenic Granuloma: Characterization of an Aggressive Multisystemic Disorder. J Pediatr 2020;226:157–66.

55. Baselga E, Wassef M, Lopez S, et al. Agminated, eruptive pyogenic granuloma-like lesions developing over congenital vascular stains. Pediatr Dermatol 2012;29(2):186–90.

56. Hoeger PH, Colmenero I. Vascular tumours in infants. Part I: benign vascular tumours other than infantile haemangioma. Br J Dermatol 2014; 171(3):466–73.

57. Benedetto C, Crasto D, Ettefagh L, et al. Development of Periungual Pyogenic Granuloma with Associated Paronychia Following Isotretinoin Therapy: A Case Report and a Review of the Literature. J Clin Aesthet Dermatol 2019;12(4):32–6.

58. Inoue A, Sawada Y, Nishio D, et al. Pyogenic granuloma caused by afatinib: Case report and review of the literature. Australas J Dermatol 2017;58(1): 61–2.

59. Groesser L, Peterhof E, Evert M, et al. BRAF and RAS Mutations in Sporadic and Secondary Pyogenic Granuloma. J Invest Dermatol 2016;136(2): 481–6.

60. Lim YH, Douglas SR, Ko CJ, et al. Somatic Activating RAS Mutations Cause Vascular Tumors Including Pyogenic Granuloma. J Invest Dermatol 2015;135(6):1698–700.

61. Pereira T, de Amorim LSD, Pereira NB, et al. Oral pyogenic granulomas show MAPK/ERK signaling pathway activation, which occurs independently of BRAF, KRAS, HRAS, NRAS, GNA11, and GNA14 mutations. J Oral Pathol Med 2019; 48(10):906–10.

62. Henning B, Stieger P, Kamarachev J, et al. Pyogenic granuloma in patients treated with selective BRAF inhibitors: another manifestation of paradoxical pathway activation. Melanoma Res 2016;26(3): 304–7.

63. Raulin C, Greve B, Hammes S. The combined continuous-wave/pulsed carbon dioxide laser for treatment of pyogenic granuloma. Arch Dermatol 2002;138(1):33–7.

64. Tay YK, Weston WL, Morelli JG. Treatment of pyogenic granuloma in children with the flashlamp-pumped pulsed dye laser. Pediatr 1997;99(3): 368–70.

65. Santa Cruz DJ, Aronberg J. Targetoid hemosiderotic hemangioma. J Am Acad Dermatol 1988; 19(3):550–8.

66. Juan YC, Chen CJ, Hsiao CH, et al. A microvenular hemangioma with a rare expression of progesterone receptor immunocreativity and a review of the literature. J Cutan Pathol 2018;45(11):847–50.

67. Bantel E, Grosshans E, Ortonne JP. [Understanding microcapillary angioma, observations in pregnant patients and in females treated with hormonal contraceptives]. Z Hautkr 1989;64(12): 1071–4. Zur Kenntnis mikrokapillarer Angiome, Beobachtungen bei schwangeren bzw. unter hormoneller Antikonzeption stehenden Frauen.

68. Hunt SJ, Santa Cruz DJ, Barr RJ. Microvenular hemangioma. J Cutan Pathol 1991;18(4):235–40.

69. Jeunon T, Sampaio AL, Caminha RC, et al. Glomeruloid hemangioma in POEMS syndrome: a report

on two cases and a review of the literature. An Bras Dermatol 2011;86(6):1167–73.

70. Yuri T, Yamazaki F, Takasu K, et al. Glomeruloid hemangioma. Pathol Int 2008;58(6):390–5.

71. Osano K, Hanai S, Takahashi K, et al. Glomeruloid Hemangioma in a Patient with TAFRO Syndrome. Intern Med 2022. https://doi.org/10.2169/internalmedicine.8888-21.

72. Shinozaki-Ushiku A, Higashihara T, Ikemura M, et al. Glomeruloid hemangioma associated with TAFRO syndrome. Hum Pathol 2018;82:172–6.

73. Chan JK, Fletcher CD, Hicklin GA, et al. A distinctive cutaneous lesion of multicentric Castleman's disease associated with POEMS syndrome. Am J Surg Pathol 1990;14(11):1036–46.

74. Roy RR, Shimada K, Hasegawa H. A Case of Oral Glomeruloid Hemangioma Without. Systemic Conditions Cureus 2022;14(1):e21705.

75. Suurmeijer AJ, Fletcher CD. Papillary haemangioma. A distinctive cutaneous haemangioma of the head and neck area containing eosinophilic hyaline globules. Histopathology 2007;51(5):638–48.

76. PM. Hemangioendotheliome vegetant intravasculaire. Bull Mem Soc Ant 1923;93:517–23.

77. Clearkin KP, Enzinger FM. Intravascular papillary endothelial hyperplasia. Arch Pathol Lab Med 1976;100(8):441–4.

78. Murugaraj V, Kingston GT, Patel M, et al. Intravascular papillary endothelial hyperplasia (Masson's tumour) of the oral mucosa. Br J Oral Maxillofac Surg 2010;48(4):e16–7.

79. Liu DT, Shields CL, Tse GM, et al. Periocular papillary endothelial hyperplasia (Masson's tumour) in Behcet's disease. Acta Ophthalmol 2012;90(5):e413–5.

80. Brenn T, Fletcher CD. Cutaneous epithelioid angiomatous nodule: a distinct lesion in the morphologic spectrum of epithelioid vascular tumors. Am J Dermatopathol 2004;26(1):14–21.

81. Al-Daraji WI, Prescott RJ, Abdellaoui A, et al. Cutaneous epithelioid angiomatous nodule: different views or interpretations in the analysis of ten new cases. Dermatol Online J 2009;15(3):2.

82. Sangueza OP, Walsh SN, Sheehan DJ, et al. Cutaneous epithelioid angiomatous nodule: a case series and proposed classification. Am J Dermatopathol 2008;30(1):16–20.

83. Cohen PR, Hinds BR. Acquired Elastotic Hemangioma: Case Series and Comprehensive Literature Review. Cureus 2017;9(12):e1994.

84. Requena L, Kutzner H, Mentzel T. Acquired elastotic hemangioma: A clinicopathologic variant of hemangioma. J Am Acad Dermatol 2002;47(3):371–6.

85. Val-Bernal JF, Hermana S, Aller L. Acquired Elastotic Hemangioma-like Change of the Vulva Associated With Lichen Sclerosus. Int J Gynecol Pathol 2021. https://doi.org/10.1097/PGP.0000000000000829.

86. Jeunon T, Carvalho Wagnes Stofler ME, Teixeira Rezende P, et al. Acquired Elastotic Hemangioma: A Case Report and Review of 49 Previously Reported Cases. Am J Dermatopathol 2020;42(4):244–50.

87. Kacerovska D, Portelli F, Michal M, et al. Acquired elastotic hemangioma-like changes and eccrine sweat duct squamous metaplasia in lichen simplex chronicus/prurigo nodularis-like lesions of the knee and elbow. J Cutan Pathol 2017;44(7):605–11.

88. Gutte RM, Joshi A. Targetoid hemosiderotic hemangioma. Indian Dermatol Online J 2014;5(4):559–60.

89. Zaballos P, Llambrich A, Del Pozo LJ, et al. Dermoscopy of Targetoid Hemosiderotic Hemangioma: A Morphological Study of 35 Cases. Dermatology 2015;231(4):339–44.

90. Ibrahim M, Shwayder T. Hobnail hemangioma in a nine-year-old boy: a rare case presented with dermoscopy. Dermatol Online J 2010;16(4):7.

91. Napekoski KM, Fernandez AP, Billings SD. Microvenular hemangioma: a clinicopathologic review of 13 cases. J Cutan Pathol 2014;41(11):816–22.

92. Maloney N, Miller P, Linos K. Papillary Hemangioma: An Under-Recognized Entity Not to Be Confused With Glomeruloid Hemangioma. Am J Dermatopathol 2020;42(3):211–4.

93. Bancalari B, Colmenero I, Noguera-Morel L, et al. Papillary hemangioma in a child and sonographic characterization. Pediatr Dermatol 2020;37(1):233–4.

94. Vieira CC, Gomes APN, Galdino Dos Santos L, et al. Intravascular papillary endothelial hyperplasia in the oral mucosa and jawbones: A collaborative study of 20 cases and a systematic review. J Oral Pathol Med 2021;50(1):103–13.

95. Vicensoto Moreira Milhan N, Cavassini Torquato L, Costa V, et al. A mixed form of intravascular papillary endothelial hyperplasia in an uncommon location: case and literature review. Dermatol Online J 2018;24(2).

96. Alvarez-Arguelles-Cabrera H, Guimera-Martin-Neda F, Carrasco JL, et al. Cutaneous epithelioid angiomatous nodule. J Eur Acad Dermatol Venereol 2008;22(11):1383–5.

97. Samal S, Monohar DB, Adhya AK, et al. Cutaneous Epithelioid Angiomatous Nodule of Breast. Indian Dermatol Online J 2019;10(4):463–6.

98. Hejnold M, Dyduch G, Mojsa I, et al. Hobnail hemangioma: a immunohistochemical study and literature review. Pol J Pathol 2012;63(3):189–92.

99. Rashmi MS, Alka KD, Seema C. Oral hobnail hemangioma–a case report. Quintessence Int 2008;39(6):507–10.

100. Thangamathesvaran L, Mirani N, Langer PD. Orbital Hobnail Hemangioma. Ophthalmic Plast Reconstr Surg 2018;34(3):e97–8.

101. Rongioletti F, Gambini C, Lerza R. Glomeruloid hemangioma. A cutaneous marker of POEMS syndrome. Am J Dermatopathol 1994;16(2):175–8.

102. Puig L, Moreno A, Domingo P, et al. Cutaneous angiomas in POEMS syndrome. J Am Acad Dermatol 1985;12(5 Pt 2):961–4.

103. Kanitakis J, Roger H, Soubrier M, et al. Cutaneous angiomas in POEMS syndrome. An ultrastructural and immunohistochemical study. Arch Dermatol 1988;124(5):695–8.

104. Tanio S, Okamoto A, Majbauddin A, et al. Intravascular papillary endothelial hyperplasia associated with hemangioma of the mandible: A rare case report. J Oral Maxillofacial Surg Med Pathol 2016; 28(1):55–60.

105. Luigi L, Diana R, Luca F, et al. Intravascular Papillary Endothelial Hyperplasia of the Mandible: A Rare Entity. J Craniofac Surg 2021. https://doi.org/10.1097/SCS.0000000000008372.

106. Shim HK, Kim MR. Intravascular Papillary Endothelial Hyperplasia of the Vocal Cord: A Case Report and Review of the Literature. Am J Case Rep 2019;20:1664–8.

107. Pavlidakey PG, Burroughs C, Karrs T, et al. Cutaneous epithelioid angiomatous nodule: a case with metachronous lesions. Am J Dermatopathol 2011;33(8):831–4.

108. Hicks T, Katz I. First description of the dermatoscopic features of acquired elastotic hemangioma- a case report. Dermatol Pract Concept 2016;6(4): 35–7.

109. Cooke P, Goldrich D, Iloreta AM, et al. Intravascular Papillary Endothelial Hyperplasia of the Maxillary Sinus in Patient with Tricuspid Atresia. Head Neck Pathol 2020;14(3):803–7.

110. Hashimoto H, Daimaru Y, Enjoji M. Intravascular papillary endothelial hyperplasia. A clinicopathologic study of 91 cases. Am J Dermatopathol 1983;5(6):539–46.

111. Al Dhaybi R, Lam C, Hatami A, et al. Targetoid hemosiderotic hemangiomas (hobnail hemangiomas) are vascular lymphatic malformations: a study of 12 pediatric cases. J Am Acad Dermatol 2012; 66(1):116–20.

112. Mentzel T, Partanen TA, Kutzner H. Hobnail hemangioma ("targetoid hemosiderotic hemangioma"): clinicopathologic and immunohistochemical analysis of 62 cases. J Cutan Pathol 1999;26(6):279–86.

113. Fernandez-Flores A. Lack of expression of podoplanin by microvenular hemangioma. Pathol Res Pract 2008;204(11):817–21.

114. Kakizaki P, Valente NY, Paiva DL, et al. Targetoid hemosiderotic hemangioma - Case report. An Bras Dermatol 2014;89(6):956–9.

115. Makos C, Nikolaidou A. Intravascular papillary endothelial hyperplasia (Masson's tumor) of the oral mucosa. Presentation of two cases and review. Oral Oncol Extra 2004;40(4–5):59–62.

116. Nakatsui TC, Schloss E, Krol A, et al. Eccrine angiomatous hamartoma: report of a case and literature review. J Am Acad Dermatol 1999;41(1):109–11.

117. Smith SD, DiCaudo DJ, Price HN, et al. Congenital eccrine angiomatous hamartoma: Expanding the morphologic presentation and a review of the literature. Pediatr Dermatol 2019;36(6):909–12.

118. Mendes SR, Gameiro AR, Cardoso JC, et al. Eccrine angiomatous hamartoma in an adult. BMJ Case Rep 2021;14(2). https://doi.org/10.1136/bcr-2020-240422.

119. Pelle MT, Pride HB, Tyler WB. Eccrine angiomatous hamartoma. J Am Acad Dermatol 2002;47(3): 429–35.

120. Gottron HA, Nikolowski W. [Extrarenal Lohlein focal nephritis of the skin in endocarditis]. Arch Klin Exp Dermatol 1958;207(2):156–76. Extrarenale Lohlein-Herdnephritis der Haut bei Endocarditis.

121. Bhatia R, Hazarika N, Chandrasekaran D, et al. Treatment of Posttraumatic Reactive Angioendotheliomatosis With Topical Timolol Maleate. JAMA Dermatol 2021;157(8):1002–4.

122. Lazova R, Slater C, Scott G. Reactive angioendotheliomatosis. Case report and review of the literature. Am J Dermatopathol 1996;18(1):63–9.

123. Wells AE, Monir RL, Bender NR, et al. Reactive angioendotheliomatosis associated with antiphospholipid syndrome. Dermatol Online J 2021;27(3).

124. Bridgewater K, Vilenchik V, Ngo D, et al. Pulsed dye laser to treat reactive angioendotheliomatosis. Lasers Med Sci 2021. https://doi.org/10.1007/s10103-021-03444-5.

125. Di Filippo Y, Cardot-Leccia N, Long-Mira E, et al. Reactive angioendotheliomatosis revealing a glomerulopathy secondary to a monoclonal gammopathy successfully treated with lenalidomide. J Eur Acad Dermatol Venereol 2021;35(2):e115–8.

126. Batsakis JG, Ro JY, Frauenhoffer EE. Bacillary angiomatosis. Ann Otol Rhinol Laryngol 1995; 104(8):668–72.

127. Helleberg M. Bacillary angiomatosis in a solid organ transplant recipient. IDCases 2019;18:e00649.

128. Zarraga M, Rosen L, Herschthal D. Bacillary angiomatosis in an immunocompetent child: a case report and review of the literature. Am J Dermatopathol 2011;33(5):513–5.

129. Morillas JA, Hassanein M, Syed B, et al. Early posttransplant cutaneous bacillary angiomatosis in a kidney recipient: Case report and review of the literature. Transpl Infect Dis 2021;23(4):e13670.

130. Zukerberg LR, Nickoloff BJ, Weiss SW. Kaposiform hemangioendothelioma of infancy and childhood.

An aggressive neoplasm associated with Kasabach-Merritt syndrome and lymphangiomatosis. Am J Surg Pathol 1993;17(4):321–8.

131. Ji Y, Chen S, Yang K, et al. Kaposiform hemangioendothelioma: current knowledge and future perspectives. Orphanet J Rare Dis 2020;15(1):39.

132. Croteau SE, Liang MG, Kozakewich HP, et al. Kaposiform hemangioendothelioma: atypical features and risks of Kasabach-Merritt phenomenon in 107 referrals. J Pediatr 2013;162(1):142–7.

133. Putra J, Gupta A. Kaposiform haemangioendothelioma: a review with emphasis on histological differential diagnosis. Pathol 2017;49(4):356–62.

134. Zhou S, Wang L, Panossian A, et al. Refractory Kaposiform Hemangioendothelioma Associated with the Chromosomal Translocation t(13;16)(q14; p13.3). Pediatr Dev Pathol 2016;19(5):417–20.

135. Ji Y, Chen S, Zhou J, et al. Sirolimus plus prednisolone vs sirolimus monotherapy for kaposiform hemangioendothelioma: a randomized clinical trial. Blood 2022. https://doi.org/10.1182/blood. 2021014027.

136. Wang Z, Li K, Yao W, et al. Steroid-resistant kaposiform hemangioendothelioma: a retrospective study of 37 patients treated with vincristine and long-term follow-up. Pediatr Blood Cancer 2015;62(4): 577–80.

137. Yao W, Li K, Wang Z, et al. Comparison of efficacy and safety of corticosteroid and vincristine in treating kaposiform hemangioendothelioma and tufted angioma: A multicenter prospective randomized controlled clinical trial. J Dermatol 2021;48(5): 576–84.

138. Wang Z, Yao W, Sun H, et al. Sirolimus therapy for kaposiform hemangioendothelioma with long-term follow-up. J Dermatol 2019;46(11):956–61.

139. Calonje E, Fletcher CD, Wilson-Jones E, et al. Retiform hemangioendothelioma. A distinctive form of low-grade angiosarcoma delineated in a series of 15 cases. Am J Surg Pathol 1994;18(2):115–25.

140. Zhang M, Yin X, Yao W, et al. Retiform hemangioendothelioma: a rare lesion of the vulva. J Int Med Res 2021; 49(8). https://doi.org/10.1177/03000605211027783. 3000605211027783.

141. Jiang J, Li X, Zhu F, et al. Retiform hemangioendothelioma of the mandible: A case report. Oral Oncol 2021;115:105120.

142. Chundriger Q, Tariq MU, Rahim S, et al. Retiform hemangioendothelioma: a case series and review of the literature. J Med Case Rep 2021;15(1):69.

143. Antonescu CR, Dickson BC, Sung YS, et al. Recurrent YAP1 and MAML2 Gene Rearrangements in Retiform and Composite Hemangioendothelioma. Am J Surg Pathol 2020;44(12):1677–84.

144. Keiler SA, Honda K, Bordeaux JS. Retiform hemangioendothelioma treated with Mohs micrographic surgery. J Am Acad Dermatol 2011;65(1):233–5.

145. Hirsh AZ, Yan W, Wei L, et al. Unresectable retiform hemangioendothelioma treated with external beam radiation therapy and chemotherapy: a case report and review of the literature. Sarcoma 2010; 2010doi.

146. Dabska M. Malignant endovascular papillary angioendothelioma of the skin in childhood. Clinicopathologic study of 6 cases. Cancer 1969;24(3): 503–10.

147. Fanburg-Smith JC, Michal M, Partanen TA, et al. Papillary intralymphatic angioendothelioma (PILA): a report of twelve cases of a distinctive vascular tumor with phenotypic features of lymphatic vessels. Am J Surg Pathol 1999;23(9): 1004–10.

148. Neves RI, Stevenson J, Hancey MJ, et al. Endovascular papillary angioendothelioma (Dabska tumor): underrecognized malignant tumor in childhood. J Pediatr Surg 2011;46(1):e25–8.

149. Fukunaga M. Expression of D2-40 in lymphatic endothelium of normal tissues and in vascular tumours. Histopathology 2005;46(4):396–402.

150. Nayler SJ, Rubin BP, Calonje E, et al. Composite hemangioendothelioma: a complex, low-grade vascular lesion mimicking angiosarcoma. Am J Surg Pathol 2000;24(3):352–61.

151. Hornick JL, Fletcher CD. Pseudomyogenic hemangioendothelioma: a distinctive, often multicentric tumor with indolent behavior. Am J Surg Pathol 2011;35(2):190–201.

152. Chan JK, Frizzera G, Fletcher CD, et al. Primary vascular tumors of lymph nodes other than Kaposi's sarcoma. Analysis of 39 cases and delineation of two new entities. Am J Surg Pathol 1992;16(4): 335–50.

153. Li WW, Liang P, Zhao HP, et al. Composite hemangioendothelioma of the spleen with multiple metastases: CT findings and review of the literature. Medicine (Baltimore) 2021;100(21):e25846.

154. El Hussein S, Omarzai Y. Multifocal Polymorphous Hemangioendothelioma of the Liver: Case Report and Review of Literature. Int J Surg Pathol 2017; 25(3):266–70.

155. Paul SR, Hurford MT, Miettinen MM, et al. Polymorphous hemangioendothelioma in a child with acquired immunodeficiency syndrome (AIDS). Pediatr Blood Cancer 2008;50(3):663–5.

156. Rokni GR, Montazer F, Sharifian M, et al. Composite hemangioendothelioma of the forehead and right eye; a case report. BMC Dermatol 2017; 17(1):15.

157. Trombetta D, Magnusson L, von Steyern FV, et al. Translocation t(7;19)(q22;q13)-a recurrent chromosome aberration in pseudomyogenic hemangioendothelioma? Cancer Genet 2011;204(4):211–5.

158. Panagopoulos I, Lobmaier I, Gorunova L, et al. Fusion of the Genes WWTR1 and FOSB in

Pseudomyogenic Hemangioendothelioma. Cancer Genomics Proteomics 2019;16(4):293–8.

159. Utas S, Canoz O, Ferahbas A, et al. Composite cutaneous haemangioendothelioma treated with interferon. J Eur Acad Dermatol Venereol 2008; 22(4):503–5.

160. Ross RA, Monteith PR, McAdam JG. Case report: polymorphous haemangioendothelioma, a rare cause of persistent lymphadenopathy. J R Nav Med Serv 1993;79(2):80–2.

161. Nascimento AG, Keeney GL, Sciot R, et al. Polymorphous hemangioendothelioma: a report of two cases, one affecting extranodal soft tissues, and review of the literature. Am J Surg Pathol 1997; 21(9):1083–9.

162. Kaposi. Idiopathisches multiples Pigmentsarkom der Haut. Archiv für Dermatologie und Syphilis 1872;4:265–73.

163. Lazova R, McNiff JM, Glusac EJ, et al. Promontory sign–present in patch and plaque stage of angiosarcoma. Am J Dermatopathol 2009;31(2):132–6.

164. Schwartz RA, Micali G, Nasca MR, et al. Kaposi sarcoma: a continuing conundrum. J Am Acad Dermatol 2008;59(2):179–206. quiz 207-8.

165. Etemad SA, Dewan AK. Kaposi Sarcoma Updates. Dermatol Clin 2019;37(4):505–17.

166. Marcoval J, Bonfill-Orti M, Martinez-Molina L, et al. Evolution of Kaposi sarcoma in the past 30 years in a tertiary hospital of the European Mediterranean basin. Clin Exp Dermatol 2019;44(1):32–9.

167. Parkin DM, Sitas F, Chirenje M, et al. Part I: Cancer in Indigenous Africans–burden, distribution, and trends. Lancet Oncol 2008;9(7):683–92.

168. Cahoon EK, Linet MS, Clarke CA, et al. Risk of Kaposi sarcoma after solid organ transplantation in the United States. Int J Cancer 2018;143(11): 2741–8.

169. Ramzi M, Vojdani R, Haghighinejad H. Kaposi Sarcoma After Allogeneic Hematopoietic Stem Cell Transplant: A Rare Complication. Exp Clin Transpl 2021;19(2):173–5.

170. Ursini F, Naty S, Mazzei V, et al. Kaposi's sarcoma in a psoriatic arthritis patient treated with infliximab. Int Immunopharmacol 2010;10(7):827–8.

171. Maurer T, Ponte M, Leslie K. HIV-associated Kaposi's sarcoma with a high CD4 count and a low viral load. N Engl J Med Sep 27 2007;357(13):1352–3.

172. Vangipuram R, Tyring SK. Epidemiology of Kaposi sarcoma: review and description of the nonepidemic variant. Int J Dermatol 2019;58(5):538–42.

173. Aneja KK, Yuan Y. Reactivation and Lytic Replication of Kaposi's Sarcoma-Associated Herpesvirus: An Update. Front Microbiol 2017;8:613.

174. Ye F, Zeng Y, Sha J, et al. High Glucose Induces Reactivation of Latent Kaposi's Sarcoma-Associated Herpesvirus. J Virol 2016;90(21): 9654–63.

175. Mukhtar F, Ilozumba M, Utuama O, et al. Change in Pattern of Secondary Cancers After Kaposi Sarcoma in the Era of Antiretroviral Therapy. JAMA Oncol 2018;4(1):48–53.

176. Rohrmus B, Thoma-Greber EM, Bogner JR, et al. Outlook in oral and cutaneous Kaposi's sarcoma. Lancet 2000;356(9248):2160.

177. El-Mallawany NK, McAtee CL, Campbell LR, et al. Pediatric Kaposi sarcoma in context of the HIV epidemic in sub-Saharan Africa: current perspectives. Pediatr Health Med Ther 2018;9:35–46.

178. Ackerman AB. Subtle clues to diagnosis by conventional microscopy. The patch stage of Kaposi's sarcoma. Am J Dermatopathol 1979;1(2):165–72.

179. Patel RM, Goldblum JR, Hsi ED. Immunohistochemical detection of human herpes virus-8 latent nuclear antigen-1 is useful in the diagnosis of Kaposi sarcoma. Mod Pathol 2004;17(4):456–60.

180. Dupin N. Update on oncogenesis and therapy for Kaposi sarcoma. Curr Opin Oncol 2020;32(2): 122–8.

181. Young RJ, Brown NJ, Reed MW, et al. Angiosarcoma Lancet Oncol 2010;11(10):983–91.

182. Ferrari A, Casanova M, Bisogno G, et al. Malignant vascular tumors in children and adolescents: a report from the Italian and German Soft Tissue Sarcoma Cooperative Group. Med Pediatr Oncol 2002;39(2):109–14.

183. Fury MG, Antonescu CR, Van Zee KJ, et al. A 14-year retrospective review of angiosarcoma: clinical characteristics, prognostic factors, and treatment outcomes with surgery and chemotherapy. Cancer J 2005;11(3):241–7.

184. Rouhani P, Fletcher CD, Devesa SS, et al. Cutaneous soft tissue sarcoma incidence patterns in the U.S. : an analysis of 12,114 cases. Cancer 2008;113(3):616–27.

185. Huang J, Mackillop WJ. Increased risk of soft tissue sarcoma after radiotherapy in women with breast carcinoma. Cancer 2001;92(1):172–80.

186. Gaballah AH, Jensen CT, Palmquist S, et al. Angiosarcoma: clinical and imaging features from head to toe. Br J Radiol 2017;90(1075):20170039.

187. West JG, Weitzel JN, Tao ML, et al. BRCA mutations and the risk of angiosarcoma after breast cancer treatment. Clin Breast Cancer 2008;8(6):533–7.

188. Ronchi A, Cozzolino I, Zito Marino F, et al. Primary and secondary cutaneous angiosarcoma: Distinctive clinical, pathological and molecular features. Ann Diagn Pathol 2020;48:151597.

189. Motaparthi K, Lauer SR, Patel RM, et al. MYC gene amplification by fluorescence in situ hybridization and MYC protein expression by immunohistochemistry in the diagnosis of cutaneous angiosarcoma: Systematic review and appropriate use criteria. J Cutan Pathol 2021;48(4):578–86.

190. Sheu TG, Hunt KK, Middleton LP. MYC and NOTCH1-positive postradiation cutaneous angiosarcoma of the breast. Breast J 2021;27(3):264–7.

191. Vargas AC, Grimison P, Joy C, et al. Chromosome 8 Polysomy Accounting for MYC Over-Expression in Angiosarcoma Arising as Somatic-Type Malignancy in Metastatic Teratoma. Case Rep Int J Surg Pathol. 2021. https://doi.org/10.1177/10668969211067762. 10668969211067762.

192. Webb C, Partain N, Koduru P, et al. Secondary Angiosarcoma With C-MYC Amplification Following Prophylactic Bilateral Mastectomy and Autologous Breast Reconstruction: Report of a Case and Review of the Literature. Int J Surg Pathol 2021;29(2):205–10.

193. Florou V, Wilky BA. Current and Future Directions for Angiosarcoma Therapy. Curr Treat Options Oncol 2018;19(3):14.

194. Sardaro A, Bardoscia L, Petruzzelli MF, et al. Epithelioid hemangioendothelioma: an overview and update on a rare vascular tumor. Oncol Rev 2014;8(2):259.

195. Weiss SW, Enzinger FM. Epithelioid hemangioendothelioma: a vascular tumor often mistaken for a carcinoma. Cancer 1982;50(5):970–81.

196. Rosenberg A, Agulnik M. Epithelioid Hemangioendothelioma: Update on Diagnosis and Treatment. Curr Treat Options Oncol 2018;19(4):19.

197. Rosenbaum E, Jadeja B, Xu B, et al. Prognostic stratification of clinical and molecular epithelioid hemangioendothelioma subsets. Mod Pathol 2020;33(4):591–602.

198. Jang JK, Thomas R, Braschi-Amirfarzan M, et al. A review of the spectrum of imaging manifestations of epithelioid hemangioendothelioma. AJR Am J Roentgenol 2020;215(5):1290–8.

199. Bagan P, Hassan M, Le Pimpec Barthes F, et al. Prognostic factors and surgical indications of pulmonary epithelioid hemangioendothelioma: a review of the literature. Ann Thorac Surg 2006;82(6):2010–3.

200. Kitaichi M, Nagai S, Nishimura K, et al. Pulmonary epithelioid haemangioendothelioma in 21 patients, including three with partial spontaneous regression. Eur Respir J 1998;12(1):89–96.

201. Deyrup AT, Tighiouart M, Montag AG, et al. Epithelioid hemangioendothelioma of soft tissue: a proposal for risk stratification based on 49 cases. Am J Surg Pathol 2008;32(6):924–7.

202. Anderson T, Zhang L, Hameed M, et al. Thoracic epithelioid malignant vascular tumors: a clinicopathologic study of 52 cases with emphasis on pathologic grading and molecular studies of WWTR1-CAMTA1 fusions. Am J Surg Pathol 2015;39(1):132–9.

203. Stacchiotti S, Provenzano S, Dagrada G, et al. Sirolimus in advanced epithelioid hemangioendothelioma: a retrospective case-series analysis from the italian rare cancer network database. Ann Surg Oncol 2016;23(9):2735–44.

204. Zheng Z, Wang H, Jiang H, et al. Apatinib for the treatment of pulmonary epithelioid hemangioendothelioma: A case report and literature review. Med (Baltimore) 2017;96(45):e8507.

205. Lerut JP, Orlando G, Adam R, et al. The place of liver transplantation in the treatment of hepatic epithelioid hemangioendothelioma: report of the European liver transplant registry. Ann Surg 2007;246(6):949–57 [discussion: 957].

206. Puls F, Niblett A, Clarke J, et al. YAP1-TFE3 epithelioid hemangioendothelioma: a case without vasoformation and a new transcript variant. Virchows Arch 2015;466(4):473–8.

207. Lee SJ, Yang WI, Chung WS, et al. Epithelioid hemangioendotheliomas with TFE3 gene translocations are compossible with CAMTA1 gene rearrangements. Oncotarget 2016;7(7):7480–8.

Capillary Malformations

Karla Escobar, BS, Karan Pandher, MD, Marla N. Jahnke, MD*

KEYWORDS

- Capillary malformations • Dermatology • Pediatric • Port-wine stain • Skin • vascular anomalies

KEY POINTS

- Capillary malformations are the most common type of vascular malformation.
- Most capillary malformations are non-syndromic and benign.
- Recognizing the uncommon occurrence of syndromic or high risk capillary malformations is critical.

INTRODUCTION

Capillary malformations (CMs) are the most common type of vascular malformation (VM). They are slow flow, composed of enlarged capillaries and venules with thickened perivascular cell coverage in skin and mucous membranes.[1] They occur in approximately 0.3% to 0.5% of the population with an equal sex distribution.[1–3]

While most CMs occur as isolated skin findings, a wide range of disorders feature CMs. The clinical presentation, systemic associations, genetic mutations, and prognosis vary greatly within and between disorders; therefore, identifying a disorder clinically can be difficult. Genotype–phenotype correlation aids in diagnosis and is important in better classifying syndromic CMs.

This article provides an overview of the clinical features, genetics, and current classifications of CMs and associated syndromes. Additionally, it clarifies the ambiguous nomenclature present in the existing literature.

Clinical Characteristics

CMs are slow-flow VMs, which may appear anywhere on the body. They present at birth and grow proportionately with the individual. Coloring ranges from vibrant pinks to reds to purples (Fig. 1). CMs most commonly appear on the head and neck[1–3] and may extend to the lips, gingiva, or oral mucosa.[4] On the face, CMs often follow a dermatomal distribution respecting the midline; in some cases, however, they can involve neighboring dermatomes. In the early neonatal period, distinguishing CMs from an infantile hemangioma can be difficult; infantile hemangiomas, however, tend to darken and thicken over days to weeks, whereas CMs exhibit little change.

In most affected individuals, CMs are isolated and not associated with any underlying abnormalities or genetic syndromes. Nonetheless, local complications may occur including hyperkeratosis and soft tissue hypertrophy, especially in facial lesions. Other complications in lesions of any site include pyogenic granuloma-like proliferations, which may ooze and bleed (Fig. 2). Eczematous dermatitis overlying a CM, termed the Meyerson phenomena, can lead to pruritus (Fig. 3). Additionally, stigmatization and disfigurement may contribute to significant morbidity in some patients. In more rare cases, CMs occur in association with genetic disorders with additional features as discussed in this article.

Pathogenesis

An error in vascular development during embryogenesis causes CMs.[4] Histopathological examination is rarely performed in CMs, and only clinically difficult cases are biopsied. Most of the involved vessels are located in the papillary and reticular dermis with the number of anomalous vessels decreasing with increasing depth.[4] Lesions in a V3 dermatome, neck, and trunk regions are more superficial in comparison to the V2 dermatomal area and distal extremities that have more deeply placed vessels.[4,5] This becomes clinically relevant with regard to laser treatment.

Mutations causing CMs are usually sporadic. Several genes have been identified with both

Department of Dermatology, Henry Ford Health, 3031 E Grand Blvd, Detroit, MI 48202, USA
* Corresponding author.
E-mail address: mjahnke1@hfhs.org

Dermatol Clin 40 (2022) 425–433
https://doi.org/10.1016/j.det.2022.06.005
0733-8635/22/© 2022 Elsevier Inc. All rights reserved.

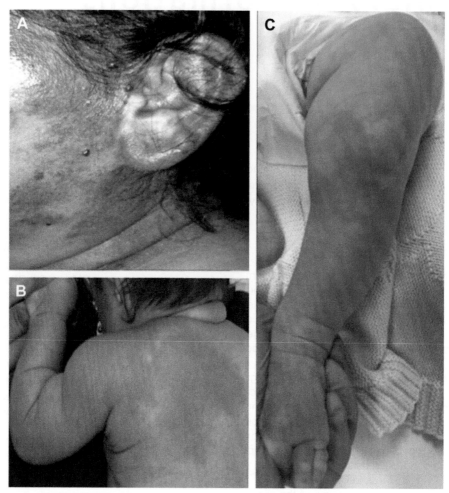

Fig. 1. Various port-wine birthmarks on different skin tones. Vascular blebs can be seen in image A in an adult patient.

isolated and syndromic lesions (see Genetics chapter for additional details).

Nevus Simplex/salmon Patch - "angel kiss," "stork bite"

Nevus simplex (NS), often called salmon patch, "angel kiss," or "stork bite," are common vascular

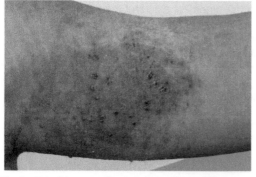

Fig. 2. CM with pyogenic granuloma-like proliferations.

lesions of childhood. They are seen in up to 82% of newborns at birth or soon after as a pale pink to red, ill-defined patch(es).[6–8] They are often seen on the mid-forehead, upper eyelids, philtrum, and nape of the neck. Less common sites include the occipital scalp, parietal scalp, and upper back.[6] The lumbosacral spine can also be affected (**Fig. 4**). When lesions are extensive, the term NS complex is used. NS complex is benign, however, a thorough physical examination to seek out additional signs of spinal dysraphism is required as NS with additional signs, such as an atypical pit, lipoma, aplasia cuti, sinus tract, localized hypertrichosis, or tag, may identify cases of dysraphism.[8]

Although NS are considered CMs by the International Society for the Study of Vascular Anomalies (ISSVA), NS are caused by dilated capillaries within the papillary dermis and are likely due to a lack of autonomic regulation of local vessels in the affected skin as opposed to being true CMs.[1] The vast majority of NS over the eyelids and

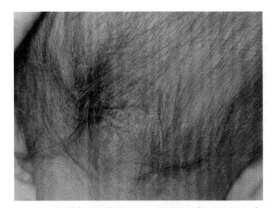

Fig. 3. CM with overlying eczematous dermatitis, also known as the Meyerson phenomena.

forehead fade over time, whereas those located at the nape of the neck tend to persist into adulthood albeit without significant darkening. Additionally, unlike true CMs, NS on the face does not follow a dermatomal distribution and are not associated with Sturge–Weber syndrome (SWS).

Large, persistent facial NS can be associated with underlying syndromes such as Beckwith–Wiedemann syndrome (BWS) and macrocephaly-CM syndrome (M-CM).[1,9] BWS is the most frequent genetic overgrowth syndrome, characterized by pre and postnatal overgrowth, macrosomia, macroglossia, a persistent NS, abdominal wall defects, neonatal hypoglycemia, and renal anomalies. Wilms tumors and other malignancies are also a feature, especially in early childhood. Persistent NS is also seen in megalencephaly–CM–polymicrogyria syndrome (MCAP), nova syndrome, odontodysplasia, M-CM, and Roberts syndrome.[1,6]

CUTANEOUS AND/OR MUCOSAL CAPILLARY MALFORMATIONS - "PORT-WINE STAIN"

PWS or nevus flammeus, seen in 3 to 5 per 1000 live births, refers to a well-demarcated pink-red patch.[6,8] The classic presentation is a unilateral patch with a segmental distribution and midline demarcation, most frequently located on the face.[6,10] A bilateral distribution may also be seen. Although most CMs are stable over time, PWS can darken and form nodules. In 55% to 70% of cases, progressive hypertrophy of the soft tissue or underlying bones is observed, especially if the CMs are located on the lip or cheek (within the V2 distribution).[8,11,12] PWS are caused by a sporadic somatic mosaic activating mutation in GNAQ or GNA11 as well as a defective expression of smooth muscle actin (SMA) in the pericytes.[10]

Capillary Malformations with Central Nervous System and/or Ocular Anomalies – Sturge–Weber Syndrome

SWS is a sporadic neurocutaneous syndrome that occurs in 1/50,000 infants, characterized by a triad of facial CMs, ipsilateral leptomeningeal angiomatosis, and glaucoma with bone and/or soft tissue involvement (**Fig. 5**).[6,11,13] Most of the cases are caused by a somatic activating mutation in GNAQ or GNA11.[13,14] A relatively recent study clarified that facial CMs are defined by embryonic craniofacial vascular patterns of development rather than trigeminal innervation, a long-held notion.[6,11] Infants with facial CMs at higher risk of suffering from this syndrome are those for which

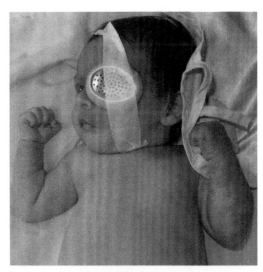

Fig. 5. A 1-month-old infant with Sturge–Weber syndrome with extensive facial, trunk, and extremity port wine birthmark with her eye patched due to glaucoma surgery.

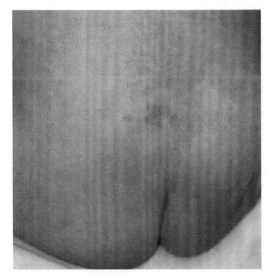

Fig. 4. Nevus simplex of lumbosacral spine.

the PWS affects the frontonasal placode (forehead, hemifacial or median phenotype).[13] This frontonasal distribution is common to nearly all patients with SWS and a multidermatomal lesion and/or bilateral distribution place a patient at higher risk.[15,16]

Children with SWS are at risk for seizures, stroke-like episodes, and cognitive delays due to the vascular stasis and poor perfusion in the cortex beneath the leptomeningeal CMs. Further, ipsilateral CMs can occur in the choroid plexus, leading to glaucoma, retinal detachment, and choroidal bleeding.[11] Leptomeningeal angioma are mostly situated over occipital and posterior parietal lobes. Laminar cortical necrosis and calcification develop due to stasis and ischemia of the neighboring leptomeningeal angiomatosis. Dental issues are also common such as gum hypertrophy and overgrowth of the maxilla.[2,3,17]

A multidisciplinary approach including dermatology, neurology, and ophthalmology with the inclusion of additional specialists is required to monitor and treat patients with SWS.

Diffuse Capillary Malformations with Overgrowth

Diffuse capillary malformation with overgrowth (DCMO) is characterized by multiple and/or extensive CMs associated with overgrowth.[18,19] Overgrowth typically involves the soft tissue or bone of an extremity and does not necessarily correlate with the location or severity of the CMs.[20] Overgrowth may affect only one extremity, ipsilateral or contralateral to the CM, or less often, an entire side of the body and is proportionate over time.[8] The CMs in DCMO are usually reticulate, pale, diffuse, involve multiple anatomic regions, and are stained contiguously (**Fig. 6**).[20] Patients with DCMO may have prominent subcutaneous veins and varicosities, but they do not have lymphatic

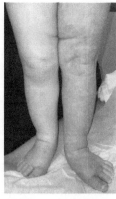

Fig. 6. Image of DCMO with GNAQ mutation.

anomalies.[8] DCMO may arise as a consequence of somatic activating mutations in PIK3CA, GNAQ and GNA11.[14,21] Many patients with DCMO are on the PIK3CA-related overgrowth spectrum (PROS) and share several features seen in other PROS conditions such as multiple CMs, facial asymmetry, limb overgrowth, and hand/foot anomalies such as macrodactyly and syndactyly.[19] Similar to other PROS phenotypes, the association with Wilms tumor continues to be under investigation. A recent retrospective review of 89 patients with DCMO did not identify any cases of Wilms tumor.[20] Thus, a diagnosis of DCMO generally portends a favorable prognosis with most complications arising from potential leg length discrepancy and those seen with extensive PWS.

RETICULATE CAPILLARY MALFORMATIONS
Capillary Malformations of Microcephaly-capillary Malformation

Microcephaly-capillary malformation syndrome (MIC-CAP) is a rare neurologic and vascular disorder characterized by congenital and progressive microcephaly, profound developmental delay, intractable epilepsy, optic atrophy causing blindness, small CMs on the skin, and poor somatic growth.[6,21,22] MIC-CAP is caused by homozygous or compound heterozygous mutations in the STAM-binding protein gene (STAMBP). Patients with MIC-CAP display reduced STAMBP expression, accumulation of ubiquitin-conjugated protein aggregates, elevated apoptosis, and insensitive activation of the RAS-MAPK and PI3K-AKT-mTOR pathways.[23]

Capillary Malformations of Megalencephaly-capillary Malformation-polymicrogyria

Patients with MCAP present with congenital or early postnatal megalencephaly, segmental overgrowth, reticulated or confluent CMs, and polymicrogyria.[2,21] Often there is a prominent midline facial CMs and segmental reticulated CMs on the body, with overgrowth and polydactyly or syndactyly.[6] Other neurologic manifestations include ventriculomegaly and cerebellar tonsillar ectopia, which may be complicated by hydrocephalus and Chiari malformation, respectively.[20] Neurologic involvement can manifest as developmental delay and seizures.[6] Patients should be followed for MCAP is caused by an activating somatic mutation in the PIK3CA gene.[2]

Capillary Malformations of CM-AVM

Capillary Malformations-Arteriovenous Malformation (CM-AVM) affects 1/100,000 individuals.[4]

CM-AVM is characterized by CMs associated with high-flow AVMs or arteriovenous fistulas (AVFs). Unique to CM-AVM is that new CMs may develop over time. CMs are usually multiple, multifocal, small (ranging from <1 cm to 3 cm in diameter), round to oval in shape, and pink to dull red annular macules or papules.[2,3,6,24] The pinkish macules can exhibit a brownish hue, a perilesional whitish halo of vasoconstriction, and hypotrichosis. The white halo suggests vascular steal and shows high flow or a bruit on Doppler ultrasound.[1,24] These pink macules are considered to be cutaneous micro-AVMs.[24] CMs can be present with or without AVMs and AVFs.[3] AVM/AVF occur in the skin, muscles, and bones of the face, ears, thorax, and extremities, as well as in the brain and spine.[2,3] It is essential to perform ultrasound Doppler if any warmth or palpable thrill is noted in a vascular lesion. Genetic counseling and magnetic resonance angiography (MRA) screening for high-flow brain or spinal AVMs may be helpful.[6] In approximately one-third of individuals with CM-AVM with AVMs, the AVM involves the bone and soft tissue of the leg; these patients have Parkes Weber Syndrome (PKWS) as part of CM-AVM.[3,25]

CM-AVM is an autosomal dominant disorder caused by germline heterozygous inactivating mutations in the RASA1 gene (p120-rasGAP) located on chromosome 5.[3,10] A second-hit somatic mutation in endothelial cells is responsible for the complete inactivation of RASA1, which is necessary for both skin lesions and high-flow lesions to develop.[10,25] Although the penetrance of this condition is greater than 95%, the number of CMs and the presence of AVMs is variable among affected family members.[3,25] Mutations in the EPHB4 gene cause a similar vascular disorder to that caused by RASA1 mutations, hence, the terms CM-AVM1 and CM-AVM2 syndrome are designated for patients with mutations in RASA1 and EPHB4, respectively.[9]

CUTIS MARMORATA TELANGIECTATICA CONGENITA

Cutis marmorata telangiectatica congenita (CMTC) is an uncommon, distinctive cutaneous VM noted at or very soon after birth with an unknown cause.[1,26] Violaceous, reticulated or mottled patches resemble physiologic cutis marmorata but are persistent despite local warming and may exhibit atrophy (Fig. 7).[1,10] Lesions tend to lighten gradually over the first few years of life. Patches may be limited to one or several extremities or may be much more extensive but typically demonstrate demarcation at the midline. Ulceration may occur. Affected limbs can display limb

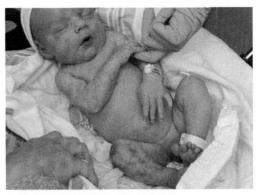

Fig. 7. CMTC in infant.

hypoplasia although hyperplasia is also seen. The most common associated finding is limb asymmetry (33%-68%), requiring orthopedic surgery involvement when limb length discrepancy becomes substantial.[26] Other organ systems may be involved (eyes, CNS, heart, and so forth) but systemic involvement is thought to be rare and seen only in those with very extensive skin lesions. Patients with CMTC should undergo a careful physical examination to assess for other congenital anomalies.[26] CMTC may be mistaken for reticulate PWS and, although no gene has been identified for CMTC, this is one reason genetic evaluation may be sought.

PHAKOMATOSIS PIGMENTOVASCULARIS

Phakomatosis pigmentovascularis (PPV) is a neurocutaneous syndrome consisting of CMs in addition to melanocytic lesions (Fig. 8). The melanocytic lesions may be dermal melanocytosis (Mongolian spots), nevus spilus, and/or nevus of Ota.[27] The classification system for PPV has changed throughout the years, but more recently a four-type scheme, created by Rudolf Happle, is utilized.[28] Type 1 PPV (phakomatosis cesio flammea) is characterized by the coexistence of dermal melanocytosis and a nevus flammeus. Type 2 PPV (phakomatosis spilorosea) is characterized by the association of a nevus spilus and a pale-pink nevus. Type 3 PPV or phakomatosis cesio marmorata is the coexistence of dermal melanocytosis with CMTC and the last group is unclassifiable PPVs.[27,29] The pathogenesis behind PPV is activating GNAQ/GNA11 mutations; these mutations were also detected in ocular melanoma.[30,31] This syndrome can also be associated with other complications such as SWS, ocular melanosis, Klippel–Trenaunay syndrome (KTS), overgrowth, leg-length discrepancy, iris mammillations, iris hamartomas, glaucoma, epilepsy, scoliosis, and others.[27]

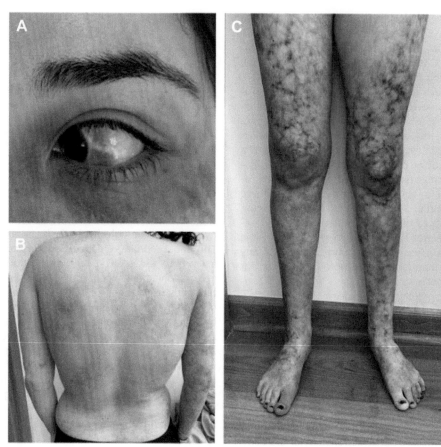

Fig. 8. 21-year-old woman with violaceous reticulated confluent patches and slight unilateral overgrowth of left limb compared to right.

Therefore, these patients require ophthalmology consultation and other specialists depending on additional features.[32]

TELANGIECTASIA
Hereditary Hemorrhagic Telangiectasia

Hereditary hemorrhagic telangiectasia (HHT), also known as Osler–Rendu–Weber syndrome, is a genetically heterogeneous, autosomal dominant disorder with high penetrance but considerable intrafamilial variability.[2,26] Incidence is estimated at 1/8000.[2,33] HHT is characterized by mucocutaneous and visceral telangiectasias and AVMs that also affect internal organs. Patients typically present in the first 2 decades of life.[26] Initial manifestations include recurrent epistaxis, which can be severe, and cutaneous or mucosal CMs that rupture and bleed after minor trauma.[2] Telangiectasias are frequently located on the lips, oral mucosa, upper extremities, nail beds, tongue, ears, and conjunctivae. In adulthood, telangiectasias develop in the gastrointestinal mucosa and result in significant bleeding in 16% of patients.[2,26] HHT can frequently be complicated by the presence of clinically significant AVMs in the lungs and brain, leading to respiratory and neurologic complications, including emboli, stroke, migraines and seizures.[13,26]

Commonly mutated genes in HHT are ENG, ACVRL1, GDF2, and SMAD4. All genes are members of the same signaling pathway (TFG-β) and various alterations in this pathway may lead to different variants of the disease. Mutations in ENG gene encoding for endoglin, a receptor for TGF-β signaling proteins, correlate with HHT type 1. Mutations in the ACVRL1 gene encoding for the anaplastic lymphoma receptor tyrosine kinase, correlate with HHT type 2. Mutations in SMAD4 may result in HHT as well as the autosomal dominant cancer predisposition syndrome, juvenile polyposis syndrome.[2]

CAPILLARY MALFORMATIONS ASSOCIATED WITH OTHER ANOMALIES
Klippel Trenaunay–Weber Syndrome

KTS is traditionally defined by the triad of CMs, venous malformation, bone and/or soft-tissue hypertrophy of the affected limb. Additional features may include LM or VLM, and varicose veins with or without deep venous anomalies.[1,6,20,26] KTS has likely been vastly overdiagnosed as features greatly overlap with other CMs syndromes including DCMO. The ability to genotype patients with VMs has improved diagnostic certainty. KTS is caused by a somatic activating mutation in PIK3CA, which regulates cell survival and growth through the activation of the mTOR1-ATK pathway.[20] KTS is associated with limb overgrowth and significant arteriovenous shunting of the involved limb.[26] The findings in KTS are classically isolated to a lower extremity, with extension onto the lower trunk.[20] The CMs are often sharply circumscribed, geographic violaceous plaques, often with visible nodules (lymphatic blebs), which become thicker over time and bleed as the patient matures.[1,4,26] Geographic lesions are often located on the lateral aspect of the thigh, knee, and lower leg.[20,26] Nongeographic CMs are pink to red and scattered over the affected limb. In patients with nongeographic CMs, other KTS symptoms (varicose veins and overgrowth) manifest later in life than in patients affected with a geographic one, whose KTS is usually obvious at birth.[26] Reticulate or blotchy CMs on the extremities can also be associated with overgrowth and venous varicosities but are less likely to demonstrate extensive underlying LM. In KTS, progressive worsening of the venous stasis and/or lymphedema is inevitable, and ulceration, pain, coagulopathy, thrombosis, pulmonary emboli, and pulmonary artery hypertension are all potential comorbidities.[1]

Parkes Weber Syndrome

Parkes Weber syndrome (PKWS) is a congenital disorder caused by a mutation in RASA1, defined by the presence of cutaneous VMs including capillary, venous, lymphatic, and AVFs.[13] Patients present with cutaneous red or pink large patches with underlying quiescent AVMs and extremity overgrowth affecting bones and soft tissue.[2] It may affect either the upper or lower extremities, including pelvic vessels, but the lower extremities are more often affected than the upper extremities.[2,13] PKWS is often distinguished from KTS by the presence of multiple high-flow vascular lesions in the affected limb. A lymphatic component may be present in some patients and congenital VMs are common. Heart failure due to arteriovenous shunting, as well as ischemic pain, ulceration, and edema, may rarely occur.[34]

Congenital Lipomatous Overgrowth, Vascular Malformations, Epidermal Nevis, Spinal/Skeletal Anomalies/Scoliosis Syndrome

Congenital lipomatous asymmetric overgrowth of the trunk with lymphatic, capillary, venous, and combined-type vascular malformations, epidermal nevi, scoliosis/skeletal and spinal anomalies (CLOVES) is a PIK3CA nonprogressive overgrowth syndrome.[6] CMs tend to show a deep purple hue and their arrangement is usually lateralized.[7] The CMs are often geographic, however, distinctive findings include primarily thoracic lipomatous masses mixed with LMs, venous malformations, AVMs of the spine, soft overgrowth of feet and/or hands, macrodactyly of the third finger, sandal gap deformity of the toes and/or cubital deviation of the fingers, and a high risk of coagulopathy. The lipomatous lesions may infiltrate the retroperitoneum, mediastinum, pleura, and paraspinal spaces.[6]

Proteus Syndrome

Proteus syndrome is characterized by asymmetric overgrowth, connective tissue nevi, epidermal nevi, cranial hyperostosis, visceral hamartomas, and vascular anomalies, including CMs. The most characteristic manifestations are plantar cerebriform connective tissue nevi.[13,26] Proteus syndrome is caused by a somatic activating mutation of AKT.[6] This syndrome is associated with a high risk of pulmonary abnormalities such as thrombosis, pulmonary embolism (the leading cause of death in affected patients), and pulmonary cysts which may be rapidly progressive, and lead to recurrent infections.[13,26]

Capillary Vascular Malformation of the Lower Lip, Lymphatic Malformations of the Head and Neck, Asymmetry, and Partial or Generalized Overgrowth Syndrome

Capillary malformations of the lower lip, LM of the face and neck, asymmetry, and partial/generalized overgrowth (CLAPO) is a rare syndrome. CLAPO is characterized by midline symmetric lower lip CMs associated with facial or cervical LMs that are sometimes accompanied by asymmetric overgrowth.[35] CMs of the lower lip are present in 100% of CLAPO cases. LMs may not be evident at birth. CLAPO may arise sporadically as a consequence of somatic activating mutations in PIK3CA.[36]

SUMMARY

CMs are complex congenital slow-flow VM of dermal capillaries and postcapillary venules. In most cases, a diagnosis can be made on clinical appearance and patient history. While CMs are often isolated skin anomalies, they are rarely associated with complex malformation syndromes, some of which may be subtle. Identifying these syndromes is vitally important as the clinician can differentiate benign, innocuous CMs from those associated with life-threatening tumors, coagulopathies, AVMs, and more. Genotyping can be an extremely helpful tool when needed. Imaging studies are not routinely performed on routine CMs, but ultrasonography or magnetic resonance may be necessary for the evaluation of associated syndromes.[7,26]

Furthermore, even small, isolated CMs can be disfiguring and a source of significant psychological stress for patients.[37] The goals of treatment (discussed in the treatment section) are aimed at reducing skin discoloration and preventing complications such as thickening, nodularity, or ulceration.

CMs present both a diagnostic and therapeutic challenge to physicians. Overlapping clinical features can be observed in many cases of syndromic CMs. The classifications presented here can aid clinicians in better identifying CMs and provide consistent terminology to facilitate the interdisciplinary management of the diverse vascular anomalies.

CONFLICTS OF INTEREST

Dr. M. N. Jahnke has served as a consultant for Sanofi Genzyme. Dr. K. Pandher and Karla Escobar do not have any financial or commercial interests to disclose. There were no funding sources for this article.

CLINICS CARE POINTS

- PIK3CA, GNAQ and GNA11 mutations are the most common mutations in CMs.
- Most CMs of the face (PWS) are not associated with SWS, however, those involving the frontonasal placode and are bilateral convey the highest risk.
- Although CMs are generally stable over time, cutaneous complications may include darkening, thickening, vascular blebs, pyogenic granuloma-like lesions and soft tissue hypertrophy.
- Due to the autosomal dominant inheritance of the RASA1 gene mutation in CM-AVM, it is one of the more common yet worrisome syndromes associated with CMs and

- recognition is critical due to the risk of internal AVMs and AVFs.
- HHT presents with CMs and extensive telangiectasias of the skin and muscosa with risk for GI hemorrhage and AVMs.

REFERENCES

1. Maguiness SM, Liang MG. Management of capillary malformations. Clin Plast Surg 2011;38(1):65–73.
2. Ustaszewski A, Janowska-Głowacka J, Wołyńska K, et al. Genetic syndromes with vascular malformations - update on molecular background and diagnostics. Arch Med Sci AMS 2021;17(4):965–91.
3. Orme CM, Boyden LM, Choate KA, et al. Capillary malformation–arteriovenous malformation syndrome: review of the literature, proposed diagnostic criteria, and recommendations for management. Pediatr Dermatol 2013;30(4):409–15.
4. Garzon MC, Huang JT, Enjolras O, et al. Vascular malformations: Part I. J Am Acad Dermatol 2007; 56(3):353–70. quiz 371-374.
5. Eubanks LE, McBurney EI. Videomicroscopy of port-wine stains: correlation of location and depth of lesion. J Am Acad Dermatol 2001;44(6):948–51.
6. McCuaig CC. Update on classification and diagnosis of vascular malformations. Curr Opin Pediatr 2017;29(4):448–54.
7. Happle R. Capillary malformations: a classification using specific names for specific skin disorders. J Eur Acad Dermatol Venereol JEADV 2015;29(12):2295–305.
8. Rozas-Muñoz E, Frieden IJ, Roé E, et al. Vascular Stains: Proposal for a Clinical Classification to Improve Diagnosis and Management. Pediatr Dermatol 2016;33(6):570–84.
9. Gonzalez ME, Burk CJ, Barbouth DS, et al. Macrocephaly-capillary malformation: a report of three cases and review of the literature. Pediatr Dermatol 2009;26(3):342–6.
10. Valdivielso-Ramos M, Torrelo A, Martin-Santiago A, et al. Histopathological hallmarks of cutaneous lesions of capillary malformation-arteriovenous malformation syndrome. J Eur Acad Dermatol Venereol JEADV 2020;34(10):2428–35.
11. Bichsel C, Bischoff J. A somatic missense mutation in GNAQ causes capillary malformation. Curr Opin Hematol 2019;26(3):179–84.
12. Mulliken JB. Capillary Malformations, Hyperkeratotic Stains, Telangiectasias, and Miscellaneous Vascular Blots. In: Mulliken JB, Burrows PE, Fishman SJ, editors. Mulliken and Young's vascular anomalies. Oxford University Press; 2013. p. 508–61. https://doi.org/10.1093/med/9780195145052.003.0013.
13. Martinez-Lopez A, Salvador-Rodriguez L, Montero-Vilchez T, et al. Vascular malformations syndromes: an update. Curr Opin Pediatr 2019;31(6):747–53.

14. Couto JA, Huang L, Vivero MP, et al. Endothelial Cells from Capillary Malformations Are Enriched for Somatic GNAQ Mutations. Plast Reconstr Surg 2016;137(1):77e–82e.

15. Sujansky E, Conradi S. Outcome of Sturge-Weber syndrome in 52 adults. Am J Med Genet 1995; 57(1):35–45.

16. Tallman B, Tan OT, Trainor S, et al. Location of Port-Wine Stains and the Likelihood of Ophthalmic and/or Central Nervous System Complications. Pediatrics 1991;87(3):323–7.

17. Dowling MB, Zhao Y, Darrow DH. Orodental manifestations of facial port-wine stains. J Am Acad Dermatol 2012;67(4):687–93.

18. Lee MS, Liang MG, Mulliken JB. Diffuse capillary malformation with overgrowth: a clinical subtype of vascular anomalies with hypertrophy. J Am Acad Dermatol 2013;69(4):589–94.

19. Goss JA, Konczyk DJ, Smits P, et al. Diffuse capillary malformation with overgrowth contains somatic PIK3CA variants. Clin Genet 2020;97(5):736–40.

20. Hughes M, Hao M, Luu M. PIK3CA vascular overgrowth syndromes: an update. Curr Opin Pediatr 2020;32(4):539–46.

21. Amyere M, Revencu N, Helaers R, et al. Germline Loss-of-Function Mutations in EPHB4 Cause a Second Form of Capillary Malformation-Arteriovenous Malformation (CM-AVM2) Deregulating RAS-MAPK Signaling. Circulation 2017;136(11):1037–48.

22. Pavlović M, Neubauer D, Al Tawari A, et al. The microcephaly-capillary malformation syndrome in two brothers with novel clinical features. Pediatr Neurol 2014;51(4):560–5.

23. McDonell LM, Mirzaa GM, Alcantara D, et al. Mutations in STAMBP, encoding a deubiquitinating enzyme, cause microcephaly-capillary malformation syndrome. Nat Genet 2013;45(5):556–62.

24. Valdivielso-Ramos M, Martin-Santiago A, Azaña JM, et al. Capillary malformation-arteriovenous malformation syndrome: a multicentre study. Clin Exp Dermatol 2021;46(2):300–5.

25. Eerola I, Boon LM, Mulliken JB, et al. Capillary malformation-arteriovenous malformation, a new clinical and genetic disorder caused by RASA1 mutations. Am J Hum Genet 2003;73(6):1240–9.

26. Garzon MC, Huang JT, Enjolras O, et al. Vascular malformations. Part II: associated syndromes. J Am Acad Dermatol 2007;56(4):541–64.

27. Dutta A, Ghosh SK, Bandyopadhyay D, et al. Phakomatosis Pigmentovascularis: A Clinical Profile of 11 Indian Patients. Indian J Dermatol 2019;64(3):217–23.

28. Happle R. Phacomatosis pigmentovascularis revisited and reclassified. Arch Dermatol 2005;141:385–8.

29. Nanda A, Al-Abdulrazzaq HK, Habeeb YKR, et al. Phacomatosis pigmentovascularis: Report of four new cases. Indian J Dermatol Venereol Leprol 2016;82(3):298–303.

30. Shields CL, Kligman BE, Suriano M, et al. Phacomatosis pigmentovascularis of cesioflammea type in 7 patients: combination of ocular pigmentation (melanocytosis or melanosis) and nevus flammeus with risk for melanoma. Arch Ophthalmol Chic Ill 1960 2011;129(6):746–50.

31. Van Raamsdonk CD, Bezrookove V, Green G, et al. Frequent somatic mutations of GNAQ in uveal melanoma and blue naevi. Nature 2009;457(7229):599–602.

32. Thomas AC, Zeng Z, Rivière JB, et al. Mosaic Activating Mutations in GNA11 and GNAQ Are Associated with Phakomatosis Pigmentovascularis and Extensive Dermal Melanocytosis. J Invest Dermatol 2016;136(4):770–8.

33. Olitsky SE. Hereditary hemorrhagic telangiectasia: diagnosis and management. Am Fam Physician 2010;82(7):785–90.

34. Carqueja IM, Sousa J, Mansilha A. Vascular malformations: classification, diagnosis and treatment. Int Angiol 2018;37(2). https://doi.org/10.23736/S0392-9590.18.03961-5.

35. Ivars M, Doixeda P, Triana P, et al. Clinical overlap between CLAPO syndrome and macrocephaly-capillary malformation syndrome. JDDG J Dtsch Dermatol Ges 2020;18(5):479–82.

36. Rodriguez-Laguna L, Ibañez K, Gordo G, et al. CLAPO syndrome: identification of somatic activating PIK3CA mutations and delineation of the natural history and phenotype. Genet Med Off J Am Coll Med Genet 2018;20(8):882–9.

37. Lanigan SW, Cotterill JA. Psychological disabilities amongst patients with port wine stains. Br J Dermatol 1989;121(2):209–15.

Venous Malformations
A Journey Through Their Multifaceted Clinical Presentations

Maria Gnarra Buethe, MD, PhD[a], Susan J. Bayliss, MD[b],
Leonid Shmuylovich, MD, PhD[b],*

KEYWORDS

- Venous malformations • Vascular malformations • Localized intravascular coagulopathy
- Thrombosis

KEY POINTS

- Venous malformations (VMs) are the most common congenital vascular malformation.
- VMs are the result of smooth muscle cell defects during angiogenesis.
- VMs have a broad clinical presentation from isolated asymptomatic lesions to severe diffuse extension.
- Pain and localized intravascular coagulopathy are the most common complications.

INTRODUCTION

Venous malformations (VMs) are both the most common type of slow-flow congenital vascular malformation and the most common reason for referral to specialty vascular anomalies centers.[1] VMs result from congenital defects in the development of smooth muscle cells during angiogenesis leading to abnormally dilated venous channels. Although locally abnormal angiogenesis is present at birth, VMs may only become apparent after some period of growth in early childhood. VMs show no ethnic or gender predilection and occur with an incidence of 1 in 2000 to 5000 births.[2] According to the 2018 International Society for the Study of Vascular Anomalies classification,[3] VMs include several distinct types: (1) Common focal and multifocal VMs, (2) Familial cutaneomucosal VMs (VMCM), (3) VMs associated with blue rubber bleb nevus syndrome (BRBNS), (4) Glomuvenous

malformations (GVM), (5) Cerebral cavernous malformations (CCM), (6) Familial intraosseous vascular malformations (VMOSs), and (7) Verrucous venous malformations (VVM). In some cases, VMs occur in the context of other cutaneous or systemic findings that comprise rare genetic syndromes like Maffucci syndrome, Proteus syndrome, PIK3CA-related overgrowth syndrome (PROS), and PTEN syndrome.

Although VMs may be small and asymptomatic, they also can be large and complicated by localized coagulopathy as well as by continued growth, which can lead to pain, functional impairment, and disfigurement. Therapeutic options often require a multidisciplinary approach, including interventional radiology, surgery, and oncology. Discoveries of the genetic basis of VMs have led to new targeted medical treatment options.

The clinical management of patients with large and complex VMs can be a challenge. VMs may

Author Contributions: All authors contributed to the planning, writing, and editing of the article. S.J. Bayliss and L. Shmuylovich provided patient photographs.
Conflicts of Interest: None.
Funding: None.
[a] Department of Dermatology, SUNY Downstate Health Sciences University, 450 Clarkson Avenue, Brooklyn, NY 11203, USA; [b] Division of Dermatology, Department of Medicine, Washington University in St. Louis School of Medicine, 660 South Euclid, MSC 8123-29-10014, Saint Louis, MO 63110, USA
* Corresponding author.
E-mail address: shmuylol@wustl.edu

Dermatol Clin 40 (2022) 435–443
https://doi.org/10.1016/j.det.2022.06.001

range from asymptomatic to debilitating or may represent a clue to an underlying genetic syndrome with significant extracutaneous manifestations that require specialty care. Understanding the typical clinical presentation of VMs, syndromes associated with VMs, and clinical mimics of VMs can help guide clinicians as to which patients require referral to specialty vascular anomaly clinics. Therefore, in this work, the authors review the clinical features of VMs with a particular focus on presentation and differential diagnosis.

Clinical Presentation

More than 90% of VMs present as isolated focal lesions, whereas the remainder are multifocal or diffuse.[4] More than 40% of VMs occur in the head and neck region,[5] and the remainder are more likely to present on the extremities than the trunk. Clinically, VMs appear as blue to purple subcutaneous compressible nodules with rapid refilling following compression (**Fig. 1**). This characteristic bluish discoloration can be difficult to appreciate in patients with darker skin color, making accurate diagnosis more challenging in this patient population. A subcutaneous VM is characterized by a deep swelling without any superficial color change.

VMs can fluctuate in size with positional changes. For example, a patient may report that a head and neck VM feels larger when laying down compared with sitting up, and observing this behavior during the physical examination can assist with diagnosis. A Valsalva maneuver can also induce VM enlargement. VMs are not characterized by a thrill or increased warmth as would be expected in high-flow vascular malformations, such as arteriovenous malformations.

Compression of a VM does not typically induce pain, although painful phleboliths may develop within longstanding VMs.

VVMs are a subtype of VM that presents with hyperkeratotic red-purple papules and plaques often in streaks. On dermoscopy, they resemble angiokeratomas with dark lacunae and a blue-white veil.[6] **Fig. 2** demonstrates a clinical photograph and dermoscopic images of a VVM on the ankle that partially recurred after surgery, which is unfortunately a typical outcome after surgery.

GVMs are a variant of VMs that, unlike common VMs, are painful to palpation.[7] On physical examination, GVMs are segmental or multifocal pink (at birth) to purple cobblestone-like scattered papules that can rarely involve the mucosa (**Fig. 3**). Suspicion of GVM should prompt further inquiry into affected family members, as it can have an autosomal dominant inheritance pattern.

Multiple VMs are uncommon and may have extracutaneous manifestations. Patients with multiple common mucosal and cutaneous VMs with affected family members may have a rare subtype called familial cutaneo-mucosal VMs,[2] which typically is autosomal dominant.

The presence of multiple VMs plus hematochezia or melena should prompt consideration of BRBNS, which is characterized by tens to hundreds of small cutaneous and mucosal VMs affecting the gastrointestinal (GI) tract.[8] These cutaneous VMs show a predilection for palms and soles (**Fig. 4**), whereas the mucosal VMs can be throughout the GI tract and can cause chronic GI bleeding. BRBNS lesions rarely involve the liver, spleen, bladder, kidneys, lung, and brain.[9]

Patients presenting with cutaneous lesions resembling a VM with a history of seizures or strokes should prompt consideration of a rare

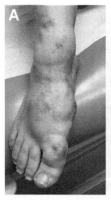
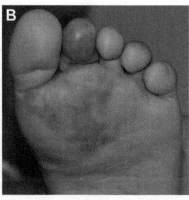
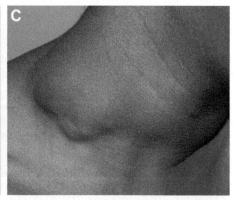

Fig. 1. (*A*) Nodular blue and purple compressible VM affecting the ankle and foot. (*B*) VM affecting the plantar surface, demonstrating less nodularity than (*A*), appearing more as a vascular plaque than nodule. (*C*) VM in an adolescent with pigmented skin. Note the more subtle nature of the blue/purple subcutaneous mass affecting the neck.

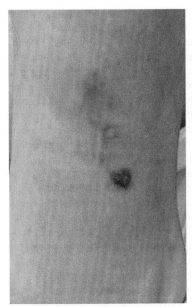
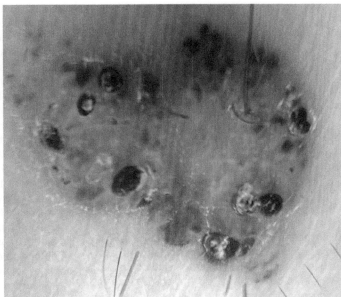

Fig. 2. VVM. Clinical and dermoscopic images of a recurrent VVM on the lateral ankle in an adolescent several years after initial surgical excision.

type of VM called cerebral cavernous malformation. CCMs are lesions in the central nervous system consisting of malformed fragile capillaries and veins with increased risk of hemorrhage, which can cause headache, seizure, focal neurological deficits, and rarely, death. Most patients with CCM remain asymptomatic throughout life and do not have cutaneous findings. About 10% of patients with CCM may have cutaneous vascular lesions, including lesions that resemble a superficial hyperkeratotic VM (**Fig. 5**).[10]

Diagnosis of VMs is based on complete physical examination, family history, and relevant review of systems. In some cases, additional workup is warranted, for example, colonoscopy if BRBNS is suspected. Histopathological confirmation is often not required, although given recent discoveries in the genetic basis of many vascular malformations, genetic sequencing of affected tissue can provide diagnostic confirmation and can guide clinical management. Imaging with contrast-enhanced MRI and Doppler ultrasound can help confirm the diagnosis and is particularly important when planning interventional treatment.[11]

NATURAL HISTORY

Although VMs are present at birth, they may not be noticed until childhood or early adulthood. This

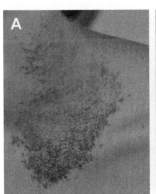
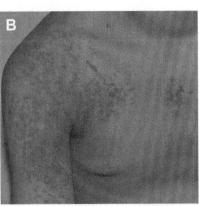
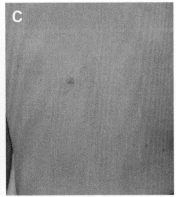

Fig. 3. GVMs can have a variety of presentations. (*A*) A confluent cobblestone-like plaque affecting the neck and anterior chest. (*B*) A segmental presentation affecting the chest shoulder and upper extremity. (*C*) Few scattered multifocal blue papules affecting the back.

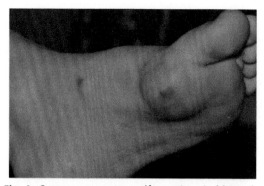

Fig. 4. Cutaneous venous malformations in blue rubber bleb syndrome on the sole.

reflects the fact that the aberrant cells driving VMs may be below a detectable threshold at birth and only become clinically apparent with continued growth. VMs grow slowly, do not show signs of spontaneous regression, and may remain asymptomatic for years. Deep VMs without obvious cutaneous findings may not be noticed until pain or swelling develops. Asymptomatic lesions may enlarge with triggers, such as hormonal changes during puberty or pregnancy.[12] VM growth is slow but can be disfiguring and functionally

debilitating, resulting in morbidity with significant impact on quality of life.[13] Compression of surrounding structures in the VMs can lead to pain, functional impairment, or even life-threatening complications. For example, in a rare subtype of VM called familial intraosseous vascular malformation, there is progressive expansion of intraosseous VMs within the mandibular, maxillary, and cranial regions, which leads to life-threatening increased intracranial pressure and bleeding. Extensive head and neck VM can create challenges for chewing and swallowing[5] and have been associated with migraine headaches.[12]

GI lesions with subsequent GI bleeding, as is seen in BRBNS, can cause severe anemia with coagulopathy,[14] requiring iron supplementation or blood transfusions.[15] GI tract VMs affect the small intestine, where they can cause intussusception, volvulus, and intestinal infarction.[16]

VMs are composed of dilated vessels, which interfere with normal venous flow, leading to stagnant blood that is prone to recurrent local infection and local coagulopathy. This localized intravascular coagulopathy (LIC)[17] consists of recurrent cycles of coagulation cascade activation and affects half of VM patients. As a result, many patients develop painful organized thrombi, called

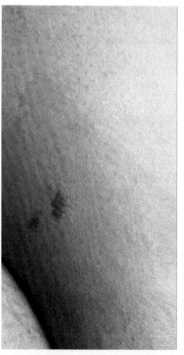
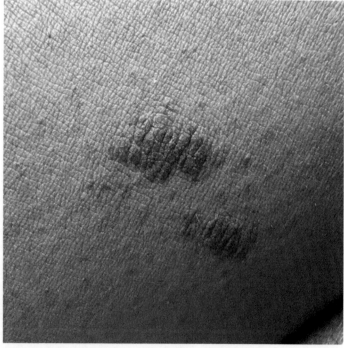

Fig. 5. Cutaneous vascular lesions resembling hyperkeratotic VM on the left inner thigh of an adolescent with pigmented skin. Lesions were present at birth, thought to be benign birthmarks. Patient developed seizures at 5 years of age and was subsequently found to have KRIT1 germline variant, which established a diagnosis of cerebral cavernous malformation.

phleboliths, which can calcify. Phleboliths can be very hard and painful on palpation and can be seen on imaging.[18] Pain associated with VM-associated coagulopathy is usually more severe in the morning, likely because of increased blood stasis overnight.[19] The extent of LIC is highly variable and can be assessed by elevation of D-dimer levels (>0.5 μg/mL). Some patients may have a few phleboliths within a VM that are mildly painful with exertion; some may have numerous phleboliths associated with debilitating chronic pain, and rarely, some patients may have a degree of LIC that predisposes them to disseminated intravascular coagulopathy (DIC) following trauma or procedures.[20] Patients with extensive VMs should be screened for risk of DIC prior to undergoing surgical procedures. In these cases, referral to hematology for risk assessment of hypercoagulability with an anticoagulation plan can be helpful. Finally, acute pain and expansion of a VM should prompt investigation for acute venous thrombosis.[21]

Pathogenesis

Studies have demonstrated that constitutive activation of endothelial cell growth through activating mutations in the *TIE2/PI3K/AKT/mTOR* pathway underlie the pathogenesis of many types of VMs.[22] These mutations lead to unregulated endothelial cell growth and defects in the smooth muscle cells that comprise venous walls, which results in dilated ectatic vasculature.[23] More than half of VMs express an activating mutation in TEK, which encodes for the tunica internal endothelial cell kinase (*TIE2*) tyrosine kinase receptor on endothelial cells, whereas a minority of VMs show a mutation in the *PIK3CA* gene.[24] Although an autosomal dominant inheritance pattern with germline *TIE2* variants has been reported in some cases of diffuse cutaneous-mucosal VMs (VMCM),[24] more than 90% of mutations are thought to be sporadic.[25] Unifocal VMs have been found to have single somatic mutations in *TIE2*, whereas patients with multiple VMs, including multifocal VMs, BRBNS, and some nongermline cases of VMCM, have been found to harbor double mutations in *TIE2*.[15]

Not all types of VM are caused by direct mutations in the *TIE2/PI3K/AKT/mTOR* pathway. A GVM is caused by abnormal proliferation of a type of smooth muscle cell called a glomus cell. GVMs are inherited in an autosomal dominant pattern and are caused by loss-of-function (LOF) mutations in the glomulin gene, which may result in mTOR activation.[26] Autosomal recessive VMOSs are caused by LOF mutations in *ELMO-2*, leading to defective vascular smooth muscles

and decreased RAC-1 signaling.[27] CCM can be sporadic or inherited. Familial cases are due to LOF mutations in *CCM1/KRIT1*, *CCM2/Malcavernin*, and *CCM3/PDCD10*, whereas somatic mutations include *MAP3K3* and GJA4.[28,29] VVMs are caused by sporadic somatic mutations in *MAP3K3*,[30] and like infantile hemangiomas (IHs), show GLUT1+ staining on histopathology.

Venous Malformations Associations

VMs are present in genetic syndromes, which are reviewed in **Table 1** with clinical features specific to each syndrome.

Other rare associations include Servelle-Martorell syndrome characterized by associated bone undergrowth,[36] and Bockenheimer syndrome associated by intra-articular infiltration of the affected limb.[37]

Differential diagnosis
VMs can be confused with other vascular lesions.

- *Lymphatic malformations* (LMs) are slow-flow malformations of the lymphatic system. They may be misdiagnosed as VMs because of their similar appearance of soft subcutaneous blue masses. In addition, hemorrhage into the lymphatic cysts often results in overlying bluish discoloration, making the diagnosis more challenging (**Fig. 6**A).[38] Doppler ultrasound or MRI with contrast confirms the diagnosis. LMs consist of hypoechoic or anechoic cysts with thick septa and fluid levels. Tissue biopsy will show positive D2-40 staining (podoplanin) of lesional tissue.[39] Because combined LMs/VMs are common, it is often difficult to confirm purely lymphatic involvement.[40]
- *Subcutaneous IHs* appear as a bluish soft subcutaneous mass, thus mimicking VMs. IHs are the most common vascular tumors of the infancy. Superficial IHs present as bright red lesions, and subcutaneous IHs can mimic VMs (**Fig. 6**B).[41] Unlike VMs, IHs have a characteristic natural evolution. They appear at birth or shortly after birth as a red patch with a pale halo and undergo rapid growth in the first 2 months of life, followed by a plateau phase and slow involution, which can last years. Doppler ultrasound can aid in the differential diagnosis by differentiating fast-flow IHs from slow-flow VMs.[42] Unlike VMs, IH histopathology will show GLUT-1 positivity.
- *Congenital hemangioma* presents as soft and compressible red-purple nodules. There is a rapidly involuting variant rapidly involuting

Table 1
Other syndromes associated with venous malformations

Syndrome	Gene	Clinical Features (in Addition to VMs)

Maffucci syndrome	IDH1/IDH2	• Enchondromas
		  ○ Often affecting hands and feet
		  ○ Potential malignant degeneration to chondrosarcoma[31]
		• Spindle cell hemangioendotheliomas

Proteus syndrome	AKT1	• Cerebriform connective tissue nevi ○ Often affecting palms and soles • Hemihyperplasia affecting head, face, digits, or limbs • CMs, LMs, epidermal nevi, lipomas, café-au-lait macules[32]
PTEN hamartoma tumor syndrome (Bannayan-Riley-Ruvalcaba, Cowden syndrome)	PTEN	• Genital lentiginosis • Macrocephaly • Intestinal polyposis • Facial, acral, oral verrucous papules, keratoses, papillomas • Lipomatous overgrowth often affecting trunk & extremities • Flexural acrochordons • Café-au-lait macules[33]
PROS	PIK3CA (mosaic)	• Spectrum of disorders including CLOVES and KTS • CLOVES: LMs, CMs, lipomatous overgrowth, epidermal nevi, spinal/skeletal anomalies, often affecting trunk[34] • KTS: CMs, LMs, asymmetric limb overgrowth ○ Often involving lower extremities,[35] knee joint in particular

Abbreviations: CLOVES, congenital, lipomatous; overgrowth, vascular malformations, epidermal nevi, and spinal/skeletal anomalies and/or scoliosis; CMs, capillary malformations; KTS, Klippel-Trenaunay syndrome.

congential hemangioma (RICH) that can be associated with a transient coagulopathy and noninvoluting variant noninvoluting congenital hemangioma (NICH), which often has a characteristic peripheral pallor. Of note, histopathology will not show GLUT-1 positivity.[43]

- *Kaposiform hemangioendothelioma (KHE)* is rare congenital vascular tumor that presents as a solitary violaceous deep plaque (**Fig. 6**C), which can be associated with Kasabach-Merritt Phenomenon (KMP), with a rapid growth of the lesion, new onset of overlying purpura, thrombocytopenia, and consumptive coagulopathy.[44] KHE is considered by many on a spectrum with tufted angioma (TA).
- *TA* may present either at birth or, in the majority of the cases, in early childhood. TA tends to

stabilize and persist after initial growth, but cases of partial or complete regression have been reported. TA appears as a painful violaceous plaque or nodule. Acute worsening pain may signal the onset of KMP, although KMP occurs more commonly in KHE than TA.[45]

Therapeutic approach
Although small isolated VMs may be asymptomatic and warrant observation only, treatment is indicated for any lesions causing pain on posing a risk of functional impairment or disfigurement. VMs management requires a multidisciplinary approach.[46] Therapeutic options include compression garments, sclerotherapy, surgical excision, and laser therapy.[47] Recurrence following surgical excision is common. In conditions like BRBNS where there may be hundreds

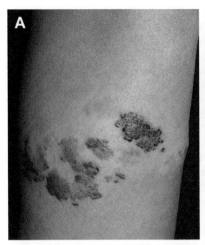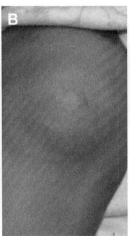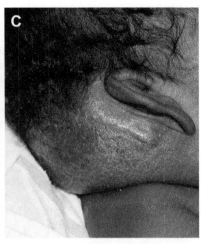

Fig. 6. (*A*) Hemorrhage into superficial blebs of an LM can result in the appearance of a purple plaque, which can be mistaken for a VM. In addition, many LMs likely have both lymphatic and venous components. (*B*) A deep IH, particularly in a patient with pigmented skin, can be difficult to distinguish from a subcutaneous VM. Unlike IHs, however, VMs do not typically regress. (*C*) KHE presents as a red violaceous (particularly in patients with pigmented skin) subcutaneous plaque. The natural history of KHE, in particular, the risk of KMP, is one factor that distinguishes these lesions from VMs.

of lesions, interventional treatments are often not practical. In deeper conditions like CCM of VMOS, the malformations may be surgically inaccessible, where they affect bones and brain. For patients with painful VMs and suspected phleboliths, a daily low dose of aspirin may be helpful in improving pain and swelling.[48] Low-molecular-weight heparin may be useful in managing severe pain associated with VMs complicated by LIC or can be used perioperatively for patients at high risk of DIC. Studies have also shown that rivaroxaban may effectively control VM-associated consumptive coagulopathy.[49]

Medical therapy targeting genetic mutations holds promise. Sirolimus (rapamycin), an mTOR inhibitor, has shown efficacy for slow-flow vascular malformations. Although some patients with VMs will experience improvement in symptoms with sirolimus, the response rate appears to be higher for patients with LMs.[50,51] Additional targeted medical treatment options, including the recently Food and Drug Administration–approved PI3Kα-specific inhibitor Alpelisib, may one day prove to be more efficacious than sirolimus for patients with VMs.[52]

SUMMARY

VMs embody a broad spectrum of slow-flow vascular malformations ranging from isolated to diffuse skin lesions that can affect bone, GI tract, and central nervous system. Based on the size, location, and extension, symptoms and complications are highly variable and can range from no

symptoms to painful, functionally impaired, disfigured lesions with life-threatening hemorrhage and coagulopathy. An interdisciplinary team composed of dermatologists, surgeons, interventional radiologists, and hematologists helps ensure that the medical needs of patients with VMs are met.

CLINICS CARE POINTS

- Isolated asymptomatic lesions can be managed with observation only, reserving treatment for symptomatic lesions.

- Complete physical examination is essential to help determine if the venous malformation is isolated or part of a more extensive syndrome.

- If syndromic association is suspected, referral to vascular anomaly specialty clinic is appropriate.

- Assessment of pain and other associated symptoms, including joint impairment, is important to help prevent complications.

- Localized pain is often the result of phlebolith formation. Daily aspirin can help, but in some settings, more aggressive anticoagulation may be warranted.

- Genetic testing has transformed the understanding of venous malformations. Targeted treatment is now available and should be considered in severe cases.

REFERENCES

1. Hage AN, Chick JFB, Srinivasa RN, et al. Treatment of venous malformations: the data, where we are, and how it is done. Tech Vasc Interv Radiol 2018; 21(2):45–54. Epub 2018 Mar 8. PMID: 29784122.

2. Boon LM, Mulliken JB, Enjolras O, et al. Glomuvenous malformation (glomangioma) and venous malformation: distinct clinicopathologic and genetic entities. Arch Dermatol 2004;140:971–6.

3. ISSVA Classification of Vascular Anomalies ©2018 International Society for the Study of Vascular Anomalies. Available at: issva.org/classification. Accessed April 07, 2022.

4. Mulliken JB, Burrows PE, Fishman SJ. Mulliken & Young's vascular anomalies: hemangiomas and malformations. 2nd edition. Oxford: Oxford University Press; 2013.

5. Seront E, Vikkula M, Boon LM. Venous malformations of the head and neck. Otolaryngol Clin North Am 2018;51(1):173–84. PMID: 29217061.

6. Dhanta A, Chauhan P, Meena D, et al. Linear verrucous hemangioma-a rare case and dermoscopic clues to diagnosis. Dermatol Pract Concept 2018; 8(1):43–7.

7. Brouillard P, Boon LM, Mulliken JB, et al. Mutations in a novel factor, glomulin, are responsible for glomuvenous malformations ("glomangiomas"). Am J Hum Genet 2002;70(4):866–74. PMID: 11845407; PMCID: PMC379115.

8. Bean WT, Charles C III. Vascular spiders and related lesions of the skin. Oxford: Blackwell Scientific Publications; 1959.

9. Wassef M, Vanwijck R, Clapuyt P, et al. [Vascular tumours and malformations, classification, pathology and imaging]. Ann Chir Plast Esthet 2006;51: 263.

10. Sirvente J, Enjolras O, Wassef M, et al. Frequency and phenotypes of cutaneous vascular malformations in a consecutive series of 417 patients with familial cerebral cavernous malformations. J Eur Acad Dermatol Venereol 2009;23:1066–72.

11. Expert Panel on Vascular Imaging, Obara P, McCool J, et al. ACR Appropriateness Criteria® Clinically Suspected Vascular Malformation of the Extremities. J Am Coll Radiol 2019;16:S340.

12. Duyka LJ, Fan CY, Coviello-Malle JM, et al. Progesterone receptors identified in vascular malformations of the head and neck. Otolaryngol Head Neck Surg 2009;141:491–5.

13. Nguyen HL, Bonadurer GF 3rd, Tollefson MM. Vascular Malformations and Health-Related Quality of Life: A Systematic Review and Meta-analysis. JAMA Dermatol 2018;154(6):661–9. PMID: 29562060; PMCID: PMC5876813.

14. Apak H, Celkan T, Ozkan A, et al. Blue rubber bleb nevus syndrome associated with consumption coagulopathy: treatment with interferon. Dermatology 2004;208(4):345–8. PMID: 15178920.

15. Fishman SJ, Smithers CJ, Folkman J, et al. Blue rubber bleb nevus syndrome: surgical eradication of gastrointestinal bleeding. Ann Surg 2005;241:523.

16. Soblet J, Kangas J, Nätynki M, et al. Blue Rubber Bleb Nevus (BRBN) Syndrome Is Caused by Somatic TEK (TIE2) Mutations. J Invest Dermatol 2017;137(1):207–16. Epub 2016 Aug 9. PMID: 27519652.

17. Mazoyer E, Enjolras O, Bisdorff A, et al. Coagulation disorders in patients with venous malformation of the limbs and trunk: a case series of 118 patients. Arch Dermatol 2008;144(7):861–7. PMID: 18645137.

18. Legiehn GM, Heran MK. Venous malformations: classification, development, diagnosis, and interventional radiologic management. Radiol Clin North Am 2008;46(3):545–97.

19. Casanova D, Boon LM, Vikkula M. Les malformations veineuses: aspects cliniques et diagnostic différentiel [Venous malformations: clinical characteristics and differential diagnosis]. Ann Chir Plast Esthet 2006;51(4–5):373–87. French. Epub 2006 Sep 27. PMID: 17007984.

20. Dompmartin A, Acher A, Thibon P, et al. Association of localized intravascular coagulopathy with venous malformations. Arch Dermatol 2008;144(7):873–7. PMID: 18645138; PMCID: PMC5572565.

21. Mavrikakis I, Heran MK, White V, et al. The role of thrombosis as a mechanism of exacerbation in venous and combined venous lymphatic vascular malformations of the orbit. Ophthalmology 2009; 116:1216–24.

22. Vikkula M, Boon LM, Mulliken JB. Molecular genetics of vascular malformations. Matrix Biol 2001;20: 327–35.

23. Dompmartin A, Vikkula M, Boon LM. Venous malformation: update on aetiopathogenesis, diagnosis and management. Phlebology 2010;25(5):224–35. PMID: 20870869; PMCID: PMC3132084.

24. Vikkula M, Boon LM, Carraway KL 3rd, et al. Vascular dysmorphogenesis caused by an activating mutation in the receptor tyrosine kinase TIE2. Cell 1996;87(7):1181–90.

25. Wouters V, Limaye N, Uebelhoer M, et al. Hereditary cutaneomucosal venous malformations are caused by TIE2 mutations with widely variable hyperphosphorylating effects. Eur J Hum Genet 2009;18: 414–20.

26. Kunimoto K, Yamamoto Y, Jinnin M. ISSVA Classification of Vascular Anomalies and Molecular Biology. Int J Mol Sci 2022;23(4):2358. PMID: 35216474; PMCID: PMC8876303.

27. Cetinkaya A, Xiong JR, Vargel I, et al. Loss-of-Function Mutations in ELMO2 Cause Intraosseous Vascular Malformation by Impeding RAC1 Signaling. Am J Hum Genet 2016;99:299–317.

28. Weng J, Yang Y, Song D, et al. Somatic MAP3K3 mutation defines a subclass of cerebral cavernous malformation. Am J Hum Genet 2021;108:942–50.

29. Ugwu N, Atzmony L, Ellis KT, et al. Cutaneous and hepatic vascular lesions due to a recurrent somatic GJA4 mutation reveal a pathway for vascular malformation. HGG Adv 2021;2(2):100028.

30. Couto JA, Vivero MP, Kozakewich HP, et al. Somatic MAP3K3 Mutation Is Associated with Verrucous Venous Malformation. Am J Hum Genet 2015;96: 480–6.

31. Enjolras O, Wassef M, Merland JJ. Syndrome de Maffucci: une fausse malformation veineuse? Un cas avec hémangioendothéliome à cellules fusiformes [Maffucci syndrome: a false venous malformation? A case with hemangioendothelioma with fusiform cells]. Ann Dermatol Venereol 1998; 125(8):512–5. French. PMID: 9747318.

32. Turner JT, Cohen MM Jr, Biesecker LG. Reassessment of the Proteus syndrome literature: application of diagnostic criteria to published cases. Am J Med Genet A 2004;130A(2):111–22. PMID: 15372514.

33. Latiff ZA, Atmawidjaja RW, RajaLope RJ, et al. Bannayan Riley Ruvalcaba syndrome. Ann Acad Med Singap 2010;39(7):578–82. PMID: 20697678.

34. Kurek KC, Luks VL, Ayturk UM, et al. Somatic mosaic activating mutations in PIK3CA cause CLOVES syndrome. Am J Hum Genet 2012;90(6): 1108–15. Epub 2012 May 31. PMID: 22658544; PMCID: PMC3370283.

35. Vahidnezhad H, Youssefian L, Uitto J. Klippel-Trenaunay syndrome belongs to the PIK3CA-related overgrowth spectrum (PROS). Exp Dermatol 2016; 25:17.

36. Ada F, Aslan C. Surgical treatment of Servelle-Martorell syndrome. Turk Gogus Kalp Damar Cerrahisi Derg 2018;26(2):301–4. PMID: 32082751; PMCID: PMC7024127.

37. Ali B, Panossian A, Taghinia A, et al. Diffuse venous malformations of the upper extremity (Bockenheimer Disease): diagnosis and management. Plast Reconstr Surg 2020;146(6):1317–24. PMID: 33234962.

38. Colbert SD, Seager L, Haider F, et al. Lymphatic malformations of the head and neck – current concepts in management. Br J Oral Maxillofac Surg 2013;51:98–102.

39. Wassef M, Vanwijck R, Clapuyt P, et al. Tumeurs et malformations vasculaires, classification anatomo-pathologique et imagerie [Vascular tumours and malformations, classification, pathology and imaging]. Ann Chir Plast Esthet 2006;51(4–5):263–81. French. Epub 2006 Sep 26. PMID: 17005309.

40. Galambos C, Nodit L. Identification of lymphatic endothelium in pediatric vascular tumors and malformations. Pediatr Dev Pathol 2005;8(2):181–9. Epub 2005 Feb 23. PMID: 15719202.

41. Drolet BA, Esterly NB, Frieden IJ. Hemangiomas in children. N Engl J Med 1999;341:173–81.

42. Paltiel HJ, Burrows PE, Kozakewich HP, et al. Soft-tissue vascular anomalies: utility of US for diagnosis. Radiology 2000;214(3):747–54. PMID: 10715041.

43. Lee PW, Frieden IJ, Streicher JL, et al. Characteristics of noninvoluting congenital hemangioma: a retrospective review. J Am Acad Dermatol 2014; 70(5):899–903.

44. Drolet BA, Trenor CC, Brandão LR, et al. Consensus-derived practice standards plan for complicated Kaposiform hemangioendothelioma. J Pediatr 2013; 163(1):285–91.

45. Osio A, Fraitag S, Hadj-Rabia S, et al. Clinical spectrum of tufted angiomas in childhood: a report of 13 cases and a review of the literature. Arch Dermatol 2010;146(7):758–63.

46. Enjolras O. Classification and management of the various superficial vascular anomalies: hemangiomas and vascular malformations. J Dermatol 1997;24(11):701–10. PMID: 9433027.

47. van der Vleuten CJ, Kater A, Wijnen MH, et al. Effectiveness of sclerotherapy, surgery, and laser therapy in patients with venous malformations: a systematic review. Cardiovasc Intervent Radiol 2014;37(4): 977–89. Epub 2013 Nov 7. PMID: 24196269.

48. Nguyen JT, Koerper MA, Hess CP, et al. Aspirin therapy in venous malformation: a retrospective cohort study of benefits, side effects, and patient experiences. Pediatr Dermatol 2014;31(5):556–60. Epub 2014 Jul 21. PMID: 25040175.

49. Mack JM, Richter GT, Crary SE. Effectiveness and safety of treatment with direct oral anticoagulant rivaroxaban in patients with slow-flow vascular malformations: a case series. Lymphat Res Biol 2018; 16(3):278–81. Epub 2018 Mar 27. PMID: 29583078.

50. Hammer J, Seront E, Duez S, et al. Sirolimus is efficacious in treatment for extensive and/or complex slow-flow vascular malformations: a monocentric prospective phase II study. Orphanet J Rare Dis 2018;13(1):191. PMID: 30373605; PMCID: PMC6206885.

51. Maruani A, Tavernier E, Boccara O, et al. Sirolimus (Rapamycin) for slow-flow malformations in children: the observational-phase randomized clinical PERFORMUS trial. JAMA Dermatol 2021;157(11): 1289–98. PMID: 34524406; PMCID: PMC8444064.

52. Kangas J, Nätynki M, Eklund L. Development of molecular therapies for venous malformations. Basic Clin Pharmacol Toxicol 2018;123(Suppl 5):6–19. Epub 2018 May 29. PMID: 29668117.

Arteriovenous Malformations

Shomoukh AlShamekh, MD*

KEYWORDS

- Vascular malformations • Arteriovenous malformations • AVMs
- International Society for the Study of Vascular Anomalies • Steal syndrome

KEY POINTS

- Standardized nomenclature and classifications should be used to describe these malformations.
- Multi-disciplinary management is key as there is no single best modality of treatment.

INTRODUCTION

As classified by the International Society for the Study of Vascular Anomalies, arteriovenous malformations (AVMs) refer to a group of high-flow congenital vascular malformations.[1,2] They are characterized by abnormal shunting of the blood supply from high-flow feeding arteries to low-resistance veins via a cluster of aberrant blood vessels termed a central nidus; by doing so, they bypass the normal capillary bed. Arteriovenous fistulas (AVFs) are also high-flow vascular malformations; however, they differ by directly connecting an artery and a vein without a nidus. AVFs may be congenital or iatrogenic, whereas AVMs are predominately congenital.[1-3]

CLINICAL FINDINGS AND NATURAL HISTORY

The pathophysiology of AVMs is still poorly understood. Although most AVMs are sporadic, they can present with associated syndromes, suggesting a genetic pathway; some of these syndromes include Parkes Weber, COBB syndrome, capillary malformation-arteriovenous malformation (CM-AVM), hereditary hemorrhagic telangiectasia (HHT), and PTEN hamartoma tumor syndrome.[4-7] Genes that may play a role in the formation of AVMs and associated syndromes are reviewed in Dov Charles Goldenberg and Rafael Ferreira Zatz's "Surgical Treatment of Vascular Anomalies", in this issue.

AVMs are perhaps the most complex vascular malformation to diagnose and manage and often lead to significant morbidity and mortality.[3,8] Although AVMs are primarily congenital, only 50% of children have visible defects at birth, and approximately 80% will become evident around puberty.[9-11] In many cases, the clinically inapparent fast-flow nature of the malformation delays diagnosis. Early detection of AVMs through recognizing the early subtle clinical features and referral to a multidisciplinary team of experienced physicians is essential for the best possible outcome.

AVMs may occur anywhere in the body, including the skin, muscle, bone, internal organs, and the central nervous system; the brain is the most common location.[1,9] Extracranial AVMs, also termed peripheral AVMs, are most frequently located in the head and neck (47.4%), followed by the extremities (28.5%).[3,8] In this article, the author focuses solely on peripheral AVMs.

DIAGNOSIS

Most AVMs are diagnosed through a thorough history and physical examination. An innocuous pink or red vascular patch may be seen anywhere on the skin or mucosa in childhood. Despite its quiescent appearance at this stage, a hand-held Doppler will detect high flow, which helps differentiate it from the more common capillary malformation and allows for earlier diagnosis.[3,12,13] These

Disclosures: None.
Department of Dermatology, Children's Hospital of Philadelphia, Philadelphia, PA, USA
* 2431 Bainbridge Street, Philadelphia, PA 19146, USA
E-mail address: Shomoukh.s@gmail.com

Dermatol Clin 40 (2022) 445–448
https://doi.org/10.1016/j.det.2022.06.012

Table 1
The Schobinger clinical classification of arteriovenous malformations

Stage	Description
I (quiescence)	Pink bluish stain, warmth, and arteriovascular shunting
II (expansion)	Enlargement, pulsations, thrill, bruit, and tortuous/tense veins
III (destruction)	Dystrophic skin changes, ulceration, bleeding, persistent pain, or tissue necrosis
IV (decompensation)	High-output cardiac failure

lesions eventually evolve later in childhood or adolescence into bulkier, pulsatile, painful vascular masses with a palpable thrill. AVM growth is thought to be triggered by hormonal stimulation, such as puberty or pregnancy as well as trauma; this explains why most AVMs are diagnosed later in life, usually in the second or third decade.[3,14]

Symptoms vary widely from being asymptomatic to life-threatening hemorrhage in very large AVMs. Location, magnitude, and the number of the AVMs determine the clinical findings and outcome. Focal AVMs usually have a favorable prognosis with appropriate management. However, diffuse lesions have multiple feeding vessels, resulting in high recurrence rates despite treatment.[9,15] Recurrence rate is decreased in AVMs managed in early stages, further emphasizing the importance of early diagnosis.[15]

In syndromes with central nervous system and other visceral involvement AVMs, cutaneous findings may be the initial clue to detecting those at risk and potentially preventing disastrous outcomes. In CM-AVM, patients present with multiple rust-colored, well-demarcated, round vascular patches, often with a surrounding halo, and some patches may also exhibit fast flow on Doppler. There will frequently be a family history of similar stains and/or a history of a hemorrhagic stroke.[6] In HHT, the Curaçao clinical criteria are used for diagnosis. The 4 criteria include multiple mucocutaneous telangiectasias, with the hands and mouth being classic locations, recurrent epistaxis, visceral AVMs, and a first-degree relative with HHT. A diagnosis is considered definite if 3 or more criteria are present and probable if 2 criteria are present.[16]

The severity of symptoms is variable and directly related to the chronic hemodynamic effects caused by shunting from the high-flow feeding arteries to the low-resistance veins leading to venous hypertension. Reduced perfusion of adjacent structures leads to ischemia via steal phenomenon; this causes pain, ulceration, and visual loss if the ophthalmic artery is involved. If the AVM is large enough, high-output cardiac failure may rarely develop. Thick telangiectasias in active AVMs will frequently bleed, and even the most minor bleeding site will classically lead to forceful pulsatile bleeding that is diffuse, prolonged, and hard to control.[3,9–11,15] In a cohort of patients younger than 21 years old admitted with complications from vascular anomalies, Kim and colleagues[17] found that children with AVMs had the highest rate of in-hospital mortality and almost twice the medical cost when compared with other vascular anomalies.

CLASSIFICATION OF ARTERIOVENOUS MALFORMATIONS
Clinical Classification

Schobinger's clinical classification is a scoring system that measures the severity of AVMs and outlines the natural history of the malformation (**Table 1**). Stage I is quiescent. Stage II is expansion, whereby the lesion becomes larger and

Table 2
Cho-Do angiographic classification of arteriovenous malformations

Type	Nidus Structure	Description
I	Arteriolo-venular	Less than 4 arteries or shunt into a single vein
II	Arteriolo-venular	Multiple arterioles shunt into a single vein
IIIa	Nondilated arteriolo-venular	Numerous delicate/fine shunts between arterioles and venules
IIIb	Dilated arteriolo-venular	Numerous dilated shunts between arterioles and venules

Table 3
Yakes arteriovenous malformation angiographic classification system

Type	Morphology
Ia	Direct shunting between arteriovenous fistulas
IIa	Typical AVM nidus
IIb	Typical AVM nidus with aneurysmal vein outflow
IIIa	Nidus is an aneurysmal vein wall
IIIb	Same as type IIIa but with multiple vein walls acting as a nidus
IV	AVM infiltrating tissue via innumerable microfistulas

develops the more identifiable characteristics of AVM, such as bruit and thrill. In stage III, destruction ensues with ulceration, necrosis, and bony lytic lesions; finally, high-output heart failure ensues in stage IV.[15] Liu and colleagues[15] reviewed 272 children with peripheral AVMs; 82.6% of stage I AVMs progressed before adulthood, with an average age of 12.7 years. Only 1.4% of patients reached stage 4, which is heart failure.

Angiographic Classification

The Cho-Do classification was described in 2006 and divides AVMs into 4 types based on the angioarchitecture of the nidus, summarized in **Table 2**. Most patients, 77%, were found to have type IIIb AVMs (dilated arteriolo-venular) either isolated or in combination with other types.[18] The Yakes classification, developed later, describes the nidus in addition to more specific morphologic measures, including the quantity and size of the draining veins[19] (**Table 3**). This aims to guide further the best treatment modality, reviewed in later articles.

CLINICS CARE POINTS

Arteriovenous malformations are highly aggressive, complex, high-flow vascular anomalies that are difficult to manage and lead to significant morbidity, including tissue and bone necrosis, ulceration, and deformity.

These lesions often present in early childhood as a red or pink vascular patch, mainly on the head, neck, ears, and extremities. These are often misdiagnosed as other vascular malformations until early adulthood when puberty

triggers growth to the more classic-appearing arteriovenous malformations.

Doppler ultrasound can detect high flow in the earliest stages of arteriovenous malformations. Utilizing this for indeterminate and suspicious vascular patches is an excellent noninvasive method for early detection.

Recurrences in arteriovenous malformations are common. Management in the earlier stages by a multidisciplinary team of knowledgeable physicians reduces this risk and results in optimal outcomes.

REFERENCES

1. Mulliken JB, Burrows PE, Fishman SJ. Mulliken and Young's vascular anomalies hemangiomas and malformation. Oxford Med Online; 2013.
2. International Society for the Study of Vascular Anomalies. ISSVA classification for vascular anomalies—2018. ISSVA; 2018.
3. Greene AK, Orbach DB. Management of arteriovenous malformations. Clin Plast Surg 2011;38(1): 95–106.
4. Tan W, Baris HN, Burrows PE, et al. The spectrum of vascular anomalies in patients with PTEN mutations: implications for diagnosis and management. J Med Genet 2007;44:594–602.
5. Revencu N, Boon LM, Mulliken JB, et al. Parkes Weber syndrome, vein of Galen aneurysmal malformation, and other fast-flow vascular anomalies are caused by RASA1 mutations. Hum Mutat 2008;29:959–65.
6. Revencu N, Boon LM, Mendola A, et al. RASA1 mutations and associated phenotypes in 68 families with capillary malformation-arteriovenous malformation. Hum Mutat 2013;34(12):1632–41.
7. Thiex R, Mulliken JB, Revencu N, et al. A novel association between RASA1 mutations and spinal arteriovenous anomalies. AJNR Am J Neuroradiol 2010; 31(4):775–9.
8. Uller W, Alomari AI, Richter GT. Arteriovenous malformations. Semin Pediatr Surg 2014;23(4):203–7.
9. Kohout MP, Hansen M, Pribaz JJ, et al. Arteriovenous malformations of the head and neck: Natural history and management. Plast Reconstr Surg 1998;102:643–54.
10. Kim JB, Lee JW, Choi KY, et al. Clinical Characteristics of Arteriovenous Malformations of the Head and Neck. Dermatol Surg 2017;43:526–33.
11. Schimmel K, Ali MK, Tan SY, et al. Arteriovenous malformations—current understanding of the pathogenesis with implications for treatment. Int J Mol Sci 2021;22:9037.
12. Galligan ER, Baselga E, Frieden IJ, et al. Characterization of vascular stains associated with high flow. J Am Acad Dermatol 2021;84(3):654–60.

13. Esposito F, Ferrara D, Di Serafino M, et al. Classification and ultrasound findings of vascular anomalies in pediatric age: the essential. J Ultrasound 2019; 22(1):13–25.

14. Kulungowski AM, Hassanein AH, Nosé V, et al. Expression of androgen, estrogen, progesterone, and growth hormone receptors in vascular malformations. Plast Reconstr Surg 2012;129:919e–24e.

15. Liu AS, Mulliken JB, Zurakowski D, et al. Extracranial arteriovenous malformations: natural progression and recurrence after treatment. Plast Reconstr Surg 2010;125(4):1185–94.

16. McDonald J, Bayrak-Toydemir P, DeMille D, et al. Curaçao diagnostic criteria for hereditary hemorrhagic telangiectasia is highly predictive of a pathogenic variant in ENG or ACVRL1 (HHT1 and HHT2). Genet Med 2020;22(7):1201–5.

17. Kim J, Sun Z, Leraas HJ, et al. Morbidity and health-care costs of vascular anomalies: a national study. Pediatr Surg Int 2016;33(2):149–54.

18. Cho SK, Do YS, Shin SW, et al. Arteriovenous Malformations of the Body and Extremities: Analysis of Therapeutic Outcomes and Approaches According to a Modified Angiographic Classification. J Endovasc Ther 2006;13(4):527–38.

19. Yakes WF, Yakes AM. The Yakes AVM classification system: therapeutic implications. In: Mattassi R, Loose DA, Vaghi M, editors. Atlas of hemangiomas and vascular malformations. 2nd edition. Milan: Springer Italia; 2015. p. 263–76.

Genetic Causes of Vascular Malformations and Common Signaling Pathways Involved in Their Formation

Aubrey L. Rose, MS, CGC*, Sara S. Cathey, MD

KEYWORDS

- Vascular • Venous • Capillary • AVM • Lymphatic • Somatic • Germline • PI3K-AKT-mTOR

KEY POINTS

- Genetic causes of vascular malformations include mutations in overlapping gene signaling pathways involved in vasculogenesis, lymphangiogenesis, and angiogenesis. Imbalances in the RAS-MAPK and PI3K-AKT-mTOR signaling pathways are drivers in the development of many vascular malformations.
- Identification of a genetic diagnosis impacts treatment and management for patients and, in the case of germline variants, for their family members.
- Identification of somatic variants requires different testing strategies than identification of germline variants.

Congenital lesions that occur in lymphatic vessels, arteries, veins, capillaries, or in combinations of these tissues are broadly called vascular malformations. The underlying genetic causes of many vascular malformations have been recently discovered as improved characterization of the gene signaling pathways involved in vasculogenesis, lymphogenesis, and angiogenesis has converged with rapid advances in genetic testing technologies.

Taxonomy of vascular malformations based on clinical phenotype has historically "split" into separate categories what common molecular signaling pathways "lump." Molecular diagnosis of vascular malformations is becoming complimentary to clinical diagnosis. The emergence of targeted therapies for vascular malformations necessitates awareness of the gene pathways and appropriate genetic testing to reach molecular diagnosis.

Pathogenic variants associated with vascular lesions may be germline or somatic. Germline variants may be inherited from a parent or arise de novo in either gamete or early zygote. Germline variants are in all cells and therefore identifiable in DNA extracted from white blood cells in peripheral blood samples or buccal cells in saliva samples. Somatic mutations are not inherited but arise postzygotically, and identification of somatic mutations in vascular malformations often requires skin/surgical biopsy of affected tissue. Somatic mutations may be absent or present at only very low levels in peripheral blood/saliva DNA. Next-generation sequencing technologies allow identification of lower level mosaic mutations than was achievable with standard Sanger sequencing. Best practice strategies to identify underlying genetic mutations in vascular malformations are influenced by the tissues involved and the type of vascular lesion.

Normal vascular system development and ongoing regulation require continual choreography of positive and negative drivers. The RAS-MAPK and PI3K-AKT-mTOR signaling pathways

Greenwood Genetic Center, 3520 West Montague Avenue, #104, North Charleston, SC 29418, USA
* Corresponding author.
E-mail address: arose@ggc.org

Dermatol Clin 40 (2022) 449–459
https://doi.org/10.1016/j.det.2022.07.002
0733-8635/22/© 2022 Elsevier Inc. All rights reserved.

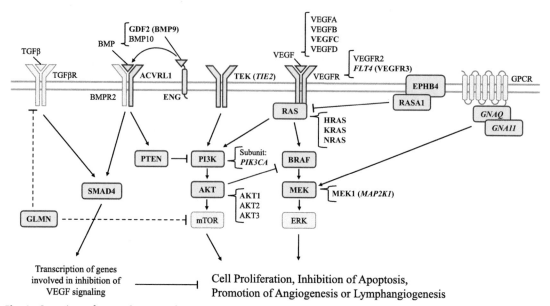

Fig. 1. Overview of normal protein functions within the PI3K-AKT-mTOR, RAS-MAPK, and TGF-β pathways. Genes that cause disorders involving vascular malformations are shown in blue and in bold text. Arrows indicate activation of a pathway, and "T"s indicate inhibition of a pathway. Dotted lines represent pathways that are under investigation.

have emerged as major influencers in the formation of vascular malformations. These well-studied signal transduction pathways are crucial in cell growth, differentiation, and angiogenesis. Dysregulation of these interconnected pathways is implicated in multiple congenital anomaly syndromes, oncogenesis, and also vascular malformations.[1,2] **Fig. 1** depicts theses signaling cascades and additional influencing upstream and downstream pathways. The vascular endothelial growth factor (VEGF) signaling pathway is critical in formation of new blood vessels and lymphatics in embryogenesis and later in angiogenesis. *FLT4 (VEGFR3)* is primarily involved in formation and regulation of lymphatics. *PTEN* is a negative regulator, but *TEK(TIE2)* is a positive regulator of PI3K-AKT-mTOR pathway. Loss-of-function *PTEN* mutations and activating *TEK* mutations result in loss of inhibition or constitutive activation of PI3K-AKT-mTOR and downstream cascades. Genes implicated in hereditary hemorrhagic telangiectasia diseases decrease the transforming growth factor-beta (TGF-β) bone morphogenetic protein signaling pathway (BMP9/10), leading to decreased PTEN activity and increased PI3K-AKT-mTOR. The crosstalk between signaling cascades is a complicated orchestra of synergistic and antagonizing paths. Multiple avenues for pathogenesis of vascular malformations provide multiple potential targets for treatment.

CAPILLARY MALFORMATIONS

Congenital dermal capillary malformations (CMs), also called port wine stains (PWS), can be isolated or observed as part of syndromes, such as Sturge-Weber syndrome (SWS). Widespread CMs can also be associated with soft tissue overgrowth beneath the lesion, termed diffuse capillary malformation with overgrowth (DCMO). The same pathogenic somatic variant, R183Q, in the *GNAQ* gene is identified in approximately 90% of CMs (both isolated PWS and those in SWS or DCMO). *GNAQ* encodes the Gαq subunit of heterotrimeric G-protein.[3,4] G-proteins are involved in a wide range of signaling cascades, and heterotrimeric G-protein is specifically involved in the activation of the RAS-MAPK signaling pathway.[5] The arginine to glutamine change at residue 183 of the Gαq protein (p.R183Q) causes instability in the activation of heterotrimeric G-protein, leading to increased activation of the MAPK signaling pathway.[5,6] A closely related gene, *GNA11*, encodes a different subunit of the heterotrimeric G-protein; *GNA11* mutations have also been reported in patients with isolated CMs, SWS, and DCMO.[6,7] In both isolated CMs and SWS or DCMO, variants in *GNAQ* and *GNA11* occur as mosaic somatic variants, present only in affected cells. Genetic diagnosis requires biopsy of affected tissue and testing designed to identify somatic mutations present at low levels.

Table 1
Capillary Malformations

Gene	Inheritance	Dermatologic Features	Syndromic Features	Tissue Type	Details
GNAQ *GNA11*	N/A (somatic)	Port wine stains, DCMO, or dermal melanocytosis with phakomatosis pigmentovascularis	In Sturge-Weber syndrome: seizures, glaucoma, intellectual disability	Biopsy of affected tissue	p.R183Q in 90% Codon 183 hotspot
RASA1 or *EPHB4*	Autosomal dominant	1- to 2-cm pink or tan round lesions ± surrounded by white halo	CM-AVM syndrome 30% with AVM or AVF in CNS, face, extremities	Blood/saliva	
STAMBP	Autosomal recessive	Small capillary malformations across the body	MIC-CAP syndrome Microcephaly, developmental delay, seizures	Blood/saliva	Exonic and intronic mutations reported

Mosaic pathogenic variants in *GNAQ* and *GNA11* have also been identified in dermal melanocytosis with or without phakomatosis pigmentovascularis lesions. The commonly observed SWS *GNAQ* variant, p.R183Q, was identified in several reported patients, but other *GNAQ* and *GNA11* variants were also identified. *GNAQ* or *GNA11* variants were mosaic, found only in affected tissue and undetectable in blood.[8]

The CMs that characterize capillary malformation-arteriovenous malformation (CM-AVM) syndrome are different than the common CMs. In CM-AVM, the skin lesions are small, round/oval, pink to tan, and may be surrounded by a pale halo. More skin lesions are noted over time. Patients may also have larger (5–22 cm) CMs that are more irregularly shaped and/or very small, pinpoint lesions surrounded by a white halo.[9] As opposed to PWS, which are typically slow flow, these malformations are multifocal and fast flow.[4] Approximately 30% of affected individuals have AVM/AVF in the brain, spine, face, or extremities.[9,10] Identification of CM-AVM syndrome allows for screening and early management of these associated findings.

CM-AVM syndrome is inherited in an autosomal-dominant manner and is caused by germline variants in *RASA1* (50%) or *EPHB4* (10%).[10] *RASA1* and *EPHB4* are involved in the regulation of the RAS-MAPK signaling pathway, functioning as inhibitors of the pathway. Loss-of-function variants in these genes lead to upregulation of the MAPK pathway and the development of CMs and AVMs.[11]

Approximately 40% of patients with CM-AVM syndrome do not have an identifiable variant in *RASA1* or *EPHB4*. The inheritance pattern in these families is still apparently autosomal dominant. It should be presumed that a pathogenic variant is present and currently unidentifiable. CNS imaging for AVM/AVF is recommended in all patients suspected to have CM-AVM syndrome to detect and therefore treat these abnormalities before symptoms arise.[12]

Microcephaly-capillary malformation syndrome (MIC-CAP) is a severe neurodevelopmental disorder that presents at birth with microcephaly and generalized CMs varying from small to large. Patients have severe developmental delay, intractable epilepsy, and profound intellectual disability.[13,14] MIC-CAP is caused by pathogenic variants in the *STAMBP* gene and unlike the other disorders discussed thus far, is inherited in an autosomal recessive manner. *STAMBP* is a deubiquitinating isopeptidase that plays an important role in cell-surface receptor–mediated endocytosis. Cells with deficient *STAMBP* expression show accumulated ubiquitin-conjugated protein aggregates, increased apoptosis (the likely mechanism for the microcephaly), and persistent activation of the RAS-MAPK and PI3K-AKT-mTOR pathways (the mechanism for the CMs)[14] (**Table 1**).

VENOUS MALFORMATIONS

Venous malformations (VM) are the most common type of vascular malformation for which patients seek treatment. VM typically involve skin and mucosa, but deeper lesions in muscle, bone, and internal organs also occur. More than 90% of VM are sporadic, and causative pathogenic mutations are identified at low mutant allele levels only in affected tissue. Sporadic VM include unifocal VM, multifocal VM, and the blue rubber bleb syndrome (BRBN). Familial VM are rare, and the inherited condition called cutaneomucosal venous malformation (VMCM) accounts for just 1% to 2% of VM. Mutations in *TEK* have been found in VMCM and in each of the sporadic type of VM.[15–19] *TEK* encodes the endothelial receptor tyrosine kinase TIE2. *TEK* is an important positive regulator of the downstream PI3K-AKT-mTOR signaling pathway. Activating mutations in *TEK* lead to increased ligand-independent hyperphosphorylation of TIE2, which activates the PI3K-AKT-mTOR pathway.[20]

Single somatic TEK mutations cause 60% of sporadic unifocal VM, and somatic *PIK3CA* mutations account for another 20% of VM.[21] Double *TEK* somatic mutations (2 somatic *TEK* mutations in *cis*) are found in lesions in sporadic multifocal VM and in BRBN. Familial VMCM lesions also demonstrate double TEK mutations on the same allele but one is a germline mutation (consistent with the autosomal dominant inheritance) and the second mutation is somatic. The second hit somatic change may be different in different VM lesions on the same patient.[18,19]

In the familial disorder VMCM the most common *TEK* mutation is the germline missense change, c.2545C>T (p.R849W).[15] The most common somatic *TEK* mutation is c.2740C>T (L1914F), and it is sufficient in and of itself to cause VM.[17,18]

Glomuvenous malformations, named for the characteristic glomus cells in the walls of affected venous channels, are considered a subgroup of VM and account for 5% of VM.[2,22] Glomus cells are abnormally differentiated vascular smooth muscle cells. They are caused by loss-of-function variants, inherited in an autosomal dominant manner, in the *GLMN* gene. Affected patients have one germline variant, which is either *de novo* or inherited from a parent. Cells that acquire a second somatic "hit," or loss-of-function variant, in the *GLMN* gene give rise to glomuvenous malformations. Identification of a pathogenic *GLMN* variant in an affected patient establishes a clear diagnosis and defines recurrence risk for families. Research suggests *GLMN* may be involved in the TGF-β signaling pathway as well as regulation of downstream targets of PI3K[2] (Table 2).

ARTERIOVENOUS MALFORMATIONS

Arteriovenous malformations (AVMs) are most often sporadic. Activating somatic variants in *KRAS*, *BRAF*, and *MAP2K1* (encoding MEK1) have been identified in sporadic AVMs. These genes are involved in the RAS-MAPK signaling pathway.[1,23–25] Hereditary hemorrhagic telangiectasia (HHT) is the most common hereditary cause of AVMs. HHT is inherited in an autosomal dominant manner and is caused by pathogenic variants in *ACVRL1*, *ENG*, *GDF2*, and *SMAD4*.[26,27] These genes are all involved in TGF-β/BMP signaling pathway. BMP9/10 signaling affects endothelial cells' response to VEGF stimulation, and the PIK3 pathway is affected further downstream of VEGF.[26] Thus there are many ways imbalanced VEGF signaling contributes to the development of AVMs and other vascular malformations. The complexity and crosstalk of the pathways provides many targets for treatment. They function to either inhibit or promote VEGF signaling, which regulates angiogenesis.

HHT is characterized by multiple AVMs. The smallest present as telangiectasia of skin and mucosal membranes, many of which can be seen on the skin or form in mucosal membranes. Larger AVMs may also form in the lungs, liver, or brain.[1] Most of the patients (>90%) with HHT have pathogenic loss-of-function variants in either *ENG* or *ACVRL1*. Patients with HHT caused by pathogenic *GDF2* variants tend to have a milder clinical presentation, and patients with HHT caused by *SMAD4* variants have juvenile polyposis syndrome in addition to their features of HHT.[26] Genetic diagnosis and clarification of the causative gene in patients with HHT is crucial for clarification of other health risks. Testing for these germline mutations that cause HHT will be done on DNA from blood or saliva sample. Sequencing and deletion duplication analysis of *ENG* and *ACVRL1* is a reasonable approach.[27] However, multigene vascular malformation panels may be a better option if there is clinical uncertainty. The ideal multigene next-generation sequencing (NGS) "vascular malformations" panel includes all 4 known HHT genes plus other genes associated with inherited conditions that may present with dermal manifestations (the 3 genes associated with cerebral cavernous malformations—*KRIT1*, *CCM2*, and *PDCD10*—plus *PTEN*, *RASA1*, *EPHB4*) (Table 3).

LYMPHATIC MALFORMATIONS

The umbrella term "lymphatic malformations" (LM) applies to solitary cystic LM (microcystic, macrocystic, or mixed), primary lymphedema, and complex lymphatic anomalies involving multiple organs. The complex group includes generalized lymphatic anomaly, Gorham-Stout disease, and central conducting lymphatic anomaly.[28,29]

Table 2
Venous Malformations

Gene	Inheritance	Lesions	Tissue Type for Testing	Details
PIK3CA	N/A (somatic)	Sporadic, unifocal VM (20%)	Biopsy of affected tissue	—
TEK	N/A (somatic)	Sporadic, unifocal VM (60%)	Biopsy of affected tissue	c.2740C>T (L914F) is the most common somatic mutation
	N/A Double somatic TEK mutations in cis	Sporadic, multifocal VM	Mosaicism may be detectable in low levels in blood/saliva	
	N/A Double somatic TEK mutations in cis	BRBN Blue-rubber bleb nevus syndrome Multifocal VM in skin, soft tissues, and GI tract	Biopsy of affected tissue	
	Autosomal dominant germline mutation + somatic second mutation in cis	CMVM syndrome Multiple cutaneous and mucosal venous malformations	Germline mutation in blood/saliva Somatic mutation in lesions	c.2545C>T (R849W) is most common germline mutation
GLMN	Autosomal dominant Most cases familial	Glomuvenous malformations—bluish-purple lesions, tender and noncompressible on palpation Wide clinical variability due to possible somatic second hit	Germline mutation in peripheral DNA, somatic mutation in lesion	Incomplete penetrance, variable expressivity

Table 3
Arteriovenous Malformations

Gene	Inheritance	Lesions	Tissue Type for Testing	Details
KRAS BRAF MAP2K1	N/A (somatic)	Sporadic AVM	Biopsy of affected tissue	
ACVRL1 ENG GDF2 SMAD4	Autosomal dominant	Telangiectasias, AVM in the lungs, liver, or brain	Blood/saliva	Nosebleeds Nosebleeds, juvenile polyposis syndrome

Primary lymphedema is heterogeneous and transmitted in families in either autosomal dominant or autosomal recessive manner. Incomplete penetrance causes variable expressivity and phenotypic variability even among affected members of the same family[30] **(Table 4)**.

Lymphatic abnormalities are also common features of the chromosomal aneuploidy Turner syndrome and the RASopathies—Noonan syndrome (PTPN11, SOS1, RIT1), cardiofaciocutaneous syndrome (BRAF, KRAS), and Costello syndrome (HRAS).[32] The most severe end of the phenotypic spectrum of diseases associated with the X-linked gene IKBKG (previously called NEMO) is osteopetrosis and lymphedema-anhidrotic ectodermal dysplasia with immunodeficiency.[33]

COMPLEX VASCULAR ANOMALIES
PTEN

Germline pathogenic variants in the PTEN gene can cause a spectrum of conditions referred to as PTEN hamartoma tumor syndrome (PHTS). This spectrum includes Cowden syndrome (CS), Bannayan-Riley-Ruvalcaba syndrome (BRRS), and macrocephaly autism syndrome.[34] PTEN plays an important regulatory role in the PI3K-AKT-mTOR signaling pathway by inhibiting PI3K function. Loss of PTEN function causes increased PI3K activity. Increased activation of this important signaling pathway leads to increased cell survival, inhibition of apoptosis, and increased angiogenesis.[35]

Table 4
Lymphatic Malformations

Germline Lymphedema Disease	Inheritance	Gene
Lymphatic malformation 1/Milroy disease	AD	FLT4 (VEGFR3)
Hennekam lymphangiectasia lymphedema syndrome (HLLS) 1	AR	CCBE1
HLLS2	AR	FAT4
HLLS3	AR	ADAMST3
Lymphedema distichiasis syndrome	AR	FOXC2
Emberger syndrome/primary lymphedema with myelodysplasia	AD	GATA2
Lymphatic malformation 3	AD	GJC2
Oculodental dysplasia with lymphedema	AD	GJA1
Choanal atresia and lymphedema	AR	PTPN14
Hypotrichosis-lymphedema telangiectasia syndrome Hypotrichosis-lymphedema telangiectasia syndrome-renal defect	AR AD	SOX18
Lymphatic malformation 4/Milroy-like disease	AD	VEGFC
Microcephaly ± chorioretinopathy, lymphedema, mental retardation	AD	KIF11[30]
Primary lymphedema	AD	ANGPT2[31]

Patients with both CS and BRRS have been observed with various vascular anomalies. Tan and colleagues (2007) described vascular anomalies in a set of patients with PHTS. Fifty-four percent of the patients in this study had vascular anomalies. Radiologically, observed anomalies had features of fast-flow vascular malformations with arteriovenous shunting. When characterized with histopathology, these anomalies appeared as growths of blood vessels, adipose, and fibrous tissue. The location and appearance of these lesions varied between patients. However, all presented with skin discoloration, various degrees of swelling, or pain. About half of the patients with vascular anomalies presented with anomalies at more than one site.[36] A more recent case report characterized vascular malformations found in an adult patient with BRRS. These anomalies were also described as fast-flow with arteriovenous shunting.[37]

PIK3CA

PIK3CA encodes an important subunit of PI3-kinase (PI3K) that is involved in activation of the PI3K-AKT-mTOR pathway. Activating somatic variants in the PIK3CA gene causes a range of symptoms referred to as PIK3CA-related overgrowth spectrum (PROS).[38] Before PIK3CA was identified as the common underlying cause for symptoms, PROS conditions were separated by name into multiple conditions including megalencephaly-capillary malformation syndrome, Klippel-Trenaunay syndrome, fibroadipose vascular anomaly, and CLOVES syndrome (congenital lipomatous asymmetric overgrowth of the trunk, lymphatic, capillary, venous, and combined-type vascular malformations, epidermal nevi, skeletal, and spinal anomalies). Congenital or early onset segmental overgrowth is a main clinical feature.[21,38] The patients with PROS may present with capillary, venous, lymphatic, or mixed vascular malformations.[38,39] PIK3CA mutations are also reported in isolated vascular malformations, in the absence of syndromic overgrowth. It is estimated that 20% of unifocal venous malformations are caused by somatic pathogenic variants in PIK3CA.[18,21] Somatic mutations lead to different features in different tissues, based on when and where (cell type) the mutation occurs. Many of the hotspot mutations in vascular malformations are also common mutations in cancer.[38] Paolacci and colleagues identified the same somatic PIK3CA mutation, E545K, in lesional tissue from 5 patients with different types of vascular malformations: one patient each for lymphatic, lymphatic-venous, and capillary-venous malformations; 2 patients had venous malformations in different areas of the body.[40]

Detecting somatic PIK3CA mutations requires biopsy of affected tissue. Detection rate is affected by sample collection, sample handling, the testing used, and the interpretation of data. Patient factors or surgical considerations determine location of tissue biopsy. Whether it is best to isolate DNA directly from fresh tissue or to culture cells first is not resolved and likely is dependent on the type of tissue, the degree of mutation load, and even the type of mutation. Biopsy and testing of both affected and unaffected tissue requires two biopsies but provides evidence that the mutation is indeed associated with the disease state.[41] Testing strategy—hot spot mutation testing versus full gene analysis—affects diagnostic yield. Although there are recurrent hotspot mutations, there are also many other rare mutations outside these hotspots. Absence of an identifiable PIK3CA variant should not rule out a PROS diagnosis in patients with consistent symptoms.[38]

With new advancements, proper diagnosis of PROS can have a significant impact on treatment. A PIK3CA specifically inhibiting drug, Alpelisib, has recently emerged as a promising treatment of patients with PROS. Patients treated with this drug have observed decreases in overgrowth and improvement of associated symptoms.[39]

Proteus Syndrome

Proteus syndrome is a rare condition characterized by asymmetric disproportionate overgrowth of multiple tissues, commonly including bone, skin, adipose tissue, and the central nervous system. Overgrowth is either mild or not present at birth but presents around 6 to 18 months old and progresses rapidly during childhood as more complex features develop.[42,43] The classic feature is cerebriform connective tissue nevus.[43] Vascular malformations reported in patients with Proteus syndrome include extensive CMs or combined capillary-venous-lymphatic malformations. Arteriovenous malformation and lymphangioma were reported in one patient with Proteus syndrome.[44]

Proteus syndrome is caused by a somatic, mosaic pathogenic variant in AKT1, c.49G>A (p.E17K). Diagnosis is often made based on clinical criteria, but identification of the AKT1 variant in affected tissue can help make a diagnosis in certain cases where a diagnosis is unclear. As with other mosaic somatic variants, identification of the AKT1 p.E17K variant requires analysis of affected tissue. AKT1 plays a crucial role in the PI3K-AKT-mTOR signaling pathway, and

Table 5
Complex Vascular Anomalies

Gene	Inheritance	Dermatologic Features	Syndromic Features	Tissue Type	Details
PTEN	Autosomal dominant	Trichilemmomas, papillomatous lesions, hyperpigmented macules of glans penis, fast-flow vascular anomalies with arteriovenous shunting	Macrocephaly, various cancers, developmental delay, autism, hamartomatous intestinal polyps	Blood/saliva	—
PIK3CA	N/A (somatic)	Capillary malformations, venous malformations	Segmental overgrowth	Biopsy of affected tissue	Sequence variants
AKT1	N/A (somatic)	Capillary malformations, prominent veins, lymphatic malformations	Rapid segmental overgrowth in childhood	Biopsy of affected tissue	c.49 G > A (E17 K)
KRIT1 CCM2 PDCD10	Autosomal dominant	Hyperkeratotic capillary venous malformations, punctate capillary malformations, deep blue nodules	Cerebral cavernous malformations	Blood/saliva	Sequencing and del/dup variants

upregulation of AKT signaling leads to increased cell growth and angiogenesis.[42]

Familial Cerebral Cavernous Malformation

Various cutaneous vascular malformations may also be observed in patients with familial cerebral cavernous malformation (FCCM). Dermal lesions have been reported in approximately 9% of patients with FCCM. Lesions observed in these patients include hyperkeratotic cutaneous capillary-venous malformations, punctate CMs, and deep blue nodules. These malformations are commonly located on extremities. Individuals with FCCM have numerous cerebral cavernous malformations (CCMs), although penetrance is variable even within a family.[45]

FCCM is a dominantly inherited condition caused by pathogenic variants in KRIT1, CCM2, or PDCD10.[45–47] KRIT1 and CCM2 have been identified as playing an important role in vascular permeability, functioning to stabilize endothelial cell-cell junctions.[47] Most of the patients will have either a sequencing or del/dup variant in KRIT1. CCM2 variants are the second most common cause of FCCM, followed by PDCD10 variants. A multigene panel including these 3 genes is most practical to identify a genetic diagnosis. If no variant is identified with sequencing, del/dup analysis should also be performed. A causative variant is identified in at least 75% of families with FCCM.[46] Identification of a genetic cause in a family may aid in diagnosis, management, and treatment of family members at risk for CCMs (**Table 5**).

The identification of the genetic cause of vascular malformations is improving understanding of pathogenesis of these lesions and also informing potential opportunities for treatment. Somatic activating mutations affecting RAS/MAPK and PIK3/AKT/mTOR pathways are implicated in all types of vascular malformations. Numerous drug therapies that inhibit these pathways are in trials or have recently become clinically available. There are many challenges to identifying mosaic somatic mutations. Diagnostic yield is affected by the tissue type submitted for testing, whether DNA is isolated directly from the tissue or if the cells are cultured, the mutant variant allele frequency in the tissue, and the laboratory defined cutoffs for reporting mosaic variants. Deep NGS has allowed identification of pathogenic changes with very low mutant allele frequencies. Although NGS technology is widely available, somatic mutations show tissue heterogeneity; only affected tissues have the mutation, and if the variant allele frequency is less than the laboratory's cutoff for reporting, the mutation will be missed.

It is known that fragments of DNA may be released from cells into the circulatory system in both typical and pathologic processes. This cell-free DNA (cfDNA) can be found in plasma and other body fluids. In the field of oncology "liquid biopsies" using cfDNA isolated from plasma are increasingly used as a less invasive way to assess genetic changes in tumor cells.[48] More recently, a similar approach has been found effective in identifying somatic variants associated with vascular malformations. NGS analysis of cfDNA from plasma has been shown to identify the same somatic variants identified on tissue biopsy from arteriovenous or venous malformations. Somatic mutations identified on tissue biopsy of lymphatic malformations were found in cyst fluid cfDNA but not plasma cfDNA.[49] Palmieri and colleagues used the technique of obtaining samples for cfDNA from an efferent vein at the AVMs. This technique allowed detection of somatic *KRAS* mutations that were not found at all on peripheral cfDNA or found at a much lower variant allele frequency in one patient.[50]

In clinical practice identification of molecular causes of vascular malformations requires insight into likely pathogenesis. When a patient's diagnosis is suspected to be due to a germline mutation (primary lymphedema disorders, CMAVM, PTEN disorders, HHT, CCMs, germline *TEK* mutations in MCVM) blood or saliva sample is appropriate for DNA isolation. Because of the clinical overlap of many of the conditions NGS panels are cost-effective and offer reasonable turnaround times to results. For sporadic lesions, complex/mixed component lesions, and recognized segmental syndromes or overgrowth conditions associated with vascular malformations (Proteus, Sturge Weber, PROS) detection of somatic mutations requires a tissue biopsy of *affected* tissue. For certain sporadic lesions (AVM, VM, LM), cfDNA isolated from an efferent vein may allow for detection of somatic mutations. Tissue biopsies may be required for these lesions before clinical laboratories become well versed in the use of cfDNA liquid biopsies for vascular malformations. Clinical laboratories have to adjust bioinformatics algorithms to detect the very low allele frequency mutations. The experience of cancer genomics has demonstrated that identifying low-level somatic mutations in tissue is achievable at clinical laboratories[51]; this is vital to advancing therapy by precision medicine.

It is important for patients to understand the limitations of genetic testing before testing is ordered and the implications of genetic testing results when reported. Patients with vascular malformations who are undergoing genetic testing need to be educated about the difference between somatic and germline mutations, the likelihood of detecting causative mutations in different sample types, and the implications for recurrence risk within a family. Informed consent requires explanation of the limitations of testing, particularly in cases where somatic variants may be missed if present at a low allele frequency. When a germline condition is suspected, even negative genetic testing results do not guarantee that a condition is not hereditary. Genetic counselors are uniquely qualified to explain complicated genetic information in a way patients can understand. In any case where a genetic cause is suspected and genetic testing is pursued, genetic counseling should be offered.

CLINICS CARE POINTS

- Diagnostic DNA testing may be ordered on peripheral blood sample on patients with suspected autosomal diseases including hereditary hemorrhagic telangiectasia, CM-AVM, PTEN-related diseases, familial cerebral cavernous malformations, familial gloumulovenous disease, and primary lymphedema disorders.

- Tissue biopsy is necessary for possible molecular diagnosis in cases of sporadic or segmental vascular malformations. Mutation detection rate is affected by sample collection and handling, tissue type, mutation load, and type of mutation. Best care requires planning in coordination with the appropriate lab personnel prior to the biopsy procedure.

DISCLOSURE

The authors have nothing to disclose.

REFERENCES

1. Borst AJ, Nakano TA, Blei F, et al. A primer on a comprehensive genetic approach to vascular anomalies. Front Pediatr 2020;8:579591.

2. Fereydooni A, Dardik A, Nassiri N. Molecular changes associated with vascular malformations. J Vasc Surg 2019;70(1):314–26.e1.

3. Shirley MD, Tang H, Gallione CJ, et al. Sturge-Weber syndrome and port-wine stains caused by somatic mutation in GNAQ. N Engl J Med 2013;368(21): 1971–9.

4. Bichsel C, Bischoff J. A somatic missense mutation in GNAQ causes capillary malformation. Curr Opin Hematol 2019;26(3):179–84.

5. Nguyen V, Hochman M, Mihm MC Jr, et al. The Pathogenesis of port wine stain and Sturge Weber syndrome: complex interactions between genetic alterations and aberrant MAPK and PI3K activation. Int J Mol Sci 2019;20(9):2243.

6. Couto JA, Ugur MA, Konczyk DJ, et al. A somatic GNA11 mutation is associated with extremity capillary malformation and overgrowth. Angiogenesis 2017;20(3):303–6.

7. Polubothu S, Al-Olabi L, Carmen Del Boente M, et al. GNA11 mutation as a cause of Sturge-Weber syndrome: expansion of the phenotypic spectrum of $G_{\alpha/11}$ mosaicism and the associated clinical diagnoses. J Invest Dermatol 2020;140(5):1110–3.

8. Thomas AC, Zeng Z, Rivière JB, et al. Mosaic activating mutations in GNA11 and GNAQ are associated with phakomatosis pigmentovascularis and extensive dermal melanocytosis. J Invest Dermatol 2016;136(4):770–8.

9. Revencu N, Boon LM, Mendola A, et al. RASA1 mutations and associated phenotypes in 68 families with capillary malformation-arteriovenous malformation. Hum Mutat 2013;34(12):1632–41. https://doi.org/10.1002/humu.22431.

10. Amyere M, Revencu N, Helaers R, et al. Germline loss-of-function mutations in EPHB4 cause a second form of Capillary Malformation-Arteriovenous Malformation (CM-AVM2) deregulating RAS-MAPK signaling. Circulation 2017;136(11):1037–48.

11. Peterson K, Coffman S, Zehri A, et al. Somatic Mosaicism in the Pathogenesis of de novo Cerebral Arteriovenous Malformations: A paradigm shift implicating the RAS-MAPK signaling cascade. Cerebrovasc Dis 2021;50(2):231–8.

12. Whitaker S, Leech S, Taylor A, et al. Multifocal capillary malformations in an older, asymptomatic child with a novel RASA1 mutation. Clin Exp Dermatol 2016;41:156–8.

13. Carter MT, Geraghty MT, De La Cruz L, et al. A new syndrome with multiple capillary malformations, intractable seizures, and brain and limb anomalies. Am J Med Genet A 2011;155A(2):301–6.

14. McDonell LM, Mirzaa GM, Alcantara D, et al. Mutations in STAMBP, encoding a deubiquitinating enzyme, cause microcephaly-capillary malformation syndrome. Nat Genet 2013;45(5):556–62.

15. Vikkula M, Boon L, Carraway K III, et al. Vascular dysmorphogenesis caused by an activating mutation in the receptor tyrosine kinase TIE2. Cell 1996;(87):1181–90.

16. Limaye N, Wouters V, Uebelhoer M, et al. Somatic mutations in angiopoietin receptor gene TEK cause solitary and multiple sporadic venous malformations. Nat Genet 2009;41(1):118–24.

17. Soblet J, Limaye N, Uebelhoer M, et al. Variable somatic TIE2 mutations in half of sporadic venous malformations. Mol Syndromol 2013;4(4):179–83.

18. Soblet J, Kangas J, Nätynki M, et al. Blue Rubber Bleb Nevus (BRBN) syndrome is caused by somatic TEK (TIE2) mutations. J Invest Dermatol 2017; 137(1):207–16.

19. Queisser A, Seront E, Boon L, et al. Genetic basis and therapies for vascular anomalies. Circ Res 2021;(129):155–73.

20. Wouters V, Limaye N, Uebelhoer M, et al. Hereditary cutaneomucosal venous malformations are caused by TIE2 mutations with widely variable hyperphosphorylating effects. Eur J Hum Genet 2010; 18(4):414–20.

21. Limaye N, Kangas J, Mendola A, et al. Somatic activating PIK3CA mutations cause venous malformation. Am J Hum Genet 2015;97(6):914–21.

22. Brouillard P, Boon LM, Revencu N, et al. Genotypes and phenotypes of 162 families with a glomulin mutation. Mol Syndromol 2013;4(4):157–64.

23. Couto JA, Huang AY, Konczyk DJ, et al. Somatic MAP2K1 mutations are associated with extracranial arteriovenous malformation. Am J Hum Genet 2017;100:546–54.

24. Nikolaev SI, Vetiska S, Bonilla X, et al. Somatic activating KRAS mutations in arteriovenous malformations of the brain. N Engl J Med 2018;378(3):250–61.

25. Al-Olabi L, Polubothu S, Dowsett K, et al. Mosaic RAS/MAPK variants cause sporadic vascular malformations which respond to targeted therapy. J Clin Invest 2018;128(4):1496–508.

26. Snodgrass RO, TJA Chico, Arthur HM. Hereditary haemorrhagic telangiectasia, an inherited vascular disorder in need of improved evidence-based pharmaceutical interventions. Genes 2021;12(2):174.

27. McDonald J, Wooderchak-Donahue W, VanSant Webb C, et al. Hereditary hemorrhagic telangiectasia: genetics and molecular diagnostics in a new era. Front Genet 2015;(6):1.

28. Ozeki M, Fukao T. Generalized lymphatic anomaly and Gorham-Stout disease: overview and recent insights. Adv Wound Care (New Rochelle) 2018;8(6):230–45.

29. Makinen T, Boon L, Vikkula M, et al. Lymphatic malformations genetics, mechanisms and therapeutic strategies. Circ Res 2021;129:136–54.

30. Brouillard P, Boon L, Vikkula M. Genetics of lymphatic anomalies. J Clin Invest 2014;124(3): 898–904.

31. Leppanen VM, Brouillard P, Korhonen E, et al. Characterization of ANGPT2 mutations associated with primary lymphedema. Sci Transl Med 2020; 12(560):eaax8013.

32. Sleutjes J, Kleimeier L, Leenders E, et al. Lymphatic abnormalities in Noonan syndrome spectrum disorders: a systematic review. Mol Syndromol 2022;13: 1–11.

33. Ricci S, Romano F, Nieddu F, et al. OL-EDA-ID syndrome: a novel hypomorphic NEMO mutation associated with a severe clinical presentation and transient HLH. J Clin Immunol 2017;37:7–11.

34. Yehia L, Keel E, Eng C. The clinical spectrum of *PTEN* mutations. Annu Rev Med 2020;71:103–16.

35. Song MS, Salmena L, Pandolfi PP. The functions and regulation of the PTEN tumour suppressor. Nat Rev Mol Cell Biol 2012;13(5):283–96.

36. Tan WH, Baris HN, Burrows PE, et al. The spectrum of vascular anomalies in patients with PTEN mutations: implications for diagnosis and management. J Med Genet 2007;44(9):594–602.

37. Anusic S, Clemens RK, Meier TO, et al. Assessment of PTEN-associated vascular malformations in a patient with Bannayan-Riley-Ruvalcaba syndrome. BMJ Case Rep 2016;2016. bcr2016215188.

38. Keppler-Noreuil KM, Rios JJ, Parker VE, et al. PIK3CA-related overgrowth spectrum (PROS): diagnostic and testing eligibility criteria, differential diagnosis, and evaluation. Am J Med Genet A 2015; 167A(2):287–95.

39. Pagliazzi A, Oranges T, Traficante G, et al. *PIK3CA*-Related Overgrowth Spectrum from Diagnosis to Targeted Therapy: A case of CLOVES syndrome treated with Alpelisib. Front Pediatr 2021;9: 732836.

40. Paolacci S, Mattassi RE, Marceddu G, et al. Somatic variant analysis identifies targets for tailored therapies in patients with vascular malformations. J Clin Med 2020;9(11):3387.

41. Lalonde E, Ebrahimzadeh J, Rafferty K, et al. Molecular diagnosis of somatic overgrowth conditions: A single-center experience. Mol Genet Genomic Med 2019;7:e536.

42. Lindhurst MJ, Sapp JC, Teer JK, et al. A mosaic activating mutation in AKT1 associated with the Proteus syndrome. N Engl J Med 2011;365(7):611–9.

43. He M, Zhao W. Proteus syndrome of the foot: a case report and literature review. Exp Ther Med 2020;20: 2716–20.

44. Asilian A, Kamali AS, Riahi NT, et al. Proteus syndrome with arteriovenous malformation. Adv Biomed Res 2017;6:27.

45. Manole AK, Forrester VJ, Zlotoff BJ, et al. Cutaneous findings of familial cerebral cavernous malformation syndrome due to the common Hispanic mutation. Am J Med Genet A 2020;182(5):1066–72.

46. D'Angelo R, Marini V, Rinaldi C, et al. Mutation analysis of CCM1, CCM2 and CCM3 genes in a cohort of Italian patients with cerebral cavernous malformation. Brain Pathol 2011;21(2):215–24 [Erratum appears in Brain Pathol 2011; 21(3):360].

47. Stockton RA, Shenkar R, Awad IA, et al. Cerebral cavernous malformations proteins inhibit Rho kinase to stabilize vascular integrity. J Exp Med 2010; 207(4):881–96.

48. Palmieri M, Baldassarri M, Fava F, et al. Two-point-NGS analysis of cancer genes in cell-free DNA of metastatic cancer patients. Cancer Med 2020;9(6): 2052–61.

49. Zenner K, Jensen DM, Cook TT, et al. Cell-free DNA as a diagnostic analyte for molecular diagnosis of vascular malformations. Genet Med 2021;23(1): 123–30.

50. Palmieri M, Currò A, Tommasi A, et al. Cell-free DNA next-generation sequencing liquid biopsy as a new revolutionary approach for arteriovenous malformation. JVS Vasc Sci 2020;1:176–80.

51. Siegel D, Cottrell C, Streicher J, et al. Analyzing the genetic spectrum of vascular anomalies with overgrowth via cancer genomics. J Invest Dermatol 2017;138:957–67.

Medical Treatment of Vascular Anomalies

Alexa DeMaio, BS[a], Christina New, MD[b], Shayla Bergmann, MD[b],*

KEYWORDS

- Vascular malformation (VascM) • Vascular anomaly(ies) (VAs) • Sirolimus • mTOR

KEY POINTS

- Sirolimus for medical management of vascular malformations (VascMs)/vascular anomalies (VAs).
- Combined therapy modalities for treatment VM/VA.
- Phosphatidylinositol 3-kinase (PIK3CA)/protein kinase B/mammalian target of rapamycin pathway.
- Role of anticoagulation in VM/VA.
- Future role of MEK and PIK3CA inhibitors.

INTRODUCTION

The treatment of vascular anomalies (VAs) is often complex, combining various approaches which emphasize the art of medicine to provide best outcomes and quality of life for these patients. Treatment may include but is not limited to the following: local control with compression garments and attire, pain control, surgical procedures and debulking, laser therapy, sclerotherapy, and medical management. In this article, the authors discuss the aspects of medical management, visiting the history of medical treatment, the recent utilization and success of enzymatic pathway inhibitors, specifically sirolimus and new therapies that hold promise for the future for these patients.

COMMON MEDICAL MANAGEMENT

VAs often result in acute and sometimes lifelong clinical complications such as disfigurement, acute and chronic pain, coagulopathy, bleeding, thrombosis, organ and musculoskeletal dysfunction, and even death.[1] Medical management has been an important component of the comprehensive treatment plans for VAs (VAs). Historically, treatment of VAs was primarily surgical, composed of excision and debulking along with interventional therapies such as pulsed laser dye and sclerotherapy. Medical therapies were mainly supportive such as compression garments, nonsteroidal anti-inflammatories, and anticoagulation—all with limited utility.

Corticosteroids have been frequently used as the first-line therapy in the treatment of uncomplicated vascular malformations (VascMs), with or without other agents such as propranolol, aspirin, and antifibrinolytics—most often with varying results. The use of conventional chemotherapy (eg, vincristine, cyclophosphamide, or actinomycin-D), interferon, platelet inhibitors (clopidogrel, ticlopidine), antiangiogenetic agents (bevacizumab or Avastin), or combinations of these various agents may be considered as second-line therapy or to treat complex vascular lesions. All such treatment approaches have limited responses yet can cause serious, even potentially fatal adverse events.[2,3] Complicated VAs such as proliferative vascular tumors or refractory VMs have been treated with various approaches and combinations of medical therapies.

The recent advances of pharmacologic agents effective in treating VAs have broadened our medical therapeutic options lessening the need for invasive procedures and therefore improving patients' quality of life.[4] The discovery of sirolimus as an effective treatment has changed the

[a] Medical University of South Carolina, College of Medicine, 14 Lockwood Drive Apartment 9A, Charleston, SC 29401, USA; [b] Division of Pediatric Hematology-Oncology, Medical University of South Carolina, 125 Doughty Street, Suite 520, MSC 917, Charleston, SC 29525, USA
* Corresponding author.
E-mail address: bergmans@musc.edu

Dermatol Clin 40 (2022) 461–471
https://doi.org/10.1016/j.det.2022.06.013

management paradigm of patients with complicated VMs.[4]

Sirolimus (Rapamune or rapamycin), with its specific and potent inhibition of the mammalian target of rapamycin (mTOR), is established as a safe treatment option for several types of VMs. mTOR or FK506-binding protein 12-rapamycin-associated protein 1 (FRAP1) is a kinase important in multiple cellular functions including cellular growth and proliferation, motility, cellular transcription and protein synthesis, cellular survival, and autophagy.

Sirolimus demonstrates remarkable responses in patients with microcystic and diffuses lymphatic malformations, capillary-lymphatic-venous malformations, PTEN-associated VAs, and lymphatic-venous malformations (LVM). Many of these patients experience improvement in clinical symptoms and quality of life.[5–8]

Sirolimus was first isolated in 1972 as a product of the bacteria known as *Streptomyces hygroscopicus* in the soil of the island of Rapa Nui, also known as Easter Island.[9] Nowadays, this unique drug has a wide range of diverse potential applications. Initially, information on the compound suggested that it could function as a potent antifungal. Owing to its concurrent immunosuppressive effects, sirolimus was deemed unsuitable for antifungal use. Instead, in 1999, sirolimus was commercially marketed as an immunosuppressant prophylactic medication for the prevention of renal transplant rejection.[10]

In the years following its discovery, sirolimus's utilization has broadened to include coronary stent restenosis prevention,[11] treatment of early-stage

Alzheimer's disease,[12] and use in antiaging[13] and oncology. Although sirolimus is still currently only FDA approved as a transplant immunosuppressive, it has amassed many promising off-label uses including management of tuberous sclerosis (TS) renal angiomyolipomas,[14] lymphangioleiomyomatosis,[15,16] and TS subependymal giant cell astrocytomas.[17,18] Sirolimus has shown utility in other cutaneous conditions as well, including Kaposi sarcoma,[19,20] psoriasis,[21] and lichen planus.[22,23]

Owing to the discovery of its antiproliferative and antitumor effects, sirolimus and its derivatives have played a significant role in cancer therapy and research. These antiproliferative properties involve the inhibition of mammalian target of sirolimus (mTOR), a serinike/threonine kinase in the phosphatidylinositol 3-kinase (PI3K) pathway which is responsible for regulation of vascular and lymphatic development.[7] The PI3K/AKT/mTOR/pathway is shown in **Fig. 1**. When this pathway becomes dysregulated, an increased expression of vascular endothelial growth factor (VEGF) can lead to aberrant proliferation and tissue overgrowth resulting in a VA. Both activating mutations leading to overexpression as well as loss of function mutations in tumor expressor genes have been associated with VAs in this pathway.[7] Sirolimus, with its inhibition of the mTOR pathway, prevents cells from progressing from phase G1 to S of the cell cycle therefore preventing cell proliferation.[24]

Through the study of the mTOR pathway, sirolimus has been shown to inhibit proliferation in both benign and malignant vascular tumors.[25] The early 2010s began the exploration of sirolimus in the treatment of VAs. Several case reports brought the treatment into international focus. Much of the early data based on the isolated case reports demonstrated positive treatment responses. One early study, a retrospective review of six patients with complicated VAs found that response rates were excellent among these patients, even in cases where the lesions had been refractory to other treatments.[26] A case report in 2017 described shrinkage of a previously unresectable complex VM in response to 24 months of sirolimus allowing for successful surgical resection.[27] In fact, sirolimus was found to be quite effective in a wide variety of different types of VMs[28] as well as syndromes with VMs such as but not limited to Klippel–Trenaunay syndrome and Sturge–Weber.[29–33] Examples of the different syndromes in which sirolimus has been used are listed in **Table 1**.

Owing to the diversity of VMs as well as the genetic syndromes associated with them, more

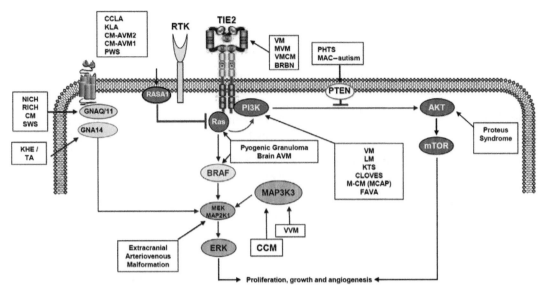

Fig. 1. Signaling pathways in vascular anomalies. CCLA, central conducting lymphatic anomaly; CM-AVM, capillary malformation-arteriovenous malformation; FAVA, fibroadipose vascular anomaly; KLA, kaposiform lymphangiomatosis; PI3K, phospoinositide-3-kinase; PWS, Prader-Willi Syndrome; RTK- Receptor tyrosine kinase; LM, Lymphatic malformation; KTS, Klippel-Trenaunay syndrome; MCAP, megalencephaly–capillary malformation syndrome; M-CM, Multifocal- capillary malformations; PHTS-PTEN Hamartoma Syndrome (PHTS); TA, Tufted angioma; SWS, Sturge-Weber syndrome; CCM, cerebral cavernous malformation; MVM, multifocal venous malformation; VMCM, inherited cutaneomucosal venous malformation; BRBN, blue rubber bleb nevus syndrome; BRAF, B-raf proto oncogene; VVM, verrucous venous malformations; NICH, noninvoluting congenital hemangioma; RICH, rapidly involuting congenital hemangioma. (*From* Adams DM, Ricci KW. Vascular Anomalies: Diagnosis of Complicated Anomalies and New Medical Treatment Options. Hematol Oncol Clin North Am. 2019 Jun;33(3):455-470.)

research is warranted in these specialized areas. The properties of VMs and the level of impairment that they may cause vary widely. Treatments are highly individualized, makings one-to-one comparisons between the effects of sirolimus on VM responses challenging. One unfortunate result of this is a lack of uniform treatment guidelines. Not every syndrome associated with a VM may respond to sirolimus. For example, early studies using sirolimus in the treatment of Maffucci Syndrome have shown conflicting results.[40,42] Thus, as more is learned about the use of sirolimus in the treatment of VMs, it is highly unlikely there will be a one size fits all approach.

In addition to efficacy, safety profiles in the use of sirolimus among different types of vascular tumors and malformations are an important area of research. Recent studies have investigated the safety and efficacy profile of sirolimus on different types of VMs such as high-flow versus low-flow lesions.[6,43,44]

Sirolimus can be administered both topically and orally. Optimum dosing has not been officially established,[45] but the most common and initial suggested oral dose is 0.8 mg/m^2 given twice daily. Once a day dosing has also been suggested and used in adolescent patients to encourage compliance. Medication dosing may range from 1 to 4 mg/m^2.[28,43] Most studies recommend that levels be maintained at 5 to 15 ng/mL.[44] This suggested level has been based on a case series of patients with astrocytoma treated with sirolimus.[46] A patient's clinical status should also be considered. Some patients may see clinical improvement of symptoms with lower trough levels. A study evaluating high-flow VMs showed clinical improvement in patients with a median trough level of 3.5 ng/dL.[43] **Fig. 2** shows the visual comparison before and after treatment. Given the long half-life of sirolimus of about 62 hours, one study recommended dose changes be done based on trough levels obtained more than 5 days apart.[47] Trough levels should be followed regularly and patients should also be monitored for hypertriglyceridemia, hyperglycemia, hypercholesterolemia, and neutropenia.[7,48] Complete blood counts, comprehensive metabolic panels, and lipid panels, specifically triglyceride levels, should be monitored at regular intervals; however, there are no formal guidelines for monitoring frequencies or intervals.

Table 1
Conditions and syndromes where use of oral sirolimus has been used for the treatment of complex vascular anomalies

Condition	Number of Case/ Type of Study	Type of Vascular Lesion(s)	Response/Result
Sturge–Weber syndrome	Retrospective chart review[32]	Port wine stain, leptomeningeal angioma	Shrinkage of lesions, improved hemifacial hypertrophy, epilepsy better controlled
	Observational study[34]	Port wine stain, leptomeningeal angioma	Improvement in cognitive function, no statistical effect on port wine stain
Proteus syndrome	Case report[35]	Capillary malformation, hemihypertrophy,	Shrinkage of a cerebriform connective tissue nevus, lipoma shrinkage
PTEN hamartoma syndrome	Case report[31]	Cavernous hemangioma	Regain of limb function, shrinkage of lesion
CLOVES syndrome	Two case reports[30]	Macrocystic lymphatic malformation	Mass reduction, absence of cutaneous lymphorrhea
Klippel-Trenaunay Syndrome	Case report[29]	Microcystic lymphatic malformation with deep vein hypoplasia	Reduction of cutaneous lymphatic infiltration and control of potentially life-threatening bleeding
Blue rubber bleb nevus syndrome case	Case report[36]	Venous malformations in the skin, soft tissue, and Gastrointestinal (GI) tract	Improvement of cutaneous lesions, decreased GI bleeding
Kaposiform hemangioendothelioma with Kasabach–Merritt phenomenon	Case report[37]	Kaposiform hemangioendothelioma	Decrease in lesion size
Gorham-Stout	Case report[38]	Bone and soft tissue lymphatic malformations	Disease remission
Kaposiform lymphangiomatosis	Retrospective chart review[39]	Generalized lymphatic anomaly	Most patients achieved stable disease or partial improvement
Maffucci syndrome	Case report[40]	Spindle cell hemangiomas	Shrinkage and softening of the vascular nodules
PHACE syndrome	Case report[41]	Extensive segmental facial infantile hemangioma	Regression of infantile hemangioma and improvement in vision in a patient who failed conventional therapy
Fibroadipose vascular anomaly	Retrospective review	Intramuscular fibrofatty infiltrative slow-flow lesion	Reduced pain and improved function

The immunosuppressive effects of sirolimus should not be overlooked. There are case reports of sirolimus-related deaths attributed to infection,[48,49] so its utilization should not be taken lightly. Given the immunosuppressant effects, providers should consider treating with prophylaxis management of Pneumocystis pneumonia with either Bactrim or pentamidine, particularly in younger patients.[50] The most reported side effects are listed in **Box 1**.

In effort to reduce systemic side effects and the risks they carry, use of topical sirolimus is also being explored. One recent retrospective study showed at least partial improvement in all 18 patients studied,[51] though the degree of response warrants further study. Topical sirolimus has also

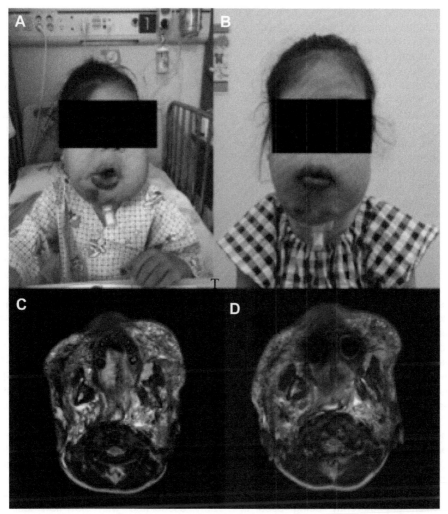

Fig. 2. Visual comparison of mandibular and submandibular/cervial areas in a patient bafore and after medical treatment of extensive large vascular malformation with sirolimus. (*From* Cho YJ, Kwon H, Kwon YJ, Kim SC, Kim DY, Namgoong JM. Effects of sirolimus in the treatment of unresectable infantile hemangioma and vascular malformations in children: A single-center experience. J Vasc Surg Venous Lymphat Disord. 2021 Nov;9(6):1488-1494.)

Box 1
Most common side effects of oral sirolimus[26,28,43]
Side Effects
Mucositis
Hypercholesterolemia
Headache
Transaminitis
Neutropenia
Upper respiratory tract infection
Hyperlipidemia

been shown to be effective in the treatment of angiofibromas in TS patients,[48,52–54] with safety and efficacy validated by a randomized controlled clinical trial. Questions remain regarding long-term treatment response duration.[55] Patient's with Sturge–Weber syndrome have seen a decrease in port wine stains when treated with topical sirolimus used in conjunction with pulse dye laser.[56]

Duration of treatment with sirolimus is not yet well established. Formal prospective studies are required to establish long-term guidelines, evaluate possible long-term effects, and establish long-term benefits of prolonged treatment. Studies have shown various responses to discontinuation of treatment with sirolimus including significant rebound growth and return of lesion-related side effects (ie, increasing size, pain, ulceration) to no change on discontinuation of the drug. Most patients who responded initially to treatment often again respond to restarting sirolimus. Less perioperative complications and bleeding with the use of sirolimus in the perioperative/periprocedural periods when undergoing surgical procedures (excision and debulking) and interventional procedures (sclerotherapy) have been reported.[57,58] In addition, multiple lesions initially deemed inoperable were able to undergo sclerotherapy or resection.[6] Safety may be a concern for long-term use, especially in the pediatric population when long-term treatment is required. Follow-up warrants close monitoring of possible side effects in addition to infectious complications. Strategies, such as dose reductions to maintain efficacy, have been used to minimize drug exposure and resultant side effects.

Everolimus is an mTOR inhibitor derived from sirolimus. It has been in use for a shorter time, and thus our knowledge on its detailed effects on patients is more limited. It has been used sporadically for the treatment of VMs, but no prospective clinical trial has yet been reported.[59,60] Whether everolimus and sirolimus have equivalent benefits as well as risk profiles remain to be studied. Although mTOR inhibitors have clearly revolutionized the therapeutic options for patients with complicated VMs, a significant proportion of patients will need treatments targeting other signaling complexes.[61]

There is a growing interest in the use of angiogenesis inhibitors to treat these vascular lesions, such as Avastin or bevacizumab and thalidomide, many of which are currently being used in oncology regimens. Several case reports have suggested bevacizumab or thalidomide may provide some benefit in intestinal vascular lesions such as HHT and other high-flow lesions, though potential for serious adverse events such as impaired wound healing resulting in lower limb amputation and even fatal adverse events raise concern.[2,3,62] In certain patients, severe symptoms, who experience refractory bleeding, are at risk for life-threatening hemorrhage or are at risk for high-output heart failure, these agents may be appropriate.[3,63] A recent meta-analysis endorsed the safety of bevacizumab in HHT treatment,[63] through more research into safety is likely warranted. It remains unclear which VMs may benefit from these targeted therapies as additional prospective studies are needed.

ROLE OF ANTICOAGULATION

In general, consumptive coagulopathy is thought to be a common mechanism for thrombocytopenia

and for coagulation factor derangement associated with VAs. Important differences between the coagulopathies encountered in patients with VMs and vascular tumors should be pointed out, as distinct therapies are required to prevent their progression. The activation of coagulation seen with VMs is relatively mild and confined primarily within the vascular lesion; it is known as localized intravascular coagulopathy (LIC).[64] In contrast, the more severe coagulopathy associated with vascular tumors, such as tufted angiomas and kaposiform hemangioendotheliomas, is designated as Kasabach–Merritt phenomenon (KMP).[64] KMP begins locally due to intra-tumoral platelet trapping, often becoming widespread and thus life-threatening. Severe thrombocytopenia, hemolytic anemia, and hypofibrinogenemia are common, and the blood smear demonstrates microangiopathy. Laboratory evaluation of pediatric patients reveal a range of abnormalities ranging from D-dimer elevation alone to hypofibrinogenemia, thrombocytopenia, and prolongation of both prothrombin and activated partial thromboplastin time, known as venous malformation-associated DIC (VM-DIC). Clinically, LIC/VM-DIC occurs in patients with slow-flow VMs including venous and combined lesions (ie, CVM, LVM). D-dimer elevation is the hallmark of LIC with a variable prevalence of LIC in children with slow-flow VAs ranging from 1% to 88%.[64]

The use of heparin has long been reported in children with coagulopathy associated with vascular lesions but without specific data to guide management of LIC.[65] As such, there is no consensus for the management of the coagulopathy associated with slow-flow lesions. Low-molecular-weight heparin (LMWH) effectively decreases thrombin activation in patients with LIC associated with VM and results in a reduction of D-dimer.[66] LMWH seems to relieve pain in these patients by reducing superficial thrombotic events within these lesions. LMWH is commonly used to manage periprocedural coagulopathy although no evidence-based guidelines exist.

In addition to LMWH, other anticoagulant therapies such as vitamin K antagonists, direct oral anticoagulants (DOACs), and antiplatelet agents may also be effective; however, there is a paucity of published experience with these agents.[64] The use of aspirin is largely anecdotal despite its common use.[67] A significant risk of venous thrombotic embolism occurs with larger low-flow lesions. The complex scenarios of thrombocytopenia and coagulopathy may be seen with complex mixed VM lesions, especially those involving both venous and capillary components.[68,69]

Chronic anticoagulation, commonly with LMWH and the recently pediatrically approved DOAC.

Dabigatran may be considered for patients who have had a history of thrombotic complications or have chronic pain. In addition, compression garments provide significant pain relief, especially in the event of symptomatic phleboliths.

FUTURE ROLE OF MEK AND PHOSPHATIDYLINOSITOL 3-KINASE INHIBITORS

It is now established that most VMs are caused by somatic or mosaic mutations that activate at least one of the two major intracellular signaling pathways: the RAS/MAPK/ERK or the phosphatidylinositol 3-kinase (PIK3CA or PI3K pathway)/protein kinase B (AKT)/mammalian target of rapamycin (mTOR) pathway.[61] The PIK3CA/AKT/mTOR pathway is implicated in many cellular processes, such as cell-cycle regulation, proliferation, protein synthesis, and cell survival, thus proclaiming it the "anti-apoptosis pathway."[61] Inhibition of PIK3CA is a promising strategy for *PIK3CA*-mutated VMs, both sporadic and associated with PIKC3A-related overgrowth syndromes (PROS). Several PIK3CA inhibitors are under development for PIK3CA-dependent tumors. BYL719 (alpelisib) is currently being investigated in clinical trials and shows a favorable tolerability profile.[70,71] Alpelisib has been tested in a clinical study treating 19 patients with PROS, 9 of 19 of which had failed sirolimus, based on the preclinical observation that this compound could prevent and improve organ dysfunction in a mouse model of PROS/CLOVES.[61,72] BYL719 treatment decreased vascular tumor size, improved congestive heart failure, reduced hemihypertrophy, and attenuated scoliosis, improving symptoms in all patients, without serious safety issues.[1,61,73]

As previously approved for PIK3CA-mutated breast cancer, in April 2022, alpelisib became the first FDA-approved treatment of PROS in patients 2 years and older. Dosing recommendation for children is 50 mg once daily with titration to 125 mg recommended in patients 6 to 18 years if incomplete response by 25 weeks. Adult dosing is recommended at 250 mg daily, although anecdotal recommendations for dose titration to this maximum exist as well. Dose reduction should be undertaken when needed for side effect management. There are reports of successful off-label use in infants. A role in VAs without documented PIK3CA mutations is also being established (personal communication). Some of the more common side effects associated with alpelisib include cutaneous eruptions, diarrhea, stomatitis, hyperglycemia, and more rarely pneumonitis.[74] A formulation for topical use is also being developed. This could allow wider use in more localized VMs with reduction of side effects. Patients with PROS/CLOVES could also be candidates for trials with other PI3K/AKT pathway inhibitors, such as ARQ 092 (miransertib), a potent, selective, allosteric, orally bioavailable, and highly selective AKT inhibitor currently under clinical development.[75,76]

Other complex VAs, such as sporadic arteriovenous malformations (AVMs), kaposiform lymphangiomatosis, and some central conducting lymphatic anomalies have been associated with somatic mutations occurring in the RAS/MAPK pathway (mosaic/somatic RASopathies). These devastating conditions may benefit from treatment with MEK inhibitors, such as trametinib.[77,78] As previously mentioned, treatment of VAs is likely to remain a highly individualized process, and much of the available literature focuses on single case reports or small case series, though several clinical trials are also ongoing.[79,80] One promising area for future research includes the treatment of capillary malformation-AVMs with trametinib.[81] Several case reports have also demonstrated reduction in the flow of spinal cord AVMs, which are specifically difficult to treat and can have devastating detrimental effects for patients.[82,83] Certain lesions may respond better than others to MEK inhibitors, which in the future may be guided by genetic testing.[84] MEK inhibitors may have significant side effects including bleeding; various degrees of skin irritation; dryness of eyes, skin, and mouth; and muscle cramping. Bevacizumab is a recombinant humanized monoclonal antibody that binds and inhibits VEGF, making it a potential treatment option to control bleeding in these patients.[61] However, the not insignificant side effects that these medications can cause including the more severe cardiac toxicities or ocular complications are not to be ignored.[83]

The immunomodulatory agent thalidomide downregulates VEGF and has been used in treatment of VA-associated gastrointestinal bleeding, such as in HHT, though it may have potential as preventative treatment of intracranial hemorrhage as shown in a mouse model study.[85,86] This suggests thalidomide may prove to be a useful therapy in treatment of CNS AVMs though more study is needed on its human efficacy. Although thalidomide is most known for its teratogenic effects, it can also cause other rare adverse events such as neutropenia and therefore patients taking the drug should be monitored with complete blood count and differential tests.

SUMMARY

Medical management plays a pivotal role in the treatment of patients with VMs and VAs, both as a single modality of therapy and combination therapies. Sirolimus proves to be safe and efficacious as medical management in a large group of VM/VAs patients. Emerging therapies provide new avenues for effective medical management of VAs and associated syndromes. Current and future studies will allow us to continue to target-specific pathways and genetic alterations in this population and establish guidelines for medical management and safety of long-term use.

CLINICS CARE POINTS

- Vascular malformations and anomalies (VascM and VAs) often result in acute and sometimes lifelong clinical complications.[1]
- Treatment options for these patients often complex combined modalities.
- Sirolimus (Rapamune or rapamycin), with its specific and potent inhibition of the mammalian target of rapamycin or mammalian target of rapamycin (mTOR), is established as a safe treatment option for several types of VMs.
- Coagulopathy is thought to be a common mechanism for thrombocytopenia and coagulation factor derangement associated with vascular lesions and clinical symptoms.
- RAS/MAPK/ERK or the phosphatidylinositol 3-kinase (PIK3CA or PI3K pathway)/protein kinase B/mTOR pathway[61]—implicated in many cellular processes poses promising strategies for targeted treatment development for VMs/VAs.

REFERENCES

1. Adams DM, Ricci KW. Vascular Anomalies: Diagnosis of Complicated Anomalies and New Medical Treatment Options. Hematol Oncol Clin North Am 2019;33(3):455–70.
2. Buscarini E, Botella LM, Geisthoff U, et al. Safety of thalidomide and bevacizumab in patients with hereditary hemorrhagic telangiectasia. Orphanet J Rare Dis 2019;14(1):28.
3. Guilhem A, Fargeton A-E, Simon A-C, et al. Intravenous bevacizumab in hereditary hemorrhagic telangiectasia (HHT): a retrospective study of 46 patients. PLoS One 2017;12(11):e0188943.
4. Ricci KW. Advances in the medical management of vascular anomalies. Semin Intervent Radiol 2017; 34(3):239–49.
5. Uno T, Ito S, Nakazawa A, et al. Successful treatment of Kaposiform hemangioendothelioma with everolimus. Pediatr Blood Cancer 2015;62(3):536–8.
6. Hammer J, Seront E, Duez S, et al. Sirolimus is efficacious in treatment for extensive and/or complex slow-flow vascular malformations: a monocentric prospective phase II study. Orphanet J Rare Dis 2018;13(1):191.
7. Adams DM, Trenor CC 3rd, Hammill AM, et al. Efficacy and safety of sirolimus in the treatment of complicated vascular anomalies. Pediatrics 2016; 137(2):e20153257.
8. Tian R, Liang Y, Zhang W, et al. Effectiveness of sirolimus in the treatment of complex lymphatic malformations: Single center report of 56 cases. J Pediatr Surg 2020;55(11):2454–8.
9. Sehgal SN, Baker H, Vezina C. Rapamycin (AY-22,989), a new antifungal antibiotic. II. Fermentation, isolation and characterization. J Antibiot (Tokyo) 1975;28(10):727–32.
10. Kahan BD, Julian BA, Pescovitz MD, et al. Sirolimus reduces the incidence of acute rejection episodes despite lower cyclosporine doses in caucasian recipients of mismatched primary renal allografts: a phase II trial.Rapamune Study Group. Transplantation 1999;68(10):1526–32.
11. Vishnevetsky D, Patel P, Tijerino H, et al. Sirolimus-eluting coronary stent. Am J Health Syst Pharm 2004;61(5):449–56.
12. Kaeberlein M, Galvan V. Rapamycin and Alzheimer's disease: Time for a clinical trial? Sci Transl Med 2019;11:476.
13. Blagosklonny MV. Fasting and rapamycin: diabetes versus benevolent glucose intolerance. Cell Death Dis 2019;10(8):607.
14. Cabrera Lopez C, Marti T, Catala V, et al. Effects of rapamycin on angiomyolipomas in patients with tuberous sclerosis. Nefrologia 2011;31(3):292–8.
15. Casanova A, Maria Giron R, Acosta O, et al. Lymphangioleiomyomatosis treatment with sirolimus. Arch Bronconeumol 2011;47(9):470–2.
16. McCormack FX, Inoue Y, Moss J, et al. Efficacy and safety of sirolimus in lymphangioleiomyomatosis. N Engl J Med 2011;364(17):1595–606.
17. Koenig MK, Butler IJ, Northrup H. Regression of subependymal giant cell astrocytoma with rapamycin in tuberous sclerosis complex. J Child Neurol 2008;23(10):1238–9.
18. Major P. Potential of mTOR inhibitors for the treatment of subependymal giant cell astrocytomas in tuberous sclerosis complex. Aging (Albany NY). Mar 2011;3(3):189–91.
19. Saggar S, Zeichner JA, Brown TT, et al. Kaposi's sarcoma resolves after sirolimus therapy in a patient with pemphigus vulgaris. Arch Dermatol 2008; 144(5):654–7.
20. Yaich S, Charfeddine K, Zaghdane S, et al. Sirolimus for the treatment of Kaposi sarcoma after renal transplantation: a series of 10 cases. Transpl Proc 2012;44(9):2824–6.

21. Ormerod AD, Shah SA, Copeland P, et al. Treatment of psoriasis with topical sirolimus: preclinical development and a randomized, double-blind trial. Br J Dermatol 2005;152(4):758–64.

22. Mahevas T, Bertinchamp R, Battistella M, et al. Efficacy of oral sirolimus as salvage therapy in refractory lichen planus associated with immune deficiency. Br J Dermatol 2018;179(3):771–3.

23. Soria A, Agbo-Godeau S, Taieb A, et al. Treatment of refractory oral erosive lichen planus with topical rapamycin: 7 cases. Dermatology 2009;218(1): 22–5.

24. Huang S, Houghton PJ. Inhibitors of mammalian target of rapamycin as novel antitumor agents: from bench to clinic. Curr Opin Investig Drugs 2002;3(2):295–304.

25. Du W, Gerald D, Perruzzi CA, et al. Vascular tumors have increased p70 S6-kinase activation and are inhibited by topical rapamycin. Lab Invest 2013; 93(10):1115–27.

26. Hammill AM, Wentzel M, Gupta A, et al. Sirolimus for the treatment of complicated vascular anomalies in children. Pediatr Blood Cancer 2011;57(6):1018–24.

27. Goldenberg DC, Carvas M, Adams D, et al. Successful Treatment of a Complex Vascular Malformation With Sirolimus and Surgical Resection. J Pediatr Hematol Oncol 2017;39(4):e191–5.

28. Al-Huniti A, Fantauzzi M, Willis L, et al. Sirolimus Leads to Rapid Improvement in Fibroadipose Vascular Anomalies: Experience in 11 Children. J Vasc Anom 2021;2(4):e030.

29. Bessis D, Vernhet H, Bigorre M, et al. Life-threatening cutaneous bleeding in childhood klippel-trenaunay syndrome treated with oral sirolimus. JAMA Dermatol 2016;152(9):1058–9.

30. de Grazia R, Giordano C, Cossio L, et al. CLOVES syndrome: Treatment with oral Rapamycin. Report of two cases. Rev Chil Pediatr 2019;90(6):662–7. Sindrome de CLOVES: Tratamiento con Rapamicina oral. Reporte de dos casos.

31. Schmid GL, Kassner F, Uhlig HH, et al. Sirolimus treatment of severe PTEN hamartoma tumor syndrome: case report and in vitro studies. Pediatr Res 2014;75(4):527–34.

32. Sun B, Han T, Wang Y, et al. Sirolimus as a potential treatment for sturge-weber syndrome. J Craniofac Surg 2021;32(1):257–60.

33. Yuksekkaya H, Ozbek O, Keser M, et al. Blue rubber bleb nevus syndrome: successful treatment with sirolimus. Pediatr 2012;129(4):e1080–4.

34. Sebold AJ, Day AM, Ewen J, et al. Sirolimus Treatment in Sturge-Weber Syndrome. Pediatr Neurol 2021;115:29–40.

35. Weibel L, Theiler M, Gnannt R, et al. Reduction of disease burden with early sirolimus treatment in a child with proteus syndrome. JAMA Dermatol 2021;157(12):1514–6.

36. AlNooh BM, AlQadri NG, Alghubayn M, et al. Sirolimus in the Management of Blue Rubber Bleb Nevus Syndrome: A Case Report and Review of the Literature. Case Rep Dermatol 2021;13(2):417–21.

37. Cabrera TB, Speer AL, Greives MR, et al. Sirolimus for Kaposiform Hemangioendothelioma and Kasabach-Merritt Phenomenon in a Neonate. AJP Rep 2020;10(4):e390–4.

38. Garcia V, Alonso-Claudio G, Gomez-Hernandez MT, et al. Sirolimus on Gorham-Stout disease. Case Report Colomb Med (Cali) 2016;47(4):213–6.

39. Eng W, Al-Sayegh H, Ma C, et al. Kaposiform Lymphangiomatosis: Update on Outcomes and Use of Sirolimus As a Therapeutic Intervention. Blood 2018;132:3734.

40. Lekwuttikarn R, Chang J, Teng JMC. Successful treatment of spindle cell hemangiomas in a patient with Maffucci syndrome and review of literatures. Dermatol Ther 2019;32(3):e12919.

41. Kaylani S, Theos AJ, Pressey JG. Treatment of Infantile Hemangiomas with Sirolimus in a Patient with PHACE Syndrome. Pediatr Dermatol 2013;30(6): e194–7.

42. Gupta V, Mridha AR, Khaitan BK. Unsatisfactory response to sirolimus in Maffucci syndrome-associated spindle cell hemangiomas. Dermatol Ther 2019;32(3):e12851.

43. Duran-Romero AJ, Hernandez-Rodriguez JC, Ortiz-Alvarez J, et al. Efficacy and safety of oral sirolimus for high-flow vascular malformations in real clinical practice. Clin Exp Dermatol 2022;47(1):57–62.

44. Freixo C, Ferreira V, Martins J, et al. Efficacy and safety of sirolimus in the treatment of vascular anomalies: A systematic review. J Vasc Surg 2020;71(1): 318–27.

45. Lee B-B. Sirolimus in the treatment of vascular anomalies. J Vasc Surg 2020;71(1):328.

46. Bevacqua M, Baldo F, Pastore S, et al. Off-Label Use of Sirolimus and Everolimus in a Pediatric Center: A Case Series and Review of the Literature. Pediatr Drugs 2019;21(3):185–93.

47. MacDonald A, Scarola J, Burke JT, et al. Clinical pharmacokinetics and therapeutic drug monitoring of sirolimus. Clin Ther 2000;22:B101–21.

48. Ying H, Qiao C, Yang X, et al. A Case Report of 2 Sirolimus-Related Deaths Among Infants With Kaposiform Hemangioendotheliomas. Pediatr Apr 2018; 141(Suppl 5):S425–9.

49. Rössler J, Baselga E, Davila V, et al. Severe adverse events during sirolimus "off-label" therapy for vascular anomalies. Pediatr Blood Cancer 2021; 68(8):e28936.

50. Shetty AK. Pneumocystis jirovecii pneumonia: a potential complication of sirolimus therapy. J Paediatrics Child Health 2019;55(4):484.

51. Dodds M, Tollefson M, Castelo-Soccio L, et al. Treatment of superficial vascular anomalies with topical

sirolimus: a multicenter case series. Pediatr Dermatol 2020;37(2):272–7.

52. DeKlotz CM, Ogram AE, Singh S, et al. Dramatic improvement of facial angiofibromas in tuberous sclerosis with topical rapamycin: optimizing a treatment protocol. Arch Dermatol 2011;147(9):1116–7.

53. Haemel AK, O'Brian AL, Teng JM. Topical Rapamycin: A Novel Approach to Facial Angiofibromas in Tuberous Sclerosis. Arch Dermatol 2010;146(7):715–8.

54. Wataya-Kaneda M, Tanaka M, Nakamura A, et al. A topical combination of rapamycin and tacrolimus for the treatment of angiofibroma due to tuberous sclerosis complex (TSC): a pilot study of nine Japanese patients with TSC of different disease severity. Br J Dermatol 2011;165(4):912–6.

55. Koenig MK, Bell CS, Hebert AA, et al. Efficacy and Safety of Topical Rapamycin in Patients With Facial Angiofibromas Secondary to Tuberous Sclerosis Complex: The TREATMENT Randomized Clinical Trial. JAMA Dermatol 2018;154(7):773–80.

56. Marqués L, Núñez-Córdoba JM, Aguado L, et al. Topical rapamycin combined with pulsed dye laser in the treatment of capillary vascular malformations in Sturge-Weber syndrome: phase II, randomized, double-blind, intraindividual placebo-controlled clinical trial. J Am Acad Dermatol 2015;72(1):151–8.e1.

57. Azouz H, Salah H, Al-Ajlan S, et al. Treatment of cystic hygroma in a young infant through multidisciplinary approach involving sirolimus, sclerotherapy, and debulking surgery. JAAD Case Rep 2016;2(4):350–3.

58. Honnorat M, Viremouneix L, Ayari S, et al. Early Adjuvant Medication With the mTOR Inhibitor Sirolimus in a Preterm Neonate With Compressive Cystic Lymphatic Malformation. Case Rep Front Pediatr 2020. https://doi.org/10.3389/fped.2020.00418.

59. Matsumoto H, Ozeki M, Hori T, et al. Successful Everolimus Treatment of Kaposiform Hemangioendothelioma With Kasabach-Merritt Phenomenon: Clinical Efficacy and Adverse Effects of mTOR Inhibitor Therapy. J Pediatr Hematol Oncol 2016;38(8):e322–5.

60. Jenkins D, McCuaig C, Drolet BA, et al. Tuberous Sclerosis Complex Associated with Vascular Anomalies or Overgrowth. Pediatr Dermatol 2016;33(5):536–42.

61. Van Damme A, Seront E, Dekeuleneer V, et al. New and Emerging Targeted Therapies for Vascular Malformations. Am J Clin Dermatol 2020;21(5):657–68.

62. Perez Botero J, Burns D, Thompson CA, et al. Successful treatment with thalidomide of a patient with congenital factor V deficiency and factor V inhibitor with recurrent gastrointestinal bleeding from small bowel arteriovenous malformations. Haemophilia 2013;19(1):e59–61.

63. Gossage JR. The Current Role of Bevacizumab in the Treatment of Hereditary Hemorrhagic Telangiectasia–Related Bleeding. Mayo Clinic Proc 2018;93(2):130–2.

64. Brandão LR, TCM. Hemostasis/Thrombosis Considerations in Vascular Anomalies. In: Trenor III C. AD-Vascular anomalies. 1 edition. Cham (Switzerland): Springer; 2020. p. 195–212. chap Hemostasis/Thrombosis Considerations in Vascular Anomalies.

65. Mazoyer E, Enjolras O, Bisdorff A, et al. Coagulation disorders in patients with venous malformation of the limbs and trunk: a case series of 118 patients. Arch Dermatol 2008;144(7):861–7.

66. Dompmartin A, Acher A, Thibon P, et al. Association of localized intravascular coagulopathy with venous malformations. Arch Dermatol 2008;144(7):873–7.

67. Mathes EFD, Haggstrom AN, Dowd C, et al. Clinical Characteristics and Management of Vascular Anomalies: Findings of a Multidisciplinary Vascular Anomalies Clinic. Arch Dermatol 2004;140(8):979–83.

68. Dompmartin A, Acher A, Thibon P, et al. Association of Localized Intravascular Coagulopathy With Venous Malformations. Arch Dermatol 2008;144(7):873–7.

69. Mazoyer E, Enjolras O, Bisdorff A, et al. Coagulation Disorders in Patients With Venous Malformation of the Limbs and Trunk: A Case Series of 118 Patients. Arch Dermatol 2008;144(7):861–7.

70. Margolin JF, Soni HM, Pimpalwar S. Medical therapy for pediatric vascular anomalies. Semin Plast Surg 2014;28(2):79–86.

71. Markham A. Alpelisib: First Global Approval. Drugs 2019;79(11):1249–53.

72. Lindhurst MJ, Yourick MR, Yu Y, et al. Repression of AKT signaling by ARQ 092 in cells and tissues from patients with Proteus syndrome. Sci Rep 2015;5:17162.

73. Morin G, Degrugillier-Chopinet C, Vincent M, et al. Treatment of two infants with PIK3CA-related overgrowth spectrum by alpelisib. J Exp Med 2022;219(3). https://doi.org/10.1084/jem.20212148.

74. Nunnery SE, Mayer IA. Management of toxicity to isoform α-specific PI3K inhibitors. Ann Oncol 2019;30(Suppl_10):x21–6.

75. Biesecker LG, Edwards M, O'Donnell S, et al. Clinical report: one year of treatment of Proteus syndrome with miransertib (ARQ 092). Cold Spring Harb Mol Case Stud 2020;6(1). https://doi.org/10.1101/mcs.a004549.

76. Ranieri C, Di Tommaso S, Loconte DC, et al. In vitro efficacy of ARQ 092, an allosteric AKT inhibitor, on primary fibroblast cells derived from patients with PIK3CA-related overgrowth spectrum (PROS). Neurogenet 2018;19(2):77–91.

77. Li D, March ME, Gutierrez-Uzquiza A, et al. ARAF recurrent mutation causes central conducting

lymphatic anomaly treatable with a MEK inhibitor. Nat Med 2019;25(7):1116–22.

78. Ozeki M, Fukao T. Generalized Lymphatic Anomaly and Gorham-Stout Disease: Overview and Recent Insights. Adv Wound Care (New Rochelle) 2019; 8(6):230–45.

79. Chowers G, Abebe-Campino G, Golan H, et al. Treatment of severe Kaposiform lymphangiomatosis positive for NRAS mutation by MEK inhibition. Pediatr Res 2022. https://doi.org/10.1038/s41390-022-01986-0.

80. Foster JB, Li D, March ME, et al. Kaposiform lymphangiomatosis effectively treated with MEK inhibition. EMBO Mol Med 2020;12(10):e12324.

81. Nicholson CL, Flanagan S, Murati M, et al. Successful management of an arteriovenous malformation with trametinib in a patient with capillary-malformation arteriovenous malformation syndrome and cardiac compromise. Pediatr Dermatol 2022. https://doi.org/10.1111/pde.14912.

82. Edwards EA, Phelps AS, Cooke D, et al. Monitoring Arteriovenous Malformation Response to Genotype-Targeted Therapy. Pediatrics 2020;146(3): e20193206.

83. Nicholson CL, Flanagan S, Murati M, et al. Successful management of an arteriovenous malformation with trametinib in a patient with capillary-malformation arteriovenous malformation syndrome and cardiac compromise. Pediatr Dermatol 2022. https://doi.org/10.1111/pde.14912.

84. Lekwuttikarn R, Lim YH, Admani S, et al. Genotype-Guided Medical Treatment of an Arteriovenous Malformation in a Child: JAMA Dermatol 2019;155(2): 256–7.

85. Ge ZZ, Chen HM, Gao YJ, et al. Efficacy of Thalidomide for Refractory Gastrointestinal Bleeding From Vascular Malformation. Gastroenterology 2011;141(5):1629–37.e4.

86. Zhu W, Chen W, Zou D, et al. Thalidomide Reduces Hemorrhage of Brain Arteriovenous Malformations in a Mouse Model. Stroke 2018;49(5):1232–40.

Surgical Treatment of Vascular Anomalies

Dov Charles Goldenberg, MD, PhD*, Rafael Ferreira Zatz, MD

KEYWORDS

- Vascular anomalies • Infantile hemangiomas • Vascular malformations • Surgery
- Multidisciplinary approach

KEY POINTS

- Surgical treatment is part of multidisciplinary approach.
- Specific skills are necessary for satisfactory outcomes.
- When deciding for surgery, check preoperative coagulation status and presence of side effect of current pharmacologic treatment.
- Define preoperatively the goal of surgical approach: curative, adjunctive or paliative.

INTRODUCTION

Recommendation for the surgical approach to vascular anomalies is rapidly evolving. From an isolated approach, surgery is best seen nowadays as an adjunctive tool in multidisciplinary management (**Box 1**). Several studies focusing on targeted therapy based on genetic findings were published, and their use in clinical practice is on the way.

Surgical removal of complex lesions is possible and routinely performed, but pharmacologic treatment has the potential to reduce stress-related technical issues. Less blood loss, diminution of collateral damage, and reduced final scars can be obtained.

On the other hand, for small or localized vascular anomalies, surgery is still the first-line treatment, with or without endovascular procedures.[1–10]

The first step, when surgery is considered, is to establish a precise diagnosis. Clinical behavior and characteristics of image diagnosis is primordial.

TREATMENT OF VASCULAR ANOMALIES BASED ON DIAGNOSIS
Treatment of Vascular Tumors

Infantile hemangiomas
Most of infantile hemangiomas (IH) have a favorable evolution toward complete regression. However, around 20% will require treatment to reach involution. The use of beta-blockers as the first-line approach reduced the indication for surgery as well as the complexity of procedures.[11–13]

In summary, indications for a surgical approach to IH are (**Fig. 1**):

A. Presence of growth-related deformity in functional facial areas (eyelids, nose, and lips)
   When an IH causes functional impairment due to visual obstruction, airways compromise, or feeding problems, an early total or partial resection is mandatory. Otherwise, the child may present long-term sequelae due to amblyopia, nasal breathing, or nutrition.
B. Failure of pharmacologic treatment with growth-related deformities in other locations
   IH that causes a significant deformity without a vital functional impairment is submitted to the clinical treatment with propranolol as first-line treatment. Few patients do not respond and need to be submitted for surgical treatment.
C. Local evolutive complications not responding to pharmacologic treatment (ulceration, bleeding, infection)

   Repetitive bleeding, local infection, or ulceration refractory to conservative measures can be treated by surgery.

D. Involuted lesions with residual deformities

Division of Plastic Surgery, Hospital das Clínicas da Faculdade de Medicina da Universidade de São Paulo, Rua Arminda 93 cj. 121, Sao Paulo, SP 04545-100, Brazil
* Corresponding author.
E-mail address: dov.goldenberg@einstein.br

Dermatol Clin 40 (2022) 473–480
https://doi.org/10.1016/j.det.2022.06.006

Alter complete involution, IH may leave excess fibroadipose tissue, cutaneous scarring, or skin atrophy. Surgical approach is then necessary to treat contour deformities and minimize scars.

In every clinical scenario, surgical treatment must respect the following technical guidelines[14–20]:

- Removal of a lesion should not result in a sequel greater than that possibly left by spontaneous involution.

- Partial resections can be performed, to solve, and emergencial problem allowing a definitive solution after subsequent involution of the lesion. Intralesional incisions for partial resection should be preferred, as the final scar will be within the IH.

- Surgical accesses for facial IH should be conducted with reduced or hidden scars, taking advantage of anatomic lines and known approaches already used in aesthetic facial surgery.

Pyogenic Granuloma

The exception to the modern treatment of vascular anomalies is the pyogenic granuloma. There is no effective drug for this benign vascular tumor; surgery is the first-line treatment in all circumstances. Usually, removal is simple and resolves the frequent bleeding. Care must be taken for complete removal.[21]

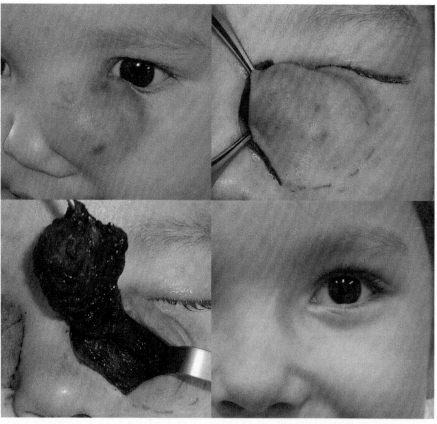

Fig. 1. A 3-year-old woman patient with a deep hemangioma in the left paranasal area, non -responsive to propranolol therapy. Indication for surgery was based on several indications: need for definitive diagnosis, growth-related deformity, absence of response to pharmacologic treatment. Upper left, reoperative aspect. Upper right: incision was positioned in the transition of nasal and cheek regions. Lower left: complete resection. Lower right: late postoperative appearance after 3 years.

Borderline and Malignant Tumors

Borderline tumors (eg, kaposiform hemangioendothelioma) should be managed with medical treatment, likely mTOR inhibitors, such as sirolimus (rapamycin). Indications include the resolution of Kasabach–Merritt phenomenon as well as volume reduction.

Surgical resection should be made in medical treatment failure or after the clinical involution of the tumor to a residual lesion.

Malignant tumors require a more aggressive posture with urgent surgical resection and oncologic neoadjuvant and adjuvant follow-up.[22–25]

TREATMENT OF VASCULAR MALFORMATIONS
Low Flow Vascular Malformations

Low flow vascular malformations (VMs) are the best examples when a multimodal approach is required.

Venous and lymphatic malformations are under the categories more frequently controlled by medical therapy. LMs are more rarely treated by surgery alone.

Systemic treatment with new pharmacologic agents (such as sirolimus and alpelisib), sclerotherapy (using sclerosing and antimetabolic drugs), and surgical resection are used in different sequences, in a case-based approach.

Regarding surgery, radical resection is not a mandatory target.

The modern approach is initiated by drug therapy or sclerotherapy, reducing lesion volume and active flow. It is believed that the effectiveness of pharmacologic treatment is better achieved in nonoperated areas. Thus, surgical resection may complete treatment instead of initiating the approach. Also, medical therapy reduces coagulation problems, very common in large malformations with venous component.

In cases responding to medical therapy, it is still unclear how long these drugs should be maintained. Surgical procedures must be applied when local control or resection is locally safe (**Fig. 2**).

After surgical procedures, pharmacologic agents can be reintroduced as well as sclerotherapy may be used to complete treatment. When a total resection is performed or when the malformation is quiescent, discontinuation of drug therapy does may be considered.[26–31]

CAPILLARY MALFORMATION

Treatment of capillary malformation (CM) is classically achieved with the use of laser therapy. However, surgical resection has some specific indications, treating hypertrophic cutaneous areas, nodular lesions, and skeletal deformities. Treatment is mainly directed to facial lesions (**Fig. 3**).

CM are mainly cutaneous and resection is usually simpler than other VM. Surgical reconstruction is performed by primary closure or using local flaps and full-thickness skin grafts.[32–35]

VENOUS MALFORMATION

Intralesional treatment with sclerosing agents (alcohol, polidocanol) and antimetabolic drugs (bleomycin) as well as medical therapy may treat deep and superficial components and usually precede surgical approach when partial resections of large VMs are planned. For smaller VMs primary treatment can be direct resection. If a small recurrence is observed, sclerotherapy may be used secondarily.

Surgical approach has a low recurrence rate, even when radical resection is not indicated. Long-term follow-up must be carried out and sequential resections over time are acceptable as a planned surgical approach[36–40] (**Fig. 4**).

LYMPHATIC MALFORMATION

Lymphatic malformations must be characterized by macrocystis and microcystic. In the first group, aspiration of the content and injection of sclerosing agents, such as bleomycin and doxycycline, have encouraging results. Surgical resection would be more aesthetic and optional, removing exceeding skin or fibro adipose tissue (**Fig. 5**).

Microcystic lymphatic malformations are often associated with venous malformations and can significantly benefit from medical treatment. The drug is used from a neoadjuvant perspective. Surgical resection aims to offer the patient a better body or face contour, always from most hidden surgical accesses.[41–45]

HIGH FLOW VASCULAR MALFORMATIONS

Arteriovenous malformations (AVMs) are the most challenging VM from the surgeon's perspective.

Today, most of the AVM are treated by a combination of embolizations and surgical resection (**Fig. 6**). The use of targeted therapy gained a new perspective with the use of MEK inhibitors (as trametinib) as many AVM do not respond well to mTor inhibitors. It is expected in the near future that combined therapy will be the first choice to control, reduce volume and allow radical resection.[46–53]

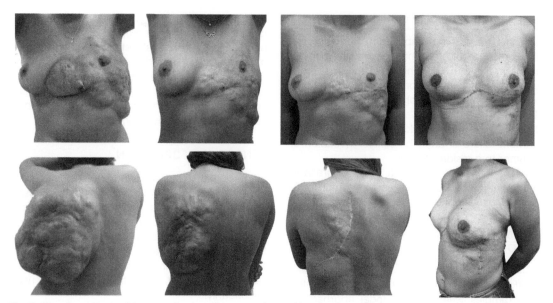

Fig. 2. Female patient with a massive low-flow vascular malformation in the back, extending to anterior chest. MRI showed the invasion of vital organs in the mediastinum and confirmed a large venous malformation. Treatment was initiated with sirolimus and a satisfactory response was obtained after 2 years. Surgical resection was performed and followed by an additional procedure for breast reconstruction with the tissue expander and breast implant.

Surgical treatment of AVMs requires specific knowledge:

- AVM must be precisely diagnosed. Other nonvascular lesions must be discarded.

- A precise clinical and radiological mapping should be held. The type of AVM, anatomic structures involved, and real extension are essential for surgical planning.

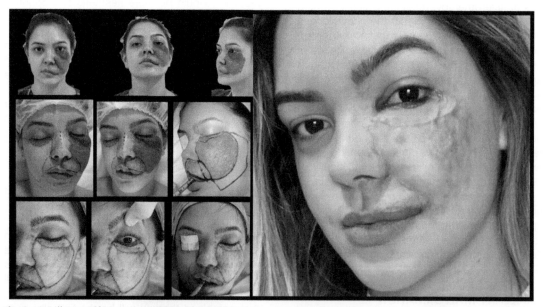

Fig. 3. Capillary malformation with increased thickness and deformity in the left cheek, eyelid, and upper lip. Surgical planning for esthetic unit removal and reconstruction with full-thickness skin grafts. The remaining lip component was partially resected in this first procedure.

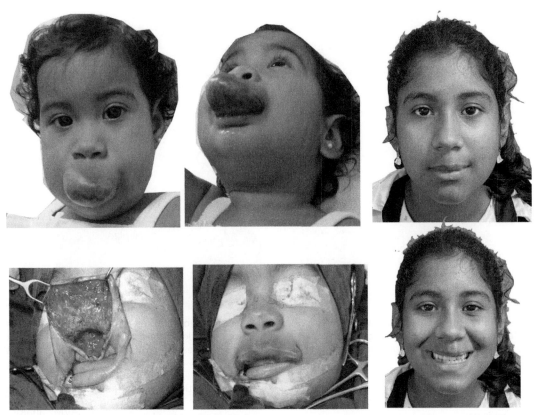

Fig. 4. A 2-year-old woman patient with a large venous malformation of the upper lip. Indication for surgery was based growth-related deformity and functional impairment. Upper left and center, preoperative aspect. Lower left, intraoperative aspect showing VM resection, preserving orbicularis oris muscle. Later in discussion, center: immediate result with the anatomic preservation of the upper lip. Upper and lower right: late postoperative appearance after 10 years.

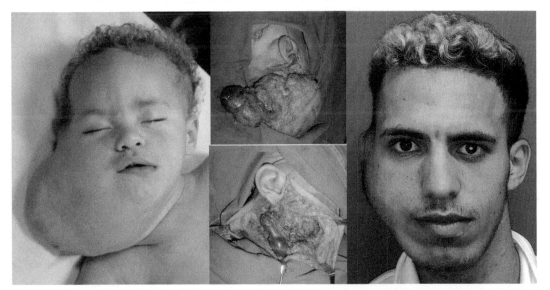

Fig. 5. Macrocystic LM can be treated by surgery, although intralesional therapy has a primary role. Clinical example of the surgical resection of a large LM (*left*), showing intraoperative aspects (*center*) and late postoperative appearance after 17 years.

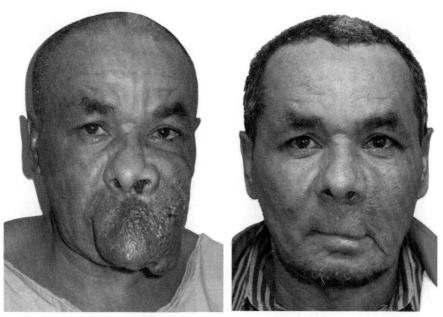

Fig. 6. Male patient with a large facial AVM (*right*). Previous embolization reduced progression but the lesion evolute with mucosal erosion. Surgical planning for radical excision considered the expansion of normal tissue to allow primary reconstruction with local flaps. Left, late postoperative appearance with no regrowth after 5 years.

- Partial resection has a higher rate of recurrence. Therefore, radical excision should be prioritized.
- Diffuse AVM with the involvement of vital structures needs an extensive discussion about the risk and benefits of the surgical procedure. Sometimes, radical resection is impossible.
- After resection, definitive reconstruction should be postponed, to guarantee no recurrence of the AVM. If a simple closure, it is not possible, a definite repair should be conducted immediately.
- The loss rate of grafts is higher in AVM lesions. Thus, flaps should be preferred as the final reconstruction.

Final Outcome

Surgical approach to all vascular anomalies should follow a specific guideline aiming at optimal functional and aesthetic results.

- Postpone surgical resection to offer a neoadjuvant treatment with medical therapy and minimally invasive procedures.
- Surgical access that offers hidden scars, often based on aesthetic procedures techniques
- Decide the extension of the resection based on the final benefit versus the iatrogenic potential of collateral damage and sequelae.

- Reconstruction is an essential part of the treatment and but must be delayed to ensure no recurrence of the malformation.

CLINICS CARE POINTS

- Surgical resection is effective.
- Type of resection varies according to diagnosis.
- Multidisciplinary approach is a key point.

DISCLOSURE

The authors have nothing to disclose.

REFERENCES

1. Burrows PE, et al. Diagnostic Imaging in the Evaluotion of Vascular Birthmarks. Dermatol Clin 1998;16:455–88.
2. Goldenberg DC, Hiraki PY, Caldas JG, et al. Surgical Treatment of Extracranial Arteriovenous Malformations after Multiple Embolizations. Plast Reconstr Surg 2015;135:543–52.
3. Mulliken JB, Enjolras O. Congenital hemangiomas and infantile hemangioma: missing links. J Am Acad Dermatol 2004;50(6):875–82.

4. Mulliken JB, Glowacki J. Hemangioma and vascular malformation in infants and children a classification based on endothelial characteristics. Plast Reconstr Surg 1982;69:412–22.

5. Mulliken JB, Burrows PE, Fishman SJ. Mulliken & Young's vascular anomalies. 2nd edition. Oxford University Press; 2013.

6. Goldenberg DC. Estudo crítico dos resultados obtidos no tratamento dos hemangiomas cutâneos cervicofaciais. Tese (mestrado), 164p. São Paulo (Brazil): Faculdade de Medicina da Universidade de São Paulo; 2002.

7. Greene AK, Goss JA. Vascular Anomalies: From a Clinicohistologic to a Genetic Framework. Plast Reconstr Surg 2018;141:709e–17e. https://doi.org/10.1097/PRS.0000000000004294. PMID: 29697621.

8. Hage AN, Chick JFB, Srinivasa RN, et al. Treatment of Venous Malformations: The Data, Where We Are, and How It Is Done. Tech Vasc Interv Radiol 2018;21:45–54. https://doi.org/10.1053/j.tvir.2018.03.001. Epub 2018 Mar 8. PMID: 29784122.

9. Haggstrom AN, Drolet BA, Baselga E, et al. Prospective Study of Infantile Hemangiomas: Clinical Characteristcs Predicting Complications and Treatment. Pediatrics 2006;118:882–7.

10. Deng W, Huang D, Chen S, et al. Management of high-flow arteriovenous malformation in the maxillofacial region. J Craniofac Surg 2010;21:916–9.

11. Bruckner AL, Frieden IJ. Hemangioma of Infancy. J Am Acad Dermatol April 2003;48:477–93.

12. Abbas, Laielly MD, Sakamoto MK, et al. Impact of Oral β-Blockers on Surgical Treatment of Infantile Hemangioma. Plast Reconstr Surg - Glob Open 2019;8S-1:64–5.

13. Bauland, Constantijn G. The Pathogenesis of Hemangiomas: A Review. Plast Reconstr Surg 2006;117:29e–35e.

14. Beck DO, Gosain AK. The presentation and management of hemangiomas. Plast Reconstr Surg 2009;123. 181e-91e.

15. Bénateau H, Labbé D, Dompmartin A, et al. Sequelae of haemangiomas: surgical treatment. Ann Chir Plast Esthet 2006;51:330–8.

16. Blei F. New clinical observation in hemangiomas. Semin Cutan Med Surg 1999;18:187–94.

17. Boye E, Jinnin M, Olsen B. Infantile Hemangioma: Challenges, New Insights, and Therapeutic Promise. J Craniofac Surg 2009;20:1.

18. Drolet BA, Esterly NB, Frieden IJ. Hemangioma in children. N Engl J Med 1999;341:173–81.

19. Goldenberg DC, Hiraki PY, Marques TM, et al. Surgical Treatment of Facial Infantile Hemangiomas: An Analysis Based on Tumor Characteristics and Outcomes. Plast Reconstr Surg 2016;136:1221–31.

20. Hiraki PY, Goldenberg DC. Diagnóstico e Tratamento do Hemangioma Infantil. Rev Bras Cir Plast 2010;25:388–97.

21. Osio A, Fraitag S, Hadj-Rabia S, et al. Clinical spectrum of tufted angiomas in childhood: a report of 13 cases and a review of the literature. Arch Dermatol 2010;146:758–63.

22. Zukerberg LR, Nickoloff BJ, Weiss SW. Kaposiform hemangioendothelioma of infancy and childhood: an aggressive neoplasm associated with Kasabach-Merritt syndrome and lymphangiomatosis. Am J Surg Pathol 1993;17:321–8.

23. Leng T, Wang X, Huo R, et al. The value of three-dimensional computed tomographic angiography in the diagnosis and treatment of vascular lesions. Plast Reconstr Surg 2008;122:1417–24.

24. Enjolras O, Wassef M, Mazoyer E, et al. Infants with Kasabach-Merritt syndrome do not have "true" hemangiomas. J Pediatr 1997;130:631–40.

25. Enjolras O, Wassef M, Maqzoyer E, et al. Infants with Kasabach-Merrit Syndrome do not have true hemangiomas. J Pediatr 1997;130:631–40.

26. Churchill P, Otal D, Pemberton J, et al. Sclerotherapy for lymphatic malformations in children: a scoping review. J Pediatr Surg 2011;46:912–22.

27. Achauer BM, Vander Kam V, Bems MW. Laser in plastic surgery and dermatology. New York: Thieme; 1992.

28. Vikkula M, Boon LM, Carraway KL III, et al. Vascular dysmorphogenesis caused by an activating mutation in the receptor tyrosine kinase TIE2. Cell 1996;87:1181–90.

29. Zorzan G, Tullio A, Baj A, et al. [Arteriovenous malformations of the head and neck. Diagnosis and methods of treatment]. Minerva Stomatol 2001;50:351–9.

30. Kang GC, Song C. Forty-one cervicofacial vascular anomalies and their surgical treatment–retrospection and review. Ann Acad Med Singapore 2008;37:165–79.

31. Einchenfield LF. Evolving knowledge of hemangiomas and vascular malformations beyond stawbwerries and port wine. Arch Dermatol 1998;134:740–2.

32. Cosman B. Clinical experience in the laser therapy of Port Wine Stain. Laser Surg Med 1980;1:133–52.

33. Mc Burney EH, Leonard GL. Argon Laser treatment of Port-Wine hemangioma: clinical and hystological correlation. South Med J 1981;74:925–9.

34. Revencu N, Boon LM, Mendola A, et al. RASA1 mutations and associated phenotypes in 68 families with capillary malformation-arteriovenous malformation. Hum Mutat 2013;34:1632–41. https://doi.org/10.1002/humu.22431. Epub 2013 Oct 10. PMID: 24038909.

35. Schwager K, Waner M, Flock S. In vivo models for studies of laser effects on blood vessels. Adv Otorhinolaryngol 1995;2:10–4.

36. Seront E, Vikkula M, Boon LM. Venous Malformations of the Head and Neck. Otolaryngol Clin North Am 2018;51:173–84. PMID: 29217061.

37. Vogel SA, Hess CP, Dowd CF, et al. Early versus later presentations of venous malformations: where and why? Pediatr Dermatol 2013;30:534–40.

38. Dompmartin A, Acher A, Thibon P, et al. Association of localized intravascular coagulopathy with venous malformations. Arch Dermatol 2008;144:873–7. PMID: 18645138 Free PMC article.

39. Razek AA, Ashmalla GA. Prediction of venous malformations with localized intravascular coagulopathy with diffusion-weighted magnetic resonance imaging. Phlebology 2019;34:156–61. PMID: 29720044.

40. Limaye N, Wouters V, Uebelhoer M, et al. Somatic mutations in angiopoietin receptor gene TEK cause solitary and multiple sporadic venous malformations. Nat Genet 2009;41:118–24. Epub 2008 Dec 14. PMID: 19079259.

41. Breugem CC, Courtemanche DJ. Portable ultrasound-assisted injection of OK-432 in lymphatic malformations by the plastic surgeon. J Plast Reconstr Aesthet Surg 2008;61:1269–70.

42. Hong JP, Lee MY, Kim EK, et al. Giant lymphangioma of the tongue. J Craniofac Surg 2009;20:252–4.

43. Zhou Q, Zheng JW, Mai HM, et al. Treatment guidelines of lymphatic malformations of the head and neck. Oral Oncol 2011;47:1105–9.

44. Närkiö-Mäkelä M, Mäkelä T, Saarinen P, et al. Treatment of lymphatic malformations of head and neck with OK-432 sclerotherapy induce systemic inflammatory response. Eur Arch Otorhinolaryngol 2011;268:123–9.

45. Wiegand S, Eivazi B, Zimmermann AP, et al. Microcystic lymphatic malformations of the tongue. Arch Otolaryngol Head Neck Surg 2009;135:976–83.

46. Goldenberg DC, Hiraki PY, Koga A. Scalp arteriovenous malformations. In: Richter GT, Suen JY, editors. Head and neck vascular anomalies: a practical case-based approach. Plural Publishing; 2015. p. 343–50. ISBN10 1597565466. ISBN13 9781597565462.

47. Chagas Ferreira MV, Charles Goldenberg D, Kharmandayan V, et al. Management of Arteriovenous Malformation of the Ear: A Protocol for Resection and Reconstruction. Laryngoscope 2020;130:1322–6.

48. Wu JK, Bisdorff A, Gelbert F, et al. Auricular arteriovenous malformation: evaluation, management, and outcome. Plast Reconstr Surg 2005;115:985–95.

49. Richter GT, Suen J, North PE, et al. Arteriovenous malformations of the tongue: a spectrum of disease. Laryngoscope 2007;117:328–35.

50. Richter GT, Suen JY. Clinical course of arteriovenous malformations of the head and neck: a case series. Otolaryngol Head Neck Surg 2010;142:184–90.

51. Weinzweig N, Chin G, Polley J, et al. Arteriovenous malformation of the forehead, anterior scalp, and nasal dorsum. Plast Reconstr Surg 2000;105:2433–9.

52. Chen WL, Ye JT, Xu LF, et al. A multidisciplinary approach to treating maxillofacial arteriovenous malformations in children. Oral Surg Oral Med Oral Pathol Oral Radiol Endod 2009;108:41–7.

53. Bradley JP, Zide BM, Berenstein A, et al. Large arteriovenous malformations of the face: aesthetic results with recurrence control. Plast Reconstr Surg 1999;103:351–61.

Laser Treatment of Vascular Anomalies

Austin N. DeHart, MD[a],*, Gresham T. Richter, MD[b]

KEYWORDS

- Laser • Vascular anomaly • Hemangioma • Capillary malformation • Venous malformation
- Arteriovenous malformation • Vascular malformation

KEY POINTS

- Lasers assist in the multimanagement of vascular anomalies with cutaneous and mucosal involvement.
- Through the process of selective photothermolysis, laser treatment preferentially targets abnormal vessels with low impact on surrounding normal tissue.
- Titrate laser settings to clinical endpoints to prevent complications.

INTRODUCTION

Vascular anomalies are a varied group of disorders involving abnormal blood vessels predominately of congenital origin. The International Society for the Study of Vascular Anomalies codified the classification system that divides these lesions into either tumors or malformations based on their clinical, imaging, and pathologic features.[1] Vascular tumors are most commonly benign infantile hemangiomas (IH), but this category does include rarer, more clinically aggressive lesions like kaposiform hemangioendothelioma. Vascular malformations are caused by abnormal blood vessel and lymphatic channel development. They are described by the predominant vessel type in the lesion and can be either capillary, venous, lymphatic, arteriovenous, or some combination. Vascular malformations often infiltrate normal tissue and bone, causing functional and aesthetic concerns. Cutaneous and mucosal manifestations can lead to ulceration, bleeding, and disfigurement.

Selective photothermolysis is the process by which laser energy preferentially targets abnormal vessels in these lesions.[2] Medical LASER (light amplification by stimulated emission of radiation) pairs wavelengths to specific chromatic targets called chromophores. By careful selection of laser parameters, the energy absorbed by a particular chromophore can induce cellular injury while minimizing damage to collateral cells.[2] During laser treatment, photons are released and absorbed by tissue, which causes rapid, localized thermal damage. This denatures enzymes and structural proteins, causing cellular injury. The target chromophore for vascular lesions is either oxygenated or deoxygenated hemoglobin, which concentrates heat energy with blood vessels.[3] Damage in the vessel leads to coagulation, closure, and obliteration of the vessel. Superficial, slow-flow, small vessels are ideally suited to concentrate thermal injury via laser energy with a better response, although high-flow vessels can respond with appropriate parameters.[4]

LASER PARAMETERS AND SELECTION

Laser selection is based on matching laser parameters with the characteristics of the targeted lesion. The wavelength of the laser determines its chromophore and depth of penetration.[2] Oxyhemoglobin has greatest absorption peaks at 418, 542, and 577 nm, so is best targeted by a wavelength of 595 nm using the pulse dye laser (PDL).[5] Deoxyhemoglobin has a maximum absorption near 750 nm and 930 nm and is best

[a] Division of Pediatric Otolaryngology-Head and Neck Surgery, Phoenix Children's Hospital, 1919 East Thomas Road, Phoenix, AZ 85016, USA; [b] Department of Pediatric Otolaryngology-Head and Neck Surgery, Arkansas Children's Hospital, University of Arkansas for Medical Sciences, 1 Children's Way, Little Rock, AR 72202, USA
* Corresponding author.
E-mail address: adehart@phoenixchildrens.com

Dermatol Clin 40 (2022) 481–487
https://doi.org/10.1016/j.det.2022.06.002
0733-8635/22/© 2022 Elsevier Inc. All rights reserved.

targeted by a wavelength of 755 nm alexandrite or 1064-nm long pulse Nd:YAG laser.[2] Longer wavelengths have an increased depth of penetration, allowing them to target deeper lesions. In addition to choosing laser wavelength, adjusting the laser pulse duration can better select for vessels of different sizes. Small vessels, with a diameter less than 100 μm, are treated with a shorter pulse duration.[4] Medium and large vessels, with a diameter of 100 to 400 μm and diameters greater than 400 μm, require longer pulse duration.[4]

Lesions with small, superficial vessels like early port-wine stains and superficial proliferating hemangiomas can be best targeted by a PDL with pulse duration of 0.45 to 1.5 milliseconds, which penetrates to a depth of 1 to 2 mm.[4] Pulse duration can affect the depth of penetration. Advanced port-wine stains and venous malformations (VM), which have larger vessel diameters and deeper extent, are better targeted by Nd:YAG lasers with longer pulse duration of 0.1 to 1 second.[4] There are multiple brands and models for each specific-wavelength laser, so it can be difficult to extrapolate laser settings across different technologies.[5] **Table 1** lists commonly used settings, but these should be applied with caution.[4] Variations in lesions and skin tone (Fitzpatrick I–V) can affect outcomes.

It is important to monitor for clinical changes reflecting tissue response and adjust settings to the desired endpoint to prevent complications.[5] With PDL, the desired endpoint is purpura (**Fig. 1**). This develops over a few minutes after pulse administration and may continue to darken slightly in the next 1 to 2 days after treatment.[6] Tissue changing gray or white can be an early hallmark of skin thermal injury. The long-pulse Nd:YAG and alexandrite lasers penetrate more deeply, so the fluence should be set at the lowest level that causes purple-blue coloration changes to avoid skin compromise.[6] Risks of laser include blistering, scarring, wound breakdown, or pigmentation changes. Adjusting a laser's power and pulse duration to these endpoints can minimize inadvertent injury. Fluence is the amount of light energy delivered to an area (measured in Watts per square centimeter), so should be started at a low setting and advanced to clinical effect.

Depending on the age of the patient, size and location of the lesion, laser therapy for vascular anomalies can be performed either in the clinic or in the office setting. It is often preferred to treat children under sedation or general anesthesia to reduce discomfort and anxiety. However, for small lesions, away from the orbit, many young children and adults can be managed in the office with or without pretreatment without sedation, using topical cutaneous local anesthetics.

LASER SAFETY

Established safety protocols are important during laser use. Appropriate protective eyeglasses that correspond to the laser type must be worn by the surgeon and staff in the room. Patients should be protected with metal corneal eye shields if performing laser around the eye or with opaque eye pads or glasses depending on the treatment site. Manufacturer guidelines should be followed. Other precautions vary by institution, but typically include door warning signs that the laser is in use, window coverings in the room, fire safety precautions if anesthesia is being used to minimize inspired oxygen levels, and appropriately trained laser safety operator staff present. Providers should confirm correct laser settings before initiating treatment. Laser test spots can be helpful to confirm safe settings, especially in darker-skinned individuals. Laser spots should be near confluent but with minimal overlap for each treatment pass.

TREATMENT AFTERCARE

After laser procedures, patients can anticipate purple skin discoloration and discomfort as the area heals. Ice packs and steroids can reduce postprocedural pain and swelling. Keep the treated area covered with petrolatum-based ointment to support healing. Pain is generally able to be controlled by over-the-counter medications. While healing, sunscreen use is recommended when outside.

LASER TREATMENT BY ANOMALY TYPE

The category of vascular anomaly encompasses many disparate pathologic conditions. Each lesion type has its own natural history and vessel composition, which should be taken into consideration for treatment.

Hemangioma

IH are common vascular tumors (**Fig. 2**). Although many IH follow a benign course and do not require treatment, "problematic" IH can lead to bleeding, ulceration, functional impairment, and disfigurement. IH that are greater than 2 cm, are segmentally distributed, or are located by the eye, mouth, or perineum are particularly high risk for complications and merit intervention.[7] Systemic propranolol is the treatment of choice for problematic hemangiomas, whereas topical treatment with timolol may be appropriate for some superficial, thin lesions.[8]

Table 1
Laser wavelengths, settings, and additional information for the most commonly treated vascular anomalies

Laser	Main Indications in Vascular Anomalies	Typical Settings	Additional Information
FPDL 595 nm	Hemangiomas, port-wine stains, and others	2 Main options: Joules: 8–15 J Duration: 0.45–1.5 ms Spot size: 7 mm Joules: 8–10 J Duration: 1.5 ms Spot size: 10 mm	Place coolant on maximum level. Joules vary based on initial skin response. 7-mm spot is most frequently used with average treatment range between 8 and 15 J. With 10-mm spot size, maximum Joule is 10 J because of the limits of the machine. The smaller the spot size, the higher the Joule maximum level
Alexandrite 755 nm	Hemangiomas, port-wine stains, and others (often used on lesions that are resistant to FPDL treatment and lesions with more purple coloration)	Joules: 60–100 J Duration: 3 ms Spot size: 8 mm Hertz: 1 Hz Coolant settings: Pre 90/ delay 80/post Off	Joule level varies with skin response. Great care should be taken when using on patients with high Fitzpatrick levels (darker skin). It will be absorbed by melanin and can result in hypopigmentation
Long pulse Nd:YAG 1064 nm	Various vascular anomalies, usually venous malformations	2 Main options: Joules: 180–220 J Duration: 20 ms Spot size: 3 mm Joules: 80–100 J Duration: 20 ms Spot size: 8 mm Constant settings: Hertz: 1 Hz Coolant settings: pre 40/ delay 30/post off	Consider this laser on darkly pigmented skin. 8-mm spot size maxes out at 120 J. Referred to as "gentle" because of the coolant spray. Same wavelength as Nd:YAG laser. Joules vary with response. Penetrates up to 8 mm to get deep venous lesions
Nd:YAG 1064 nm	Venous malformations (airway, intraoral and interstitial treatments)	Most settings are standard Watts: 15–30 W Duration: 1–2 ms	Various hand pieces and fibers exist for use to reach difficult locations. Predominately used to manage mucosal venous malformations of the aerodigestive tract. Fiber can be passed through 14-gauge 1.25 inch needle for interstitial treatment.

From Rosenberg, T.L., Richter, G.T. Lasers in the Treatment of Vascular Anomalies. *Curr Otorhinolaryngol Rep* 2, 265–272 (2014).

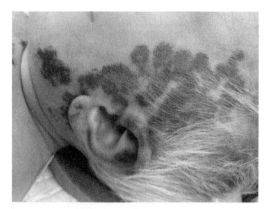

Fig. 1. PWS with purpura from laser treatment.

In the proliferative phase, laser treatment is not very effective compared with early beta-blocker use unless there is ulceration.[9–11] For hemangiomas that ulcerate, PDL laser can help facilitate healing.[12] PDL and Nd:YAG lasers can treat superficial hemangiomas and be used as an adjuvant to propranolol. This can minimize permanent skin changes after completing propranolol therapy. Starting laser treatment after hemangiomas start to involute can further improve response rates and decrease the duration of beta-blocker therapy.[13–15] Telangiectasia that persist after hemangioma involution can be treated with PDL.[16,17] Fractionated CO_2 ablative lasers can also be useful to resurface irregular skin texture or scarring.[18]

Capillary Malformation

Capillary malformation, otherwise known as port-wine birthmarks (PWB), is an congenital

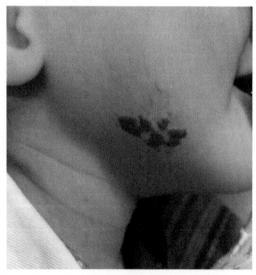

Fig. 2. Infantile hemangioma.

malformation made of small, ectatic vessels that are mostly postcapillary venules.[19] Over time, the vessels within PWB increase in diameter, causing these lesions to get darker, thicker, and hypertrophic and can contribute to soft tissue overgrowth.[20] PDL was specifically introduced into medicine for the treatment of PWB and remains the preferred treatment for these lesions.[21] Treatment with PDL is safe with a low risk of scarring, but multiple treatments are required for clinical effect. Most PWB do lighten substantially with PDL, but only 20% are completely cleared and 20% remain resistant to therapy.[21] Long term, these lesions have high recurrence rates.[22] Treatment is best started before 6 months of age to improve success.[23] If initiated early, outcomes improve to a 90% clearance rate, which is attributed to thinner dermis in infants and more complete coverage with PDL.[23]

Thicker lesions are more difficult to treat with PDL because of the persistence of blood vessels deeper in the tissue than the laser can penetrate.[3] Different laser setting variations have been explored to improve this, including "double-pass" methods. With a double-pass technique, the same area is treated sequentially with PDL at both long- and short-pulse durations to cover deeper and more superficial vessels, which show promise for resistant lesions.[24,25] The alexandrite and long-pulse Nd:YAG lasers have been used to reach deeper vessels in these lesions and are alternative options for PDL-resistant PWB.[26–28] These lasers do have narrower therapeutic margins, so caution must be used. Topical agents, including timolol, imiquimod, and rapamycin, have been trialed as adjunctive treatment for resistant PWB, but have not been shown to consistently improve disease course.[29]

Venous Malformation

VM are congenital lesions composed of thin-walled, tortuous veins. They can be characterized by spongiform, ectatic, or mixed vessels. They frequently infiltrate muscles, skin, and mucous membranes and gradually expand with patients over time. Periods of hormonal changes, especially puberty and pregnancy, can be associated with increased disease burden and symptoms.[30] VM cause symptoms owing to mass effect, distortion of normal anatomy, pressure, and bulk. They also are prone to local intravascular coagulation, where painful clots and organized phleboliths form within the malformation.[31] There are many treatment options for VM, including sclerotherapy, systemic medications, surgical resection, and laser. Because of the larger vessel size and higher

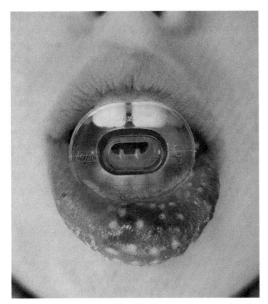

Fig. 3. VM of lower lip after treatment with fiber Nd:YAG laser.

concentration of deoxyhemoglobin in VM, the alexandrite and long-pulse Nd:YAG lasers are most commonly used. Sometime PDL can be used as an adjunct to treat lesions with a more superficial telangiectasia component or smaller vessels.[32,33]

VM involving mucosa can be treated with an Nd:YAG laser fiber. Different handpieces are available to help reach difficult to access locations, which is particularly useful for aerodigestive track or pelvic mucosal lesions.[34–36] Variation in power settings depends on the location of the lesion along the mucosa with lower settings (10–18 W) along the distal airway to 25 to 30 W for the tongue.[37] When treating mucosal disease, laser spots should be widely spaced with bridges of normal mucosa between them to prevent confluence of mucosal sloughing and ulceration[34,38] (Fig. 3). Nd:YAG can also be used interstitially under ultrasound guidance with the fiber passed through a large-bore needle to treat deeper portions of VM.[39,40] The Nd:YAG laser has a modified form with additional cooling that can be used on cutaneous VM. The cooling helps protect overlying skin from thermal injury during treatment, allowing for good clinical outcomes and a low complication rate.[41,42] For complex lesions with a deeper component, Nd:YAG laser treatment of the skin can help reduce disease volume and improve the quality of superficial tissue before future sclerotherapy or surgical resection.[43]

Arteriovenous Malformations

Peripheral arteriovenous malformations (AVM) are complex perturbations of vascular development and remodeling composed of direct arteriovenous connections without intervening capillary beds, disrupted vascular remodeling, and arterialized veins. They can occur as a part of larger inheritable syndrome capillary malformation - arteriovenous malformation (CM-AVM) or in isolation secondary to somatic mutations predominately in MAP2kinase pathway. Embolic, surgical, and now potential medical therapies may be used in their treatment. Historically, the best treatment outcomes are achieved with supraselective embolization followed by surgical resection. However, preservation of the skin and mucosa is paramount to preserve best aesthetic and functional outcomes.

Thus, AVM laser therapy, much like for VM, is used to manage cutaneous and mucosal disease. Nd:YAG laser therapy is used with fiber-directed treatment of mucosa at lower settings than used for VM (8–10 W) of these more friable vessels. This is often used for dental gingival disease that has a propensity to bleed. Cutaneous management uses PDL and cooled Nd:YAG laser to manage small and telangiectatic vessels and deeper venous outflow tracts, respectively. Again, this is performed multiple times with gradually expanding intervals between treatments.[44] Laser for peripheral/extracranial AVM is often performed in conjunction with interstitial or intraluminal sclerotherapy as a primary treatment approach. On the other hand, this can allow for skin preparation performed multiple times before a more advanced resection so that the soft tissue envelope can be preserved.

SUMMARY

Lasers are a good treatment option for the management of most vascular anomalies. Through selective photothermolysis, lasers can preferentially target hemoglobin and deoxyhemoglobin within these lesions. With repeated but gradually increasing treatment intervals, select lasers (PDL, alexandrite, and Nd:YAG) can improve the appearance of most PWB, reduce sequelae after hemangioma involution, and reduce bleeding risks, bulk, and symptoms of venous and AVM. Safety measures are important to protect patients and staff during procedures. Monitoring clinical endpoints during treatment can guide appropriate laser setting use. Complex cases should be discussed in a multidisciplinary vascular anomalies team to achieve the best possible outcomes.

CLINICS CARE POINTS

- Port-wine birthmarks (capillary malformations) can be improved in color and stain by laser treatment, although the extent of improvement can be difficult to predict and is dependent on location. Some resistant lesions may benefit from combination therapy with pulse dye laser and Nd:YAG lasers.

- Telangiectasia or cutaneous staining that persists after hemangioma involution can be treated with pulse dye laser.

- Venous and arteriovenous malformations benefit from multimodal therapy, of which treatment with Nd:YAG laser is a versatile component.

- Tailor laser treatment to clinical endpoints to minimize tissue injury.

DISCLOSURE

The authors have nothing to disclose.

REFERENCES

1. Wassef M, Blei F, Adams D, et al. Vascular Anomalies Classification: Recommendations From the International Society for the Study of Vascular Anomalies. Pediatrics 2015;136:e203–14.
2. Rox Anderson R, Parrish JA. Selective photothermolysis: precise microsurgery by selective absorption of pulsed radiation. Science 1983;220:524–7.
3. Fiskerstrand EJ, Svaasand LO, Kopstad G, et al. Photothermally induced vessel-wall necrosis after pulsed dye laser treatment: lack of response in port-wine stains with small sized or deeply located vessels. J Invest Dermatol 1996;107:671–5.
4. Rosenberg TL, Richter GT. Lasers in the Treatment of Vascular Anomalies. Curr Otorhinolaryngol Rep 2014;2:265–72.
5. Gupta D. Laser Surgery for Dermatologic Conditions in Pediatric Patients. Dermatol Clin 2022;40:215–25.
6. Wanner M, Sakamoto FH, Avram MM, et al. Immediate skin responses to laser and light treatments: Therapeutic endpoints: How to obtain efficacy. J Am Acad Dermatol 2016;74:821–33.
7. Krowchuk DP, Frieden IJ, Mancini AJ, et al. Clinical practice guideline for the management of infantile hemangiomas. Pediatrics 2019;143.
8. Ainipully A, Narayanan S, Vazhiyodan A, et al. Oral propranolol in infantile hemangiomas: Analysis of factors that affect the outcome. J Indian Assoc Pediatr Surg 2019;24:170.
9. Shen L, Zhou G, Zhao J, et al. Pulsed dye laser therapy for infantile hemangiomas: a systemic review and meta-analysis. QJM 2015;108:473–80.
10. Chinnadurai S, Sathe NA, Surawicz T. Laser treatment of infantile hemangioma: A systematic review. Lasers Surg Med 2016;48:221–33.
11. Hartmann F, Lockmann A, Gronemeyer LL, et al. Nd:YAG and pulsed dye laser therapy in infantile haemangiomas: a retrospective analysis of 271 treated haemangiomas in 149 children. J Eur Acad Dermatol Venereol 2017;31:1372–9.
12. Li Y, Hu Y, Li H, et al. Successful treatment of ulcerated hemangiomas with a dual-wavelength 595- and 1064-nm laser system. J Dermatolog Treat 2016;27:562–7.
13. Park KH, Jang YH, Chung HY, et al. Topical timolol maleate 0.5% for infantile hemangioma; it's effectiveness and/or adjunctive pulsed dye laser - single center experience of 102 cases in Korea. J Dermatolog Treat 2015;26:389–91.
14. Reddy KK, Blei F, Brauer JA, et al. Retrospective study of the treatment of infantile hemangiomas using a combination of propranolol and pulsed dye laser. Dermatol Surg 2013;39:923–33.
15. Sugimoto A, Aoki R, Toyohara E, et al. Infantile Hemangiomas Cleared by Combined Therapy With Pulsed Dye Laser and Propranolol. Dermatol Surg 2021;47:1052–7.
16. Cerrati EW, MArch TMO, Chung H, et al. Diode laser for the treatment of telangiectasias following hemangioma involution. Otolaryngol - Head Neck Surg (United States 2015;152:239–43.
17. Buckmiller LM, Munson PD, Dyamenahalli U, et al. Propranolol for infantile hemangiomas: early experience at a tertiary vascular anomalies center. Laryngoscope 2010;120:676–81.
18. Brightman LA, Brauer JA, Terushkin V, et al. Ablative fractional resurfacing for involuted hemangioma residuum. Arch Dermatol 2012;148:1294–8.
19. Braverman IM, Keh Yen A. Ultrastructure and three-dimensional reconstruction of several macular and papular telangiectases. J Invest Dermatol 1983;81:489–97.
20. Geronemus RG, Ashinoff R. The medical necessity of evaluation and treatment of port-wine stains. J Dermatol Surg Oncol 1991;17:76–9.
21. Rubin IK, Farinelli WA, Doukas A, et al. Optimal wavelengths for vein-selective photothermolysis. Lasers Surg Med 2012;44:152–7.
22. Orten SS, Waner M, Flock S, et al. Port-wine stains. An assessment of 5 years of treatment. Arch Otolaryngol Head Neck Surg 1996;122:1174–9.
23. Chapas AM, Eickhorst K, Geronemus RG. Efficacy of early treatment of facial port wine stains in

newborns: a review of 49 cases. Lasers Surg Med 2007;39:563–8.

24. Noormohammadpour P, Ehsani AH, Mahmoudi H, et al. Does Double-Pass Pulsed-Dye Laser With Long and Short Pulse Duration Increase Treatment Efficacy of Port-Wine Stain? A Randomized Clinical Trial. Dermatol Surg 2021;47:e122–6.

25. Kono T, Sakurai H, Takeuchi M, et al. Treatment of resistant port-wine stains with a variable-pulse pulsed dye laser. Dermatol Surg 2007;33:951–6.

26. Izikson L, Nelson JS, Anderson RR. Treatment of hypertrophic and resistant port wine stains with a 755 nm laser: A case series of 20 patients. Lasers Surg Med 2009;41:427–32.

27. Alster TS, Tanzi EL. Combined 595-nm and 1,064-nm laser irradiation of recalcitrant and hypertrophic port-wine stains in children and adults. Dermatol Surg 2009;35:914–9.

28. Savas JA, Ledon JA, Franca K, et al. Pulsed dye laser-resistant port-wine stains: mechanisms of resistance and implications for treatment. Br J Dermatol 2013;168:941–53.

29. Lipner SR. Topical Adjuncts to Pulsed Dye Laser for Treatment of Port Wine Stains: Review of the Literature. Dermatol Surg 2018;44:796–802.

30. Colletti G, Ierardi AM. Understanding venous malformations of the head and neck: a comprehensive insight. Med Oncol 2017;34.

31. Dompmartin A, Acher A, Thibon P, et al. Association of Localized Intravascular Coagulopathy With Venous Malformations. Arch Dermatol 2008;144: 873–7.

32. Alcántara-González J, Boixeda P, Perez-Garcia B, et al. Venous malformations treated with dual wavelength 595 and 1064 nm laser system. J Eur Acad Dermatol Venereol 2013;27.727–33.

33. Moreno-Arrones OM, Jimenez N, Alegre-Sanchez A, et al. Glomuvenous malformations: dual PDL-Nd:YAG laser approach. Lasers Med Sci 2018;33: 2007–10.

34. Glade R, Vinson K, Richter G, et al. Endoscopic management of airway venous malformations with Nd:YAG laser. Ann Otol Rhinol Laryngol 2010;119: 289–93.

35. Gurien LA, Jackson RJ, Kiser MM, et al. YAG laser therapy for rectal and vaginal venous malformations. Pediatr Surg Int 2017;33:887–91.

36. John HE, Phen HS, Mahaffey PJ. Treatment of venous lesions of the lips and perioral area with a long-pulsed Nd:YAG laser. Br J Oral Maxillofac Surg 2016;54:376–8.

37. Richter G. ND:YAG laser therapy of tongue venous malformation. CSurgeries 2013. https://doi.org/10.17797/938QZYJ3UH.

38. Miyazaki H, Ohshiro T, Romeo U, et al. Retrospective Study on Laser Treatment of Oral Vascular Lesions Using the 'Leopard Technique': The Multiple Spot Irradiation Technique with a Single-Pulsed Wave. Photomed Laser Surg 2018;36:320–5.

39. Chang CJ, Fisher DM, Chen YR. Intralesional photocoagulation of vascular anomalies of the tongue. Br J Plast Surg 1999;52:178–81.

40. Ma LW, Levi B, Oppenheimer AJ, et al. Intralesional laser therapy for vascular malformations. Ann Plast Surg 2014;73:547–51.

41. Spradley TP, Johnson AB, Wright HD, et al. YAG Laser Therapy in the Treatment of Cutaneous Venous Malformations. Facial Plast Surg Aesthet Med 2021;23:289–93.

42. Murthy AS, Dawson A, Gupta D, et al. Utility and tolerability of the long-pulsed 1064-nm neodymium: yttrium-aluminum-garnet (LP Nd:YAG) laser for treatment of symptomatic or disfiguring vascular malformations in children and adolescents. J Am Acad Dermatol 2017;77:473–9.

43. Scherer K, Waner M Nd. YAG lasers (1,064 nm) in the treatment of venous malformations of the face and neck: challenges and benefits. Lasers Med Sci 2007;22:119–26.

44. Timbang MR, Richter GT. Update on extracranial arteriovenous malformations: A staged multidisciplinary approach. Semin Pediatr Surg 2020;29.

Interventional Treatment of Vascular Anomalies

Michael J. Waters, MBBS[a], Jonathan Hinshelwood, MD[b], M. Imran Chaudry, MBBS[a],*

KEYWORDS

• Vascular anomaly • Sclerotherapy • Embolization • Interventional radiology

KEY POINTS

- Vascular anomalies require an individualized approach to treatment, with a focus on patient symptoms and quality of life.
- The antibiotic-derived sclerosants, bleomycin and doxycycline, are excellent options for the interventional treatment of head and neck venous and lymphatic malformations (LM).
- Ethanol is a potent sclerosant; however, systemic side effects can be significant, and for this reason, it should only be used when there is control of venous outflow of vascular lesions.
- Fast-flow vascular malformations usually require endovascular therapy; embolization with ethylene vinyl alcohol using balloon occlusion catheters provides a targeted therapeutic option for these lesions.

INTRODUCTION

Patients with vascular anomalies should be managed by a multidisciplinary team, with individualized treatment based on location, size, and classification of the anomaly and associated symptoms. Interventional radiology has a role in the treatment of vascular anomalies, either as a sole therapy or adjunct to surgical resection or medical therapies. An appropriate interventional treatment depends on the accurate diagnosis of the vascular anomaly using the International Society for the Study of Vascular Anomalies (ISSVA) classification, and for this reason, it is most instructional to discuss the treatment modalities based on this classification. Vascular anomalies are highly variable in their angioarchitecture, location, and flow dynamics. As such, there is not a "one fits all" approach to therapy, but rather a considered process which focuses on the individual patient and their specific vascular lesion.

Treatment of Slow-Flow Venous Malformations

Percutaneous sclerotherapy is a particularly effective treatment option for slow-flow venous and combined venolymphatic malformations, as the low flow rate allows consistent, sustained concentrations of the sclerosing agents to be delivered to the target lesion.

The aim of sclerotherapy is to reduce the size and associated symptoms of the vascular anomaly. This may take multiple procedures to achieve[1] and in complex lesions is unlikely to result in an anatomic cure. There is limited evidence to suggest efficacy of one sclerosing agent over another, and systemic reviews looking at this have been inconclusive.[2–5] There is a potential role for combining sclerotherapy with adjuvant laser therapy or surgical resection.[6] Percutaneous cryoablation under ultrasound or Computed Tomography (CT) guidance has also been described as an alternative option to sclerotherapy.[7–9]

Procedural considerations

Sclerotherapy can be performed under conscious sedation or general anesthesia, depending on the size and location of the venous malformation and patient comorbidities. Direct puncture of the venous malformation is performed with a 20- or 21G needle using ultrasound guidance. Gentle aspiration confirms placement within the

[a] Department of Neurosurgery and Neuroendovascular Surgery, Prisma Health, 701 Grove Road, Greenville, SC 29605, USA; [b] Department of Radiology, Prisma Health, 701 Grove Road, Greenville, SC 29605, USA
* Corresponding author.
E-mail address: Imran.Chaudry@prismahealth.org

Dermatol Clin 40 (2022) 489–497
https://doi.org/10.1016/j.det.2022.06.014

malformation, and the needle is connected to a transparent low-volume connecting tube to limit operator radiation exposure. Phlebography/venography using radiopaque contrast media injected into the venous malformation confirms the angioarchitecture and identifies draining veins. Multiple vascular compartments may be identified, and it may be necessary to re-puncture the lesion to optimize delivery of the sclerosing agent. The chosen sclerosant is carefully injected by hand under direct fluoroscopy, with continuous observation for extravasation or nontarget migration of the sclerosant. Where possible in peripheral lesions, application of a proximal torniquet may help in limiting passage of the sclerosing agent into the systemic circulation. An example of a peripheral venous malformation treated with sclerotherapy is shown in **Fig. 1.**

Sclerotherapy Agents

Ethanol
Mechanism: Highly concentrated ethanol acts as a sclerosant by causing protein precipitation of endothelial cells and subsequent thrombosis.[10]

Formulation: Ethanol is available in 98% to 100% concentration. It can be used as both liquid and gel formulation.

Dosing: Maximum dose 1 mL/kg body weight, limiting infusion rate to 0.1 mL/kg/10 minutes.

Complications: Common complications of ethanol include skin necrosis, local pain, and blistering.[11,12] Peripheral nerve injury adjacent to the

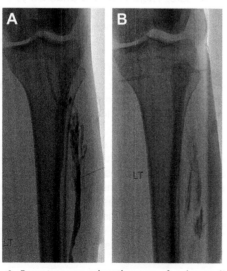

Fig. 1. Percutaneous sclerotherapy of a lower limb venous malformation with sodium tetradecyl sulfate, using proximal torniquet control. (*A*) Pre-sclerotherapy venography. (*B*) Post-sclerotherapy fluoroscopy showing the sclerosant contained within the venous malformation.

vascular anomaly can also occur.[11,13] Systemic side effects are less common but can occur if ethanol enters the systemic circulation; cardiac arrhythmia, pulmonary embolism, pulmonary hypertension, and death have all been reported.[14–17] The risk of systemic complications can be reduced by limiting the total dose of ethanol during the procedure, especially if the venous or combined venolymphatic malformation has prominent or dysplastic draining veins. Proximal tourniquets, endovascular venous balloon occlusion, or manual compression of the draining vein can also help to reduce the venous outflow and subsequent entry of ethanol into the systemic circulation. Adequate periprocedural intravenous hydration with the use of sodium bicarbonate may help to limit hemoglobinuria, but specific evidence for this is lacking.

Specific uses and comments: Ethanol is considered the most potent of sclerosing agents, with an associated higher complication rate compared with other agents.[2] It is readily available and inexpensive. It is an ideal sclerosing agent for slow-flow venous malformations. Ethanol should be used in caution in high-flow vascular lesions or if the vascular lesion is adjacent to a major peripheral nerve. We use ethanol for second-line therapy of slow-flow malformations of the face due to the higher incidence of local side effects including skin necrosis and blistering. In our experience, these side effects can usually be avoided by limiting the dose delivered to the malformation.

Sodium tetradecyl sulfate
Mechanism: A synthetic long-chain fatty acid, sodium tetradecyl sulfate (STS) acts as an anionic detergent sclerosant. Administration of STS results in destabilization of phospholipid membranes and subsequent endothelial cellular lysis and fibrosis.[18] Thrombosis can be additionally induced by a negative charge along the cell membrane at lower doses.[19]

Formulation: STS is available in a 3% solution. Concentrations ranging from 0.1% to 3% can be administered. Liquid and foam formulations are available. Administration of a foam formulation results in greater mechanical displacement of blood in the target lesion and subsequent prolonged length of exposure to the endothelium, leading to increased efficacy.[20] The foam sclerosant is produced using the Tessari technique, in which the sclerosant and room air are passed rapidly through a partially closed three-way stopcock between two syringes.[21]

Dosing: Recommended maximum dose of 10 mL per treatment (3% solution). In our experience, larger doses can be used if there is a good control of venous outflow or if STS is being used in lymphatic malformations.

Complications: Local pain, urticaria, hyperpigmentation, and skin necrosis can all occur following STS administration.[19] Anaphylaxis has been rarely reported.[22]

Specific uses and comments: Considered a less potent sclerosing agent than concentrated ethanol, STS is generally better tolerated; however, the recurrence rate may be higher.[13] Its lower complication rate, including that of tissue necrosis, when compared with ethanol, makes STS an attractive agent for facial and superficial venous malformations.

Sodium morrhuate

Mechanism: Sodium morrhuate is another anionic detergent sclerosant, with a similar mechanism of action to STS.

Formulation: Sodium morrhuate is available in a 5% solution. The Tessari technique is used to produce a foam formulation with 4:1 air-to-liquid sclerosant ratio.

Dosing: Maximum dose of 6 mL 5% sodium morrhuate solution per treatment session (corresponds to 30 mL of foam sclerosant).

Complications: Local pain and swelling are the most common side effects following sodium morrhuate injection.[23] As with other sclerosing agents, skin blistering and necrosis are possible. Systemic complications may theoretically occur if the foam sclerosant enters deep venous system and subsequently the systemic circulation.

Specific uses and comments: We find sodium morrhuate useful for superficial and facial venous malformations, with a similar profile to that of STS, but a higher rate of recurrence than ethanol or the antibiotic-derived sclerosants.

Doxycycline

Mechanism: Doxycycline is a tetracycline antibiotic, although its mechanism as a sclerosant poorly understood. Putative mechanisms include inhibition of metalloproteinases, inflammation with subsequent fibrosis, and inhibition of vascular endothelial growth factor-induced lymphangiogenesis.[24–26]

Formulation: A 10 mg/mL formulation is prepared by dissolving 100 mg of doxycycline in 10 mL of sterile saline. For better angiographic visualization, 100 mg of doxycycline can be dissolved in 5 mL of sterile water and 5 mL of contrast.

Dosing: Maximum dose of 200 mg doxycycline per treatment.

Complications: Doxycycline is generally well tolerated as a sclerosant with a low complication rate,[27] which makes it an attractive option for use in children and infants. Potential side effects include local pain, inflammation, and acidosis.[27] There is a theoretic risk of tooth discoloration in younger children; however, we are yet to encounter this given the low cumulative dose.

Specific uses and comments: Doxycycline is an excellent option for sclerotherapy of macrocystic or mixed lymphatic malformations in the pediatric population and may mitigate the need for surgical intervention.[28,29] Doxycycline is our chosen first-line agent for macrocystic lymphatic malformations of the head and neck.

Bleomycin

Mechanism: Bleomycin is a cytotoxic antibiotic derivative, produced by Streptomyces verticillus. Its cytotoxic effect is mediated by inducing single- and double-strand Deoxyribonucleic Acid (DNA) breaks.[30] At an endothelial level, this results in the destruction of tight junctions between endothelial cells, with resultant sclerosis and fibrosis.[31]

Formulation: Fifteen units (10 mg) of bleomycin can be diluted in normal saline to any concentration down to 1 unit/mL. The dilution of bleomycin is determined by the total volume of sclerosant needed for the lesion.

Dosing: Historically, a maximum of 15 units (10 mg) per session has been recommended. Others recommend a maximum dose of 1 mg/kg per treatment, with no more than 5 mg/kg lifetime dose.[32]

Complications: Bleomycin is commonly known to produce pulmonary fibrosis, in a dose-dependent fashion, with additional risk factors including advanced age and those receiving oxygen therapy.[33] Local erythema, ulceration, and hyperpigmentation can also occur; however, local inflammation and subsequent edema is seen less than with other sclerosants, particularly ethanol.[34]

Specific uses and comments: Bleomycin is an attractive agent for treatment of both venous malformations and lymphatic malformations in the region of the head and neck, where limitation of post-procedural edema is important, particular in those at risk of airway compression. Total cumulative dose is low and rarely enough to induce pulmonary fibrosis.

Treatment of Lymphatic Malformations

Sclerotherapy has a role in the treatment of macrocystic lymphatic malformations and mixed lymphatic malformations with macrocystic components.[28,35] Microcystic lymphatic malformations are difficult to treat with interventional techniques and are usually managed conservatively or with surgery. Lymphatic malformations have a predilection for the head and neck in the pediatric population and can present with airway compromise. As such, sclerosants that limit post-procedure edema are preferred, such as bleomycin and doxycycline. Sequential treatments are often necessary. STS has a limited role in the treatment of lymphatic malformations and is less effective than the antibiotic-derived sclerosants.[29] Ethanol may be associated with higher complication rates[36]; it is also limited in the pediatric population by its maximal dose of 1 mg/kg.

Procedural considerations
Procedural technique differs from that of venous malformations in a few key components. Care should be taken to cannulate each individual macrocyst of the lymphatic malformation under ultrasound guidance, and pig-tail catheters can be inserted into larger cysts. Fluid within the cysts should be fully aspirated before administration of the sclerosant, which enables a larger volume of sclerosing agent to contact the cyst wall. Care should be taken in younger pediatric patients as removal of large amounts of lymphatic fluid may result in large fluid shifts with subsequent hemodynamic compromise. Administration of the sclerosing agent is performed under fluoroscopic imaging.

Treatment of Fast-Flow Vascular Malformations

Fast-flow vascular malformations encompass both arteriovenous malformations (AVMs) and arteriovenous fistulas (AFs). In both cases, there is arteriovenous shunting, either through a distinct nidus (AVM) or through a single arterialized vein without an intervening nidus (AF).

To date, conservative and medical therapies offer little for these lesions. Compression garments may improve symptoms for those with peripheral lesions.[32] Medical therapy with mTOR inhibitors such as sirolimus has yet to show significant benefit, although new agents are showing some promise.[37] The major indications for interventional treatment are to reduce symptoms and prevent secondary complications of the fistula. In the peripheries, untreated lesions can progress to cause local compressive symptoms, distal ischemic symptoms from steal phenomenon, and less commonly skin ulceration or hemorrhage. Larger malformations may also result in high-output cardiac failure in left untreated.[38] Treatment modalities may differ depending on the classification of the malformation. Type I lesions have three or less arteries shunting into a single vein. Type II lesions have multiple arterioles draining to a single vein. Type IIIa and IIIb are more complex lesions with multiple shunting sites from multiple arterioles, with draining veins that are nondilated or dilated, respectively.[39,40]

Endovascular therapy
The aim of endovascular therapy is to completely embolize the nidus or fistulous point, resulting in cessation of arteriovenous shunting. Endovascular procedures can be performed under conscious sedation or general anesthesia. Digital subtraction angiography is performed to characterize the angioarchitecture of the vascular malformation. Transarterial embolization is most commonly performed; however, a transvenous route or combination of both can also be used. Direct puncture of the lesion with combined endovascular techniques may also be appropriate for superficial lesions.[41] The choice of embolic agent depends on the size of the nidus or fistula, the rate of arteriovenous shunting, and the nature of the venous drainage. The most common liquid embolization agents used are N-butyl cyanoacrylate (NBCA) and ethylene vinyl alcohol copolymer (EVOH). Ethanol is a potent embolic agent; however, in fast-flow lesions, its use is limited by systemic side effects related to its displacement into the systemic circulation. It has a role in lower grade malformations (types I–II), in which there is a simple pattern of venous outflow, and systemic passage of the sclerosant can be prevented. Coils and vascular plugs can be used for embolization, but rarely as the sole modality given complete occlusion of the nidus or fistulous point is required for effective treatment. They are more likely to be used as an adjuvant technique to reduce arterial inflow rates before liquid embolization or in combined transvenous/transarterial procedures to restrict venous outflow.

N-butyl cyanoacrylate
Mechanism: NBCA is a liquid adhesive agent, which polymerizes irreversibly into a firm cast on exposure to ionic solutions (including blood).

Formulation and procedural considerations: NBCA is available in 1 mL vials of 100% adhesive agent. Before use, NBCA is premixed with lipiodol, which is radiopaque, and also acts as a polymerization retardant. Different concentrations of NBCA–lipiodol are used, ranging from 1:1 to 1:5, depending on the characteristics of the malformation being treated, with increasing time to polymerization when more lipiodol is added to the formulation. Fast-flow malformations require a higher ratio of NBCA to lipiodol. Before administration through the delivery microcatheter, the catheter must be flushed with a nonionic solution, such as 50% glucose. The microcatheter must be removed immediately after delivery of the

NBCA to the vascular malformation to prevent catheter tip adhesion.

Dosage: No specific dose restrictions apply

Complications: Complications include embolization of nontarget arteries resulting in ischemia. Catheter tip adhesion following NBCA delivery can occur. Systemic embolization of NBCA through the draining veins of the vascular malformation may occur, which can result in pulmonary embolism. Embolization of superficial malformations can result in local pain, inflammation, and skin necrosis.

Ethylene vinyl alcohol copolymer

Mechanism: EVOH is a nonadhesive liquid polymer, which is stable in its liquid form when saturated with solvent. On exposure to blood and the solvent disperses, gradual polymerization occurs.[42]

Formulation and procedural considerations: EVOH is suspended in dimethyl sulfoxide (DMSO) solvent and radiopaque tantalum powder. It must be shaken vigorously before use to fully suspend the tantalum powder and ensure fluoroscopic visibility. A DMSO-compatible catheter must be used to deliver the EVOH, with consideration of a compatible dual-lumen balloon catheter, which helps to establish a proximal "plug" on EVOH delivery. Before delivery of the EVOH, the dead space of the catheter is purged with DMSO. Injection rates of EVOH should be performed slowly, at approximately 0.1 mL/min. Allowing the EVOH to precipitate around the tip of the catheter forms a proximal plug, which then helps facilitate anterograde flow of the solution on further injections. Under fluoroscopy guidance, when EVOH is seen to flow into a nontarget area, the injection is stopped. Further injection after 1 to 2 minutes using this repeated "plug and push"

method helps to penetrate the entire nidus and proximal venous outflow. **Fig. 2** shows an example of balloon microcatheter EVOH embolization of a peripheral AVM.

Dosage: Dosing and toxicity is determined by the content of DMSO, which has a maximum dose of 200 mg/kg.

Complications: Although EVOH is nonadhesive, catheter retention can occur if reflux occurs proximally along the course of the catheter, especially in tortuous vessels. Systemic embolization can also occur, especially in those vascular lesions with high flow rates and large draining veins. Rapid injection can result in endothelial necrosis.[43] The embolization of subcutaneous lesions can result in permanent black discoloration of the skin,[44] which may limit its use in superficial facial vascular malformations.

Evaluation of Therapy and Treatment Resistance

Goals of therapy should be thoroughly discussed with the patient and family. In general, complete anatomic cure of venous malformations, lymphatic malformations, and combined lesions is rare.

Sclerotherapy for venous malformations can be performed preoperatively to reduce the lesion size before resection, postoperatively to control or limit recurrent or residual lesions, and primarily in cosmetically sensitive locations or in lesions adjacent to vital structures including nerves, to control disease. In the head and neck region, goals of therapy are subjective (as a residual lesion will always be seen on follow-up imaging) and these goals should be discussed before therapy is commenced. Goals can be reduction in size, improvement in discoloration, and reduction of bleeding or pain. When reasonable goals of

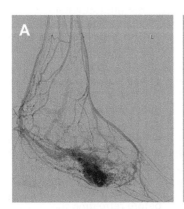 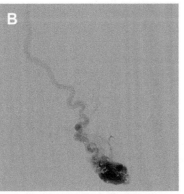 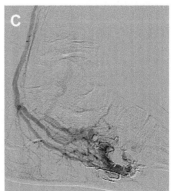

Fig. 2. (*A*) Pre-embolization angiography of a left foot arteriovenous malformation. (*B*): Super-selective balloon microcatheter angiography showing the nidus and dominant draining vein. (*C*) Post-embolization angiography showing partial embolization, with the Onyx cast visualized within the nidus.

therapy are discussed and agreed on, in our experience patient satisfaction can be achieved in approximately 90% of cases. This is consistent with a systematic review of sclerotherapy for venous malformations, which showed an overall patient satisfaction rate of 91%, with a complete cure rate of 64.7%.[5] In our experience, results are usually durable for 3 to 5 years with few patients returning for further, targeted sclerotherapy of residual lesions. Angioarchitecture plays a role in success rate; those high-grade venous malformations with outflow into venous ectasia and dysplastic veins are more likely to be treatment resistant.[45,46]

Sclerotherapy for macrocystic Lymphatic Malformation (LM) results in higher rates of subjective improvement and anatomic cure than microcystic or mixed lesions. In a systematic review looking at sclerotherapy for lymphatic malformations, a complete cure was reported in 50.5% of cases, with higher rates of cure in those with macrocystic lymphatic malformations compared with microcystic or mixed lesions and higher rates with the use of doxycycline.[47] In our experience, there is usually significant reduction in size of large macrocystic lesions so that they are no longer clinically apparent; however, repeat imaging will almost always show small residual pockets of the LM that are not clinically significant.

In fast-flow vascular malformations, the goal of therapy is anatomic cure of the arteriovenous shunting, with complete occlusion of the AVM nidus or fistulous connection. This is immediately assessable on angiography following embolization. Multiple embolization sessions are usually required for larger and more complex type IIIa and IIIb lesions.[41] Outcomes are dependent on the type of malformation; those with type III lesions are less likely to achieve anatomic cure, and agreement on subjective goals of therapy with emphasis on patient quality of life is recommended.[39,41]

At our institution, we have developed the following treatment paradigm for different subsets of vascular lesions, acknowledging that lesions are highly variable in their angioarchitecture and still require an individualized approach to therapy (Table 1).

Complication Management

Frequent post-procedural neurovascular observations should be performed on all patients, including a thorough skin assessment, looking for any evidence of necrosis. Early post-procedural mobilization is encouraged. Routine monitoring of complete blood count and urinalysis will detect post-procedural hemoglobinuria. Doppler ultrasound can be used to assess for

Table 1
Treatment paradigm for vascular anomalies based on location and classification

Vascular Lesion	First-Line Therapy	Second-Line Therapy
Head and neck venous malformations	Bleomycin sclerotherapy (2–3 sessions)	Ethanol sclerotherapy
Head and neck lymphatic malformations	Doxycycline sclerotherapy	Combination sclerotherapy, including ethanol
Peripheral venous malformations	STS sclerotherapy: 3% foam or liquid, depending on flow rate	Ethanol sclerotherapy Consider ultrasound or CT-guided cryoablation
Peripheral AVM or fistula		
Types I–II (single draining vein)	Trans-arterial EVOH with balloon occlusion catheter, combined with manual/tourniquet compression or endovascular occlusion of venous outflow	Reevaluate with angiography. Retreat with trans-arterial EVOH if required. Consider direct puncture of nidus under ultrasound or angiographic guidance as third-line therapy
Type III (multiple, dilated, or ectatic draining veins)	Trans-arterial EVOH with balloon occlusion catheter, combined with manual/tourniquet compression or endovascular occlusion of venous outflow	Reevaluate with angiography. Consider coiling of draining veins or feeding arteries before retreating the nidus trans-arterially with EVOH

deep venous thrombosis if the sclerosant or embolization liquid has entered the deep venous system.

The most common complication is postoperative pain, and for this reason, we recommend pre-emptive, regular analgesia, continuing after the procedure. The agents required will depend on the site of the procedure and the type of sclerosant used, noting that ethanol is associated with higher postoperative pain than other sclerosants.[5] Expected post-procedural swelling can be managed with oral anti-inflammatories or steroids if the vascular anomaly is located adjacent to vital structures including peripheral nerves. Neuropathic symptoms from peripheral nerve injury may settle with steroids; however, nerve decompression or grafting is required in rare cases.[48] Localized skin ulceration is managed with systemic antibiotic therapy and local wound healing measures such as silver dressings. Surgical debridement may be required for necrotic or infected tissue. Larger areas of skin ulceration may need plastic surgery input and skin grafting.[12]

SUMMARY

Interventional treatment of vascular anomalies presents a challenge to the treating team. There is a high variability in location and anatomy of these lesions. An individualized, multidisciplinary approach is required, focusing on improving patient quality of life. With appropriate percutaneous or endovascular treatment, patient satisfaction following interventional therapy is generally high, acknowledging that a complete cure may not always be possible.

CLINICS CARE POINTS

- Vascular anomalies require an individualized approach to treatment, with a focus on patient symptoms and quality of life.
- Referrals may come directly from primary care physicians, with or without imaging. The best imaging modality depends on the area being investigated; MRI with and without contrast is the most useful pretreatment investigation for lesions of the head and neck. Ultrasound may not provide additional pre-intervention information, and we think it is appropriate for primary care physicians to usually defer imaging to the treating specialist.
- The antibiotic-derived sclerosants, bleomycin and doxycycline, are excellent options for the interventional treatment of head and neck venous and lymphatic malformations

- Ethanol is a potent sclerosant; however, systemic side effects can be significant, and for this reason, it should only be used when there is a control of venous outflow of vascular lesions.
- Fast-flow vascular malformations usually require endovascular therapy; embolization with ethylene vinyl alcohol using balloon occlusion catheters provides a targeted therapeutic option for these lesions.

DISCLOSURE

The authors have nothing to disclose.

REFERENCES

1. de Lorimier AA. Sclerotherapy for venous malformations. J Pediatr Surg 1995;30:188–93.
2. van der Vleuten CJ, Kater A, Wijnen MH, et al. Effectiveness of sclerotherapy, surgery, and laser therapy in patients with venous malformations: a systematic review. Cardiovasc Intervent Radiol 2014;37: 977–89.
3. Horbach SE, Lokhorst MM, Saeed P, et al. Sclerotherapy for low-flow vascular malformations of the head and neck: a systematic review of sclerosing agents. J Plast Reconstr Aesthet Surg 2016;69: 295–304.
4. Qiu Y, Chen H, Lin X, et al. Outcomes and complications of sclerotherapy for venous malformations. Vasc Endovascular Surg 2013;47:454–61.
5. De Maria L, De Sanctis P, Balakrishnan K, et al. Sclerotherapy for venous malformations of head and neck: systematic review and meta-analysis. Neurointervention 2020;15:4–17.
6. Ranieri M, Wohlgemuth W, Muller-Wille R, et al. Vascular malformations of upper and lower extremity – from radiological interventional therapy to surgical soft tissue reconstruction – an interdisciplinary treatment. Clin Hemorheol Microcirc 2017;67:355–72.
7. Ramaswamy RS, Tiwari T, Darcy MD, et al. Cryoablation of low-flow vascular malformations. Diagn Interv Radiol 2019;25:225–30.
8. Cornelis F, Havez M, Labreze C, et al. Percutaneous cryoablation of symptomatic localized venous malformations: preliminary short-term results. J Vasc Interv Radiol 2013;24:823–7.
9. Cornelis FH, Marin F, Labreze C, et al. Percutaneous cryoablation of symptomatic venous malformations as a second-line therapeutic option: a five-year single institution experience. Eur Radiol 2017;27: 5015–23.
10. Buchta K, Sands J, Rosenkrantz H, et al. Early mechanism of action of arterially infused alcohol

U.S.P. in renal devitalization. Radiology 1982;145: 45–8.

11. Lee BB, Do YS, Byun HS, et al. Advanced management of venous malformation with ethanol sclerotherapy: mid-term results. J Vasc Surg 2003;37:533–8.

12. Lee KB, Kim DI, Oh SK, et al. Incidence of soft tissue injury and neuropathy after embolo/sclerotherapy for congenital vascular malformation. J Vasc Surg 2008; 48:1286–91.

13. Burrows PE, Mason KP. Percutaneous treatment of low flow vascular malformations. J Vasc Interv Radiol 2004;15:431–45.

14. Mason KP, Michna E, Zurakowski D, et al. Serum ethanol levels in children and adults after ethanol embolization or sclerotherapy for vascular anomalies. Radiology 2000;217:127–32.

15. Do YS, Yakes WF, Shin SW, et al. Ethanol embolization of arteriovenous malformations: interim results. Radiology 2005;235:674–82.

16. Yakes WF, Krauth L, Ecklund J, et al. Ethanol endovascular management of brain arteriovenous malformations: initial results. Neurosurgery 1997;40: 1145–52.

17. Hammer FD, Boon LM, Mathurin P, et al. Ethanol sclerotherapy of venous malformations: evaluation of systemic ethanol contamination. J Vasc Interv Radiol 2001;12:595–600.

18. Parsi K. Interaction of detergent sclerosants with cell membranes. Phlebology 2015;30:306–15.

19. Jenkinson HA, Wilmas KM, Silapunt S. Sodium tetradecyl sulfate: a review of clinical uses. Dermatol Surg 2017;43:1313–20.

20. Coleridge Smith P. Saphenous ablation: sclerosant or sclerofoam? Semin Vasc Surg 2005;18:19–24.

21. Tessari L, Cavezzi A, Frullini A. Preliminary experience with a new sclerosing foam in the treatment of varicose veins. Dermatol Surg 2001;27:58–60.

22. Goldman MP, Sadick NS. Complications and adverse sequelae of leg vein sclerotherapy. In: Nouri K, editor. Complications in dermatologic surgery. St. Louis, USA: Mosby/Elsevier; 2008. p. 219–42.

23. Zhao JH, Zhang WF, Zhao YF. Sclerotherapy of oral and facial venous malformations with use of pingyangmycin and/or sodium morrhuate. Int J Oral Maxillofac Surg 2004;33:463–6.

24. Wiegand S, Eivazi B, Zimmermann AP, et al. Sclerotherapy of lymphangiomas of the head and neck. Head Neck 2011;33:1649–55.

25. Cordes BM, Seidel FG, Sulek M, et al. Doxycycline sclerotherapy as the primary treatment for head and neck lymphatic malformations. Otolaryngol Head Neck Surg 2007;137:962–94.

26. Hurewitz AN, Wu CL, Mancuso P, et al. Tetracycline and doxycycline inhibit pleural fluid metalloproteinases. A possible mechanism for chemical pleurodesis. Chest 1993;103:1113–7.

27. Burrows PE, Mitri RK, Alomari A, et al. Percutaneous sclerotherapy of lymphatic malformations with doxycycline. Lymphat Res Biol 2008;6:209–16.

28. Nehra D, Jacobson L, Barnes P, et al. Doxycycline sclerotherapy as primary treatment of head and neck lymphatic malformations in children. J Pediatr Surg 2008;43:451–60.

29. Thomas DM, Wieck MM, Grant CN, et al. Doxycycline Sclerotherapy Is Superior in the Treatment of Pediatric Lymphatic Malformations. J Vasc Interv Radiol 2016;27:1846–56.

30. Sikic BI. Biochemical and cellular determinants of bleomycin cytotoxicity. Cancer Surv 1986;5:81.

31. Zhang W, Chen G, Ren JG, et al. Bleomycin induces endothelial mesenchymal transition through activation of mTOR pathway: a possible mechanism contributing to the sclerotherapy of venous malformations. Br J Pharmacol 2013;170:1210–20.

32. Legiehn GM, Heran MK. A step-by-step practical approach to imaging diagnosis and interventional radiologic therapy in vascular malformations. Semin Intervent Radiol 2010;27:209–31.

33. Sleijfer S. Bleomycin-induced pneumonitis. Chest 2001;120:617–24.

34. Chaudry G, Guevara CJ, Rialon KL, et al. Safety and efficacy of bleomycin sclerotherapy for microcystic lymphatic malformation. Cardiovasc Intervent Radiol 2014;37:1476–81.

35. Cahill AM, Nijs E, Ballah D, et al. Percutaneous sclerotherapy in neonatal and infant head and neck lymphatic malformations: a single center experience. J Pediatr Surg 2011;46:2083–95.

36. Alomari A, Karian VE, Lord DJ, et al. Percutaneous sclerotherapy for lymphatic malformations: a retrospective analysis of patient-evaluated improvement. J Vasc Interv Radiol 2006;17:1639–48.

37. Triana P, Dore M, Cerezo VN, et al. Sirolimus in the treatment of vascular anomalies. Eur J Pediatr Surg 2017;27:86–90.

38. Ernemann U, Kramer U, Miller S, et al. Current concepts in the classification, diagnosis and treatment of vascular anomalies. Eur J Radiol 2010;75:2–11.

39. Do YS, Park KB, Cho SK. How do we treat arteriovenous malformations (tips and tricks)? Tech Vasc Interv Radiol 2007;10:291–8.

40. Houdart E, Gobin YP, Casasco A, et al. A proposed angiographic classification of intracranial arteriovenous fistulae and malformations. Neuroradiology 1993;35:381–5.

41. Park KB, Do YS, Kim DI, et al. Endovascular treatment results and risk factors for complications of body and extremity arteriovenous malformations. J Vasc Surg 2019;69:1207–18.

42. Yamashita K, Taki W, Iwata H, et al. Characteristics of ethylene vinyl alcohol copolymer (EVAL) mixtures. AJNR Am J Neuroradiol 1994;15:1103–5.

43. Lv X, Li Y, Jiang C, et al. The incidence of trigemino-cardiac reflex in endovascular treatment of dural arteriovenous fistula with Onyx. Interv Neuroradiol 2010;16:59–63.

44. Arat A, Cil BE, Vargel I, et al. Embolization of high-flow craniofacial vascular malformations with Onyx. AJNR Am J Neuroradiol 2007;28:1409–14.

45. Hage AN, Chick JFB, Srinivasa RN, et al. Treatment of venous malformations: the data, where we are, and how it is done. Tech Vasc Interv Radiol 2018; 21:45–54.

46. Puig S, Casati B, Staudenherz A, et al. Vascular low-flow malformations in children: current concepts for classification, diagnosis and therapy. Eur J Radiol 2005;53:35–45.

47. De Maria L, De Sanctis P, Balakrishnan K, et al. Sclerotherapy for lymphatic malformations of head and neck: Systematic review and meta-analysis. J Vasc Surg Venous Lym Dis 2020;8:154–64.

48. Stuart S, Barnacle A, Smith G, et al. Neuropathy after sodium tetradecyl sulfate sclerotherapy of venous malformations in children. Radiology 2015;274:897–905.

UNITED STATES POSTAL SERVICE® Statement of Ownership, Management, and Circulation (All Periodicals Publications Except Requester Publications)

1. Publication Title	2. Publication Number	3. Filing Date
DERMATOLOGIC CLINICS	000 – 705	9/18/2022

4. Issue Frequency	5. Number of Issues Published Annually	6. Annual Subscription Price
JAN, APR, JUL, OCT	4	$429.00

7. Complete Mailing Address of Known Office of Publication (Not printer) (Street, city, county, state, and ZIP+4®)

ELSEVIER INC.
230 Park Avenue, Suite 800
New York, NY 10169

Contact Person
Malathi Samayan
Telephone (Include area code)
91-44-4299-4507

8. Complete Mailing Address of Headquarters or General Business Office of Publisher (Not printer)

ELSEVIER INC.
230 Park Avenue, Suite 800
New York, NY 10169

9. Full Names and Complete Mailing Addresses of Publisher, Editor, and Managing Editor (Do not leave blank)

Publisher (Name and complete mailing address)

DOLORES MELONI, ELSEVIER INC.
1600 JOHN F KENNEDY BLVD. SUITE 1800
PHILADELPHIA, PA 19103-2899

Editor (Name and complete mailing address)

STACY EASTMAN, ELSEVIER INC.
1600 JOHN F KENNEDY BLVD. SUITE 1800
PHILADELPHIA, PA 19103-2899

Managing Editor (Name and complete mailing address)

PATRICK MANLEY, ELSEVIER INC.
1600 JOHN F KENNEDY BLVD. SUITE 1800
PHILADELPHIA, PA 19103-2899

10. Owner (Do not leave blank. If the publication is owned by a corporation, give the name and address of the corporation immediately followed by the names and addresses of all stockholders owning or holding 1 percent or more of the total amount of stock. If not owned by a corporation, give the names and addresses of the individual owners. If owned by a partnership or other unincorporated firm, give its name and address as well as those of each individual owner. If the publication is published by a nonprofit organization, give its name and address.)

Full Name	Complete Mailing Address
WHOLLY OWNED SUBSIDIARY OF REED/ELSEVIER, US HOLDINGS	1600 JOHN F KENNEDY BLVD. SUITE 1800 PHILADELPHIA, PA 19103-2899

11. Known Bondholders, Mortgagees, and Other Security Holders Owning or Holding 1 Percent or More of Total Amount of Bonds, Mortgages, or Other Securities. If none, check box. ▶ ☐ None

Full Name	Complete Mailing Address
N/A	

12. Tax Status (For completion by nonprofit organizations authorized to mail at nonprofit rates) (Check one)
The purpose, function, and nonprofit status of this organization and the exempt status for federal income tax purposes:
☒ Has Not Changed During Preceding 12 Months
☐ Has Changed During Preceding 12 Months (Publisher must submit explanation of change with this statement)

PS Form 3526, July 2014 [Page 1 of 4 (see instructions page 4)] PSN: 7530-01-000-9931   PRIVACY NOTICE: See our privacy policy on www.usps.com.

13. Publication Title	14. Issue Date for Circulation Data Below
DERMATOLOGIC CLINICS	JULY 2022

15. Extent and Nature of Circulation		Average No. Copies Each Issue During Preceding 12 Months	No. Copies of Single Issue Published Nearest to Filing Date
a. Total Number of Copies (Net press run)		140	133
b. Paid Circulation (By Mail and Outside the Mail)	(1) Mailed Outside-County Paid Subscriptions Stated on PS Form 3541 (Include paid distribution above nominal rate, advertiser's proof copies, and exchange copies)	60	55
	(2) Mailed In-County Paid Subscriptions Stated on PS Form 3541 (Include paid distribution above nominal rate, advertiser's proof copies, and exchange copies)	0	0
	(3) Paid Distribution Outside the Mails Including Sales Through Dealers and Carriers, Street Vendors, Counter Sales, and Other Paid Distribution Outside USPS®	43	42
	(4) Paid Distribution by Other Classes of Mail Through the USPS (e.g., First-Class Mail®)	0	0
c. Total Paid Distribution (Sum of 15b (1), (2), (3), and (4))	▶	103	97
d. Free or Nominal Rate Distribution (By Mail and Outside the Mail)	(1) Free or Nominal Rate Outside-County Copies included on PS Form 3541	19	17
	(2) Free or Nominal Rate In-County Copies Included on PS Form 3541	0	0
	(3) Free or Nominal Rate Copies Mailed at Other Classes Through the USPS (e.g., First-Class Mail)	0	0
	(4) Free or Nominal Rate Distribution Outside the Mail (Carriers or other means)	0	0
e. Total Free or Nominal Rate Distribution (Sum of 15d (1), (2), (3) and (4))	▶	19	17
f. Total Distribution (Sum of 15c and 15e)	▶	122	114
g. Copies not Distributed (See Instructions to Publishers #4 (page 83))	▶	18	19
h. Total (Sum of 15f and g)	▶	140	133
i. Percent Paid (15c divided by 15f times 100)		84.42%	85.08%

* If you are claiming electronic copies, go to line 16 on page 3. If you are not claiming electronic copies, skip to line 17 on page 3.

PS Form 3526, July 2014 (Page 2 of 4)

16. Electronic Copy Circulation		Average No. Copies Each Issue During Preceding 12 Months	No. Copies of Single Issue Published Nearest to Filing Date
a. Paid Electronic Copies	▶		
b. Total Paid Print Copies (Line 15c) + Paid Electronic Copies (Line 16a)	▶		
c. Total Print Distribution (Line 15f) + Paid Electronic Copies (Line 16a)	▶		
d. Percent Paid (Both Print & Electronic Copies) (16b divided by 16c × 100)	▶		

☒ I certify that 50% of all my distributed copies (electronic and print) are paid above a nominal price.

17. Publication of Statement of Ownership

☒ If the publication is a general publication, publication of this statement is required. Will be printed in the OCTOBER 2022 issue of this publication.   ☐ Publication not required.

18. Signature and Title of Editor, Publisher, Business Manager, or Owner

Malathi Samayan

Malathi Samayan - Distribution Controller

Date 9/18/2022

I certify that all information furnished on this form is true and complete. I understand that anyone who furnishes false or misleading information on this form or who omits material or information requested on the form may be subject to criminal sanctions (including fines and imprisonment) and/or civil sanctions (including civil penalties).

PS Form 3526, July 2014 (Page 3 of 4)   PRIVACY NOTICE: See our privacy policy on www.usps.com.

Moving?

Make sure your subscription moves with you!

To notify us of your new address, find your **Clinics Account Number** (located on your mailing label above your name), and contact customer service at:

Email: journalscustomerservice-usa@elsevier.com

800-654-2452 (subscribers in the U.S. & Canada)
314-447-8871 (subscribers outside of the U.S. & Canada)

Fax number: 314-447-8029

Elsevier Health Sciences Division
Subscription Customer Service
3251 Riverport Lane
Maryland Heights, MO 63043

*To ensure uninterrupted delivery of your subscription, please notify us at least 4 weeks in advance of move.

ELSEVIER

Printed and bound by CPI Group (UK) Ltd, Croydon, CR0 4YY

08/05/2025

01864717-0010